10th Anniversary of Biomedicines—Biomarkers in Pain

10th Anniversary of Biomedicines—Biomarkers in Pain

Editors

Mats B. Eriksson
Anders O. Larsson

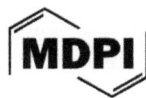

Basel • Beijing • Wuhan • Barcelona • Belgrade • Novi Sad • Cluj • Manchester

Editors
Mats B. Eriksson
Uppsala University
Uppsala, Sweden

Anders O. Larsson
Uppsala University
Uppsala, Sweden

Editorial Office
MDPI
St. Alban-Anlage 66
4052 Basel, Switzerland

This is a reprint of articles from the Special Issue published online in the open access journal *Biomedicines* (ISSN 2227-9059) (available at: https://www.mdpi.com/journal/biomedicines/special_issues/biomarker_in_pain).

For citation purposes, cite each article independently as indicated on the article page online and as indicated below:

Lastname, A.A.; Lastname, B.B. Article Title. *Journal Name* **Year**, *Volume Number*, Page Range.

ISBN 978-3-0365-9792-8 (Hbk)
ISBN 978-3-0365-9793-5 (PDF)
doi.org/10.3390/books978-3-0365-9793-5

© 2023 by the authors. Articles in this book are Open Access and distributed under the Creative Commons Attribution (CC BY) license. The book as a whole is distributed by MDPI under the terms and conditions of the Creative Commons Attribution-NonCommercial-NoDerivs (CC BY-NC-ND) license.

Contents

About the Editors vii

Preface ix

Anders O. Larsson, Emmanuel Bäckryd and Mats B. Eriksson
Biomarkers in Pain
Reprinted from: *Biomedicines* 2023, 11, 2554, doi:10.3390/biomedicines11092554 1

Emmanuel Bäckryd, Katarina Thordeman, Björn Gerdle and Bijar Ghafouri
Cerebrospinal Fluid Metabolomics Identified Ongoing Analgesic Medication in Neuropathic Pain Patients
Reprinted from: *Biomedicines* 2023, 11, 2525, doi:10.3390/biomedicines11092525 5

**Hugo Ribeiro, Raquel Alves, Joana Jorge, Ana Cristina Gonçalves,
Ana Bela Sarmento-Ribeiro, Manuel Teixeira-Veríssimo, et al.**
Platelet Membrane Proteins as Pain Biomarkers in Patients with Severe Dementia
Reprinted from: *Biomedicines* 2023, 11, 380, doi:10.3390/biomedicines11020380 15

**Hana Karpin, Jean-Jacques Vatine, Yishai Bachar Kirshenboim, Aurelia Markezana and
Irit Weissman-Fogel**
Central Sensitization and Psychological State Distinguishing Complex Regional Pain Syndrome from Other Chronic Limb Pain Conditions: A Cluster Analysis Model
Reprinted from: *Biomedicines* 2023, 11, 89, doi:10.3390/biomedicines11010089 27

**Yilong Cui, Hiroyuki Neyama, Di Hu, Tianliang Huang, Emi Hayashinaka, Yasuhiro Wada
and Yasuyoshi Watanabe**
FDG PET Imaging of the Pain Matrix in Neuropathic Pain Model Rats
Reprinted from: *Biomedicines* 2023, 11, 63, doi:10.3390/biomedicines11010063 47

**Maxim Devine, Canchen Ma, Jing Tian, Benny Antony, Flavia Cicuttini, Graeme Jones and
Feng Pan**
Association of Pain Phenotypes with Risk of Falls and Incident Fractures
Reprinted from: *Biomedicines* 2022, 10, 2924, doi:10.3390/biomedicines10112924 59

**Ahmed Chaudhry, Nur Karyatee Kassim, Siti Lailatul Akmar Zainuddin, Haslina Taib,
Hanim Afzan Ibrahim, Basaruddin Ahmad, et al.**
Potential Effects of Non-Surgical Periodontal Therapy on Periodontal Parameters, Inflammatory Markers, and Kidney Function Indicators in Chronic Kidney Disease Patients with Chronic Periodontitis
Reprinted from: *Biomedicines* 2022, 10, 2752, doi:10.3390/biomedicines10112752 69

**Valery Golderman, Shani Berkowitz, Shani Guly Gofrit, Orna Gera, Shay Anat Aharoni,
Daniela Noa Zohar, et al.**
Thrombin Activity in Rodent and Human Skin: Modified by Inflammation and Correlates with Innervation
Reprinted from: *Biomedicines* 2022, 10, 1461, doi:10.3390/biomedicines10061461 81

**Teodor Svedung Wettervik, Dick Folkvaljon, Torsten Gordh, Eva Freyhult, Kim Kultima,
Hans Ericson and Sami Abu Hamdeh**
Cerebrospinal Fluid in Classical Trigeminal Neuralgia: An Exploratory Study on Candidate Biomarkers
Reprinted from: *Biomedicines* 2022, 10, 998, doi:10.3390/biomedicines10050998 95

**Martina Morchio, Emanuele Sher, David A. Collier, Daniel W. Lambert and
Fiona M. Boissonade**
The Role of miRNAs in Neuropathic Pain
Reprinted from: *Biomedicines* **2023**, *11*, 775, doi:10.3390/biomedicines11030775 . . . . **107**

**Isabel Hong-Baik, Edurne Úbeda-D'Ocasar, Eduardo Cimadevilla-Fernández-Pola,
Victor Jiménez-Díaz-Benito and Juan Pablo Hervás-Pérez**
The Effects of Non-Pharmacological Interventions in Fibromyalgia: A Systematic Review and
Metanalysis of Predominants Outcomes
Reprinted from: *Biomedicines* **2023**, *11*, 2367, doi:10.3390/biomedicines11092367 . . . . **131**

About the Editors

Mats B. Eriksson

Mats B. Eriksson, MD and PhD, is Associate Professor at the Department of Surgical Sciences, Section of Anaesthesiology and Intensive Care Medicine at Uppsala University, Uppsala, Sweden and Affiliated Professor of Critical Care at Nova Medical School, New University of Lisbon, Portugal. He has been the principal tutor of two PhD students, who have completed their theses and contributed scientifically to several additional graduations. His research field has been sepsis and septic conditions, both from clinical and experimental aspects. Special interest has been paid to the interface between inflammation and coagulation. He has several times been invited speaker at international conferences and presented research at scientific meetings in all five major continents. He also has considerable experience from clinical trials, both as organizer and as an investigator.

Anders O. Larsson

Anders O. Larsson, MD and PhD is Professor at the Department of Medical Sciences, Section of Clinical Chemistry, Uppsala University, Sweden. He has been the principal tutor of seven PhD students that has presented their theses. His main research field is laboratory technology. A focus area within this field has been kidney function markers and especially glomerular filtration markers and tubular damage markers. Another area has been proinflammatory cytokines and cardiovascular risk. He has been involved in both clinical and experimental studies. Several of the studies have been intensive care related, looking for improved markers for acute kidney injury and infectious diseases including COVID-19. He has been participating in international collaborations such as the Global Burden of Disease consortium and determination of glomerular filtration rate consortia.

Preface

Acute and chronic pain are heavy burdens, not only to those who suffer from pain of various conditions, but also to society's health care system with expressed economic implications.

From the patient's perspective it is crucial not to be ignored or mistrusted, which may be the case, since pain is subjective and frequently difficult to demonstrate. Nobody mistrusts a trauma patient, but diffuse pain, which may be difficult to verbalize, may enhance suffering, especially if a health care provider appears to be less understanding, or even ignorant.

Chronic pain affects many people world-wide, and a link between chronic pain and the development of cardiovascular disease through activation of the sympathetic nervous system may be at hand, as pain perception contributes to sympathetic overactivation.

Opiates, one of the oldest drugs known to man, have analgesic and sedative properties. Their endogenous counterpart, opioid peptides are powerful analgesic and euphorigenic agents.

The endogenous opioid system consists of three genetically distinct families of opioid peptides (β-endorphin/Enkephalins/Dynorphin) and three various receptors μ, δ and κ. The action of endogenous opioids is regulated by their action on the specific opioid receptor. Opioid peptides and their receptors are distributed within the central and peripheral nervous systems. Each opioid peptide has pre-pro and pro-forms which are cleaved sequentially.

Phylogenetic analyses indicate that opioid receptors were already present at the origin of jawed vertebrates 450 million years ago. Hence, opioid peptides and receptors are most likely to have fundamental roles in pain transmission and reward mechanisms in mammals.

Opioid tolerance occurs when increasing doses are required to maintain the same level of analgesia. Tolerance develops quickly to analgesia, sedation, and respiratory depression.

Interestingly, genetic polymorphism is related to pain sensitivity and opioid response.

The aim of this Special Issue is to point out traceable biochemical events referring to either acute or chronic pain. Such biomarkers may be causative of pain, as in gout, where elevated levels of uric acid may clump together in sharp crystals, which can settle in joints and hereby cause a painful form of arthritis. In other conditions, the relation between a biomarker and pain is less obvious, e.g. altered relation of platelet membrane proteins. Analysis of biomarkers may also help to explain pathophysiological processes, as in classical trigeminal neuralgia, where biomarkers in the cerebrospinal fluid indicate abnormal processes in the myelin sheath. Furthermore, biomarkers may help to explain pharmacologic action of some drugs, as acetaminophen (paracetamol) is suggested to act in the CNS.

This SI addresses clinicians as well as researchers interested in pain management, its pathophysiology, and, above all biochemical process resulting in measurable analytes.

The editors express their sincere gratitude to the authors who have contributed to this SI and made its publication possible because of your efforts.

Mats B. Eriksson and Anders O. Larsson
Editors

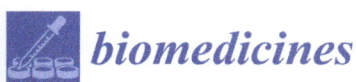

Editorial

Biomarkers in Pain

Anders O. Larsson [1], Emmanuel Bäckryd [2] and Mats B. Eriksson [3,4,*]

1. Department of Medical Sciences, Section of Clinical Chemistry, Uppsala University, 751 85 Uppsala, Sweden; anders.larsson@akademiska.se
2. Pain and Rehabilitation Center, and Department of Health, Medicine and Caring Sciences, Linköping University, 581 83 Linköping, Sweden; emmanuel.backryd@liu.se
3. Department of Surgical Sciences, Section of Anaesthesiology and Intensive Care Medicine, Uppsala University, 751 85 Uppsala, Sweden
4. NOVA Medical School, New University of Lisbon, 1099-085 Lisbon, Portugal
* Correspondence: mats.eriksson@surgsci.uu.se

The focus of this Special Issue on Biomedicines is on the value of "Biomarkers in Pain" from a broad perspective.

Pain can be viewed from different perspectives. The pain mechanism can be nociceptive, neuropathic, or nociplastic [1]. Temporally, we usually divide pain into acute and chronic conditions. Acute pain has a protective function and is part of the response to tissue damage. Although causing discomfort, acute pain is often not a major problem as this type of pain usually responds well to pharmacological treatment. In contrast, chronic pain is much more difficult to treat, and, as a rule, treatment options that relieve acute pain cannot alleviate chronic pain; hence, the latter may be regarded as a disease of its own right [2]. The International Association for the Study of Pain defines chronic pain syndromes as persistent or recurrent pain lasting ≥ 3 months [3].

Approximately 20% of the global population suffers from chronic pain [4–7], although considerably higher proportions have been described, e.g., in the UK, chronic pain affects between one third and one half of the population, which equals almost 28 million adults, a number which may continue to increase further as we face an ageing population [8]. In the United States, 100 million adults suffer from chronic pain, causing an annual economic loss that has been estimated to amount to 600 billion USD [9]. Furthermore, costs associated with pain exceed the costs of heart disease and cancer [10].

Sometimes, acute pain does not resolve. Instead, acute pain may, through hitherto largely still unknown mechanisms, sometimes shift into chronic pain. A problem with both acute and chronic pain is that it is not visible. It may therefore be overlooked or underestimated. Pain is a subjective experience and varies between individuals and different time points. At least for research purposes, it would be desirable to have a more objective way of quantifying pain in addition to a patient's description of their pain, although important ethical concerns have been raised and are worth pondering [11]. Biomarkers could also provide information of the pathophysiological mechanisms behind pain, allowing for a differentiation between different pain mechanisms and better adaptation of the treatments for each patient. This has triggered the development of potential biomarkers for pain. These biomarkers offer a way of measuring and quantifying pain, reducing the reliance on self-reported pain scales, which can be influenced by psychological and cultural factors. The impact of chronic pain on quality of life is significant, with frequent limitations in ordinary activities of daily life, as well as depression and even suicide [2].

Several previous studies have shown that pain patients' biofluids, analyzed using modern proteomic methods, exhibit biomarkers that could increase our knowledge on chronic pain and hereby guide its management (e.g., [12–15]). Such biomarkers may be valuable in order to ensure objectivity in clinical trials when new treatment options are evaluated. In the future, one may expect that biomarkers can help with the diagnosis of various pain conditions and differentiate between different types of pain.

Citation: Larsson, A.O.; Bäckryd, E.; Eriksson, M.B. Biomarkers in Pain. *Biomedicines* **2023**, *11*, 2554. https://doi.org/10.3390/biomedicines11092554

Received: 11 September 2023
Accepted: 14 September 2023
Published: 18 September 2023

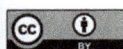

Copyright: © 2023 by the authors. Licensee MDPI, Basel, Switzerland. This article is an open access article distributed under the terms and conditions of the Creative Commons Attribution (CC BY) license (https://creativecommons.org/licenses/by/4.0/).

This issue of biomedicines focuses on "Biomarkers in Pain". It was initially discussed whether "Biomarkers of Pain" would be a more relevant title, but the latter suggestion might imply that a specific biomarker is causative of the agony and not a result of this condition, which could limit and possibly even lead to deceptive conclusions. According to the present state of knowledge, one cannot determine whether the increased levels of biomarkers that are seen in painful conditions are a cause or a consequence. It should rather be remembered that correlation does not imply causation. The relation between biomarkers and pain has previously been validated [14]. Longitudinal studies could possibly help to clarify this issue. Nevertheless, such indicators of pain may be most valuable in order to impart an agonizing process.

This Special Issue of biomedicines highlights several research articles presenting recent advances in the field of Biomarkers in Pain from a broad perspective. Displaying such biomarkers may provide pertinent information about potential new directions for interventions for chronic pain in the research realm. In addition, the review articles presented in this issue may contribute to an increased awareness of biomarkers within a broad context and from a relevant perspective.

In summary, we can expect that pain biomarkers will serve a critical role in improving the diagnosis, treatment, and management of pain conditions. They may offer more objective and precise information based on an individual's unique genetic and biological makeup, leading to better patient care, drug development, and overall understanding of pain mechanisms.

Author Contributions: All authors contributed equally to the writing and editing of this Editorial. All authors have read and agreed to the published version of the manuscript.

Conflicts of Interest: The authors declare no conflict of interest.

References

1. Kosek, E.; Cohen, M.; Baron, R.; Gebhart, G.F.; Mico, J.A.; Rice, A.S.C.; Rief, W.; Sluka, A.K. Do we need a third mechanistic descriptor for chronic pain states? *Pain* **2016**, *157*, 1382–1386. [CrossRef] [PubMed]
2. Niv, D.; Devor, M. Chronic pain as a disease in its own right. *Pain Pract.* **2004**, *4*, 179–181. [CrossRef] [PubMed]
3. Scholz, J.; Finnerup, N.B.; Attal, N.; Aziz, Q.; Baron, R.; Bennett, M.I.; Benoliel, R.; Cohen, M.; Cruccu, G.; Davis, K.D.; et al. The IASP classification of chronic pain for ICD-11: Chronic neuropathic pain. *Pain* **2019**, *160*, 53–59. [CrossRef]
4. Breivik, H.; Collett, B.; Ventafridda, V.; Cohen, R.; Gallacher, D. Survey of chronic pain in Europe: Prevalence, impact on daily life, and treatment. *Eur. J. Pain* **2006**, *10*, 287–333. [CrossRef]
5. Schopflocher, D.; Taenzer, P.; Jovey, R. The prevalence of chronic pain in Canada. *Pain Res. Manag.* **2011**, *16*, 445–450. [CrossRef] [PubMed]
6. Dzau, V.J.; Pizzo, P.A. Relieving pain in America: Insights from an Institute of Medicine committee. *JAMA* **2014**, *312*, 1507–1508. [CrossRef] [PubMed]
7. Jackson, T.; Chen, H.; Iezzi, T.; Yee, M.; Chen, F. Prevalence and correlates of chronic pain in a random population study of adults in Chongqing, China. *Clin. J. Pain* **2014**, *30*, 346–352. [CrossRef] [PubMed]
8. Fayaz, A.; Croft, P.; Langford, R.M.; Donaldson, L.J.; Jones, G.T. Prevalence of chronic pain in the UK: A systematic review and meta-analysis of population studies. *BMJ Open* **2016**, *6*, e010364. [CrossRef] [PubMed]
9. Steglitz, J.; Buscemi, J.; Ferguson, M.J. The future of pain research, education, and treatment: A summary of the IOM report "Relieving pain in America: A blueprint for transforming prevention, care, education, and research". *Transl. Behav. Med.* **2012**, *2*, 6–8. [CrossRef]
10. Smith, T.J.; Hillner, B.E. The Cost of Pain. *JAMA Netw. Open* **2019**, *2*, e191532. [CrossRef] [PubMed]
11. Kalso, E. Biomarkers for pain. *Pain* **2004**, *107*, 199–201. [CrossRef] [PubMed]
12. Moen, A.; Lind, A.L.; Thulin, M.; Kamali-Moghaddam, M.; Røe, C.; Gjerstad, J.; Gordh, T. Inflammatory Serum Protein Profiling of Patients with Lumbar Radicular Pain One Year after Disc Herniation. *Int. J. Inflamm.* **2016**, *2016*, 3874964. [CrossRef] [PubMed]
13. Lind, A.L.; Just, D.; Mikus, M.; Fredolini, C.; Ioannou, M.; Gerdle, B.; Ghafouri, B.; Bäckryd, E.; Tanum, L.; Gordh, T.; et al. CSF levels of apolipoprotein C1 and autotaxin found to associate with neuropathic pain and fibromyalgia. *J. Pain Res.* **2019**, *12*, 2875–2889. [CrossRef]

14. Bäckryd, E.; Lind, A.L.; Thulin, M.; Larsson, A.; Gerdle, B.; Gordh, T. High levels of cerebrospinal fluid chemokines point to the presence of neuroinflammation in peripheral neuropathic pain: A cross-sectional study of 2 cohorts of patients compared with healthy controls. *Pain* **2017**, *158*, 2487–2495. [CrossRef] [PubMed]
15. Gerdle, B.; Ghafouri, B. Proteomic studies of common chronic pain conditions—A systematic review and associated network analyses. *Expert. Rev. Proteom.* **2020**, *17*, 483–505. [CrossRef] [PubMed]

Disclaimer/Publisher's Note: The statements, opinions and data contained in all publications are solely those of the individual author(s) and contributor(s) and not of MDPI and/or the editor(s). MDPI and/or the editor(s) disclaim responsibility for any injury to people or property resulting from any ideas, methods, instructions or products referred to in the content.

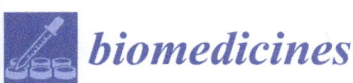

Article

Cerebrospinal Fluid Metabolomics Identified Ongoing Analgesic Medication in Neuropathic Pain Patients

Emmanuel Bäckryd *, Katarina Thordeman, Björn Gerdle and Bijar Ghafouri

Pain and Rehabilitation Center, and Department of Health, Medicine and Caring Sciences, Linköping University, Linköping, Sweden
* Correspondence: emmanuel.backryd@liu.se

Abstract: Background: Cerebrospinal fluid (CSF) can reasonably be hypothesized to mirror central nervous system pathophysiology in chronic pain conditions. Metabolites are small organic molecules with a low molecular weight. They are the downstream products of genes, transcripts and enzyme functions, and their levels can mirror diseased metabolic pathways. The aim of this metabolomic study was to compare the CSF of patients with chronic neuropathic pain ($n = 16$) to healthy controls ($n = 12$). Methods: Nuclear magnetic resonance spectroscopy was used for analysis of the CSF metabolome. Multivariate data analysis by projection discriminant analysis (OPLS-DA) was used to separate information from noise and minimize the multiple testing problem. Results: The significant OPLS-DA model identified 26 features out of 215 as important for group separation ($R^2 = 0.70$, $Q^2 = 0.42$, $p = 0.017$ by CV-ANOVA; 2 components). Twenty-one out of twenty-six features were statistically significant when comparing the two groups by univariate statistics and remained significant at a false discovery rate of 10%. For six out of the top ten metabolite features, the features were absent in all healthy controls. However, these features were related to medication, mainly acetaminophen (=paracetamol), and not to pathophysiological processes. Conclusion: CSF metabolomics was a sensitive method to detect ongoing analgesic medication, especially acetaminophen.

Keywords: acetaminophen; analgesics; biomarkers; chronic; CSF; neuropathic; metabolomics; pain

1. Introduction

To better understand the pathophysiology of chronic pain and bridge the translational gap between animals and humans [1–3], cerebrospinal fluid (CSF) is a sensible biofluid to investigate. CSF can reasonably be hypothesized to mirror central nervous system (CNS) pathology. We have previously found evidence of neuroinflammation when analyzing CSF from fibromyalgia patients [4] and neuropathic pain patients [5], compared to healthy controls. This is in line with growing evidence of an interplay between the immune and nervous systems [2,6,7]. In a CSF proteomic study, we also found that an isoform of angiotensinogen had the highest power to separate neuropathic pain patients from healthy controls in a multivariate model [8]. This finding confirmed results from animal models and clinical trials concerning the possible involvement of the renin–angiotensin system in neuropathic pain [9,10]. Hence, CSF biomarker studies seem promising for animal-to-human translation and backtranslation. However, the difficulty in sampling CSF is an obvious drawback, especially concerning healthy controls.

Neuropathic pain is caused by a lesion or disease of the somatosensory nervous system [11]. Advances in basic science using animal models have not translated into better treatments for neuropathic pain [3]. Available analgesics often have limited effects or lead to troublesome side-effects [12,13]. Current evidence indicates that at least six patients have to be treated with a first-line drug in order for one patient to obtain clinically significant pain relief [13], i.e., numbers needed to treat (NNT) ≥ 6.

Untargeted omics methods, such as proteomics [14] or metabolomics [15], can be used to explore the pathophysiological mechanisms of neuropathic pain. Metabolomics deals

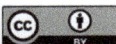

with the identification and quantification of small molecules—metabolites. Metabolites are small organic molecules with a low molecular weight. They are the downstream products of genes, transcripts and enzyme functions, and hence their levels may mirror normal or diseased metabolic pathways [15]. Knowledge about metabolic pathways activated in different chronic pain conditions can be helpful for the development of new analgesics.

Nuclear magnetic resonance (NMR) spectroscopy is a useful technique for the metabolomic study of different diseases including chronic pain conditions, such as neuropathic pain or fibromyalgia. NMR enables the detection of several hundred small molecules in body fluids such as CSF, blood or urine [15–19]. In a previous NMR metabolomic study, we compared blood from patients suffering from chronic neuropathic pain with healthy controls, finding that several of the metabolites that significantly differed between groups were involved in inflammatory processes, while others were important for CNS functioning and neural signaling [16].

The aim of this explorative, observational, cross-sectional study was to investigate the CNS pathophysiology of neuropathic pain by comparing the CSF metabolome of patients with healthy controls, using multivariate data analysis by projection (MVDA) to analyze the correlation structure of the material, thereby separating information from noise and minimizing the multiple testing problem [20,21]. We also wanted to investigate if pain intensity and/or pain duration were associated with metabolomic patterns.

2. Materials and Methods

2.1. Participants

Twelve healthy individuals were recruited as healthy controls, as described previously [8]. Chronic neuropathic pain patients ($n = 16$) were included in the study. All patients were recruited by convenience sampling from an open-label clinical trial evaluating the effect of bolus injections of ziconotide [22]. Immediately before ziconotide injection, blood and CSF samples were collected. Patients had to be refractory to conventional anti-neuropathic pain pharmacological treatment and were under consideration for spinal cord stimulation (SCS) at Linköping University Hospital, Sweden.

Inclusion criteria were as follows: patient at least 18 years of age; chronic peripheral neuropathic pain (6 months or more) caused by trauma or surgery for whom conventional pharmacological treatment had failed; average visual analogue scale (VAS) pain intensity last week of 40 mm or more; patient capable of judgement, meaning the patient was able to comprehend information about the drug, its administration and evaluation of efficacy and side effects; signed informed consent.

Exclusion criteria were: intrathecal chemotherapy; pregnant or lactating women; limited life expectancy; intracranial hypertension; known liver or kidney disease characterized by serum transaminases, total bilirubin, alkaline phosphatase or creatinine > 1.2 times above the upper normal limit; advanced cardiopulmonary disease, ongoing infection in the lumbar area (systematically or locally), coagulopathy; history of psychiatric disorder; allergy to ziconotide or any of the excipients in the ziconotide vial; participation in another clinical trial during the last 30 days.

As reported in previously published papers [8,16,22,23], the nerve injury that was deemed to cause the neuropathic pain was classified using the International Classification of Diseases version 10 (ICD-10) (see Table 1). Four patients suffered from peripheral neuropathic pain projected to the upper extremity, and twelve from peripheral neuropathic pain projected to the lower extremity. All patients included in this study described their pain as continuous. Twelve of the patients experienced an exacerbation of the pain during physical activity. Nine of the patients had concomitant diseases: hypertension ($n = 4$), polymyalgia rheumatica ($n = 1$), psoriasis ($n = 2$), fibromyalgia ($n = 1$), diabetes ($n = 1$), mild angina ($n = 2$), panic disorder ($n = 1$), mild obstructive lung disease ($n = 1$), vertebral compressions ($n = 1$), orthostatism ($n = 1$), peptic ulcer ($n = 1$), dyspepsia ($n = 1$) and anemia ($n = 1$). The use of concomitant medication including analgesics was also reported. Four of the patients no longer used any pain medication at inclusion, while three patients had a single analgesic and nine patients used two analgesics or more. The distribution of the usage of the different medications were paracetamol ($n = 7$), non-steroidal anti-inflammatory drugs (NSAID) ($n = 2$), opioids ($n = 9$), gabapentinoids ($n = 7$) and antidepressants ($n = 6$).

Table 1. Nerve injury according to the ICD-10 classification system ($n = 16$) in falling order of frequency.

ICD-10 Code	Nerve Structure	Number of Participants
S342	Root of lumbar or sacral spine	8
S142	Root of cervical spine	3
S740	Sciatic nerve at hip and thigh level	1
S549	Unspecified nerve at forearm level	1
S949	Unspecified nerve at ankle or foot level	1
S841	Peroneal nerve at lower leg level	1
S343	ICauda equina	1
G629	Polyneuropathy, unspecified	1

Participants answered questionnaires about pain and their state of health. We registered basic background information such as sex, age, weight, length, pain duration (measured in months), average pain intensity (VAS), location of pain, characterization of pain (constant, intermittent or transitory), impact of physical activity on pain, concomitant diseases and ongoing medication.

2.2. Sample Collection

A lumbar puncture was performed by an experienced anesthesiologist (EB) with a 27 GA pencil-point Whitacre needle (BD, Franklin Lakes, NJ, USA), and a 10 mL sample of CSF was drawn in five numbered syringes of 2 mL each. Each sample was immediately cooled on ice, transported to the Painomics® laboratory, Linköping University Hospital, centrifuged, divided in aliquots and stored at −70 °C.

2.3. Metabolomics Analysis

CSF samples was mixed (5:1) with phosphate buffer solution containing 1.5 M KH_2PO_4, 580 µM TSP-d4, NaN_3, D_2O, pH 7.4 and transferred to 3 mm NMR tubes. The samples were analyzed at the Swedish Nuclear Magnetic Resonance (NMR) Centre in Gothenburg using an Oxford 800 Mhz magnet equipped with a Bruker Avance III HD console, 3 mm TCI cryoprobe and a cooled Sample Jet auto sampler (Bruker BioSpin, Fällanden, Switzerland), as described previously [16]. Generated data from NMR spectrometer were processed in TopSpin3.5pl7 (Bruker BioSpin, Fällanden, Switzerland). Chenomx 9.0 (Chenomx Inc., Edmonton, AB, Canada) and the Human Metabolite Database [24] were used for identification of the metabolite signals.

2.4. Statistics

IBM SPSS Statistics (version 27.0, IBM, Armonk, NY, USA) was used for bivariate analyses. Unless stated otherwise, data are presented as median (25th–75th percentile). Mann–Whitney U test and Chi square test were used as appropriate for group comparisons. Spearman's rho was calculated for bivariate correlations. A p-value ≤ 0.05 was considered significant. To handle the multiple testing problem, a false discovery rate (FDR) at the 10% level was applied using the Benjamini–Hochberg procedure [25].

Multivariate data analysis (MVDA) by projection was performed on metabolomics data with SIMCA-P+ (v.17.0, Sartorius Stedim Biotech, Umeå, Sweden). First, principal component analysis (PCA) was used for quality control and to check for multivariate outliers (strong outliers defined as Hotelling's T2 >> T2Crit (95%) and moderate outliers as DModX > 2 *DCrit). Then, we effectuated orthogonal partial least squares—discriminant analysis (OPLS-DA)—whereby group belonging was used as the outcome variable (Y-variable) and the metabolic features as predictors (X-variables). OPLS was used instead of OPLS-DA when non-categorical variables were used as Y-variables (such as VAS pain intensity, pain duration, age or body mass index (BMI)). The parameters used for evaluation of the OPLS-DA and OPLS models were R^2 (goodness of fit), Q^2 (goodness of prediction) and cross validated analysis of variance (CV-ANOVA) which provides a familiar metric for the model as a whole (i.e., a p-value). The differences between R^2 and Q^2 should not be greater than 0.3, otherwise suggesting overfitting. The variable influence on projection (VIP) indicates the relevance of the group of X-variables that best explain Y. A backward variable elimination strategy was applied [26], whereby the 20 X-variables with the lowest VIP were eliminated and a new OPLS-DA model was built. This procedure was reiterated until Q^2 stopped increasing, indicating an optimal model. We also used p(corr) which is the loading of each variable scaled as a correlation coefficient (range from -1 to $+1$). VIP ≥ 1.0, absolute p(corr) ≥ 0.6 and CV-ANOVA ≤ 0.05 were considered as significant. The analysis and the presented parameters are in accordance with the guidelines presented by Wheelock and Wheelock [20].

2.5. Ethics

The regional ethics committee in Linköping approved the study (Dnr M136-06 and Dnr 2012/94-32). The study was conducted in accordance with the Helsinki Declaration. After verbal and written information, written informed consent was obtained from all the participants.

3. Results

3.1. Background Data

The patient group consisted of 36% females and the healthy control group of 58% females; the difference between groups was not statistically significant ($p = 0.249$). Patients were older than controls (57.5 (52.0–69.0) vs. 51.0 (27.5–54.5) years, $p = 0.005$). Patients also had a tendency towards higher BMI (26.5 (23.3–29.7) vs. 23.9 (22.0–25.4) kg/m^2, $p = 0.072$). VAS pain intensity in patients was 72 (59–82) mm and pain duration 59 (36–120) months.

3.2. Overview and Quality Control of Metabolic Data

First, an unsupervised PCA model was computed for overview and quality control of the data using 444 metabolomic features as X-variables ($n = 28$, 444 X-variables, $R^2 = 0.49$, $Q^2 = 0.27$). Two patients were identified as strong outliers and were therefore excluded from further analyses. As shown in the Supplementary Materials S1, the contribution plot of one of them revealed that the features contributing most to the position of that individual in the PCA model were almost all related to glucose—and this was indeed the patient with concomitant diabetes (see Section 2.1).

3.3. OPLS-DA Model Comparing Patients and Controls

After an initial OPLS-DA model with $n = 26$, 2 components (the first predictive and the second orthogonal), 444 X-variables, $R^2 = 0.74$, $Q^2 = 0.30$ and $p = 0.101$ by CV-ANOVA, a backward variable elimination strategy was applied, resulting in a final OPLS-DA model with $n = 26$, 2 components (the first predictive and the second orthogonal), 215 X-variables, $R^2 = 0.70$, $Q^2 = 0.42$, $p = 0.017$ by CV-ANOVA. The score plot of the model is depicted in Figure 1, illustrating clear group separation. The model was additionally validated using a permutation plot (Supplementary Materials S2). In total, 26 features had an absolute p(corr) ≥ 0.6 for the first predictive component, indicating that they, when taking the whole correlation structure of the material into consideration, were the most important variables for group separation (Table 2). Twenty-one out of twenty-six features were statistically significant when comparing the two groups by univariate statistics (Table 2), and all twenty-one remained significant when a FDR of 10% was applied. Notably, for six out of the top ten metabolomic features listed Table 2, the features were absent in *all* healthy controls. The six features only identified in patients were 26_C, 41_C, 40_C, 29_C, 30_C and 36_C.

Table 2. Cerebrospinal metabolomic features separating chronic neuropathic pain patients ($n = 14$) from healthy controls ($n = 12$).

Feature ID	Tentative Annotation	Pain Patients Intensity	Healthy Controls Intensity	p(corr)	VIP	p-Value
_43_C	Tyrosine + acetaminophen	46,954 (40,742–58,404)	36,427 (34,508–40,219)	0.81	1.48	0.041 *
_26_C	Acetaminophen	35,906 (0–59,894)	0 (0–0)	0.79	1.48	0.001 *
_44_C	Acetaminophen + tyrosine	54,407 (17,385–86,355)	15,232 (11,381–16,918)	0.79	1.47	0.005 *
_41_C	Acetaminophen	14,400 (0–26,768)	0 (0–0)	0.76	1.42	0.005 *
_40_C	Acetaminophen	42,075 (0–66,636)	0 (0–0)	0.76	1.42	0.005 *
_29_C	Acetaminophen	34,118 (0–59,041)	0 (0–0)	0.76	1.42	0.005 *
_30_C	Acetaminophen	5111 (0–14,300)	0 (0–0)	0.73	1.35	0.010 *
_450_C	Unknown singlet; acetamide?	58,600 (43,259–65,879)	39,481 (34,774–43,149)	0.73	1.34	0.005 *
_36_C	Unknown; diclofenac?	10,885 (0–16,224)	0 (0–0)	0.73	1.33	0.005 *
_503_C	Unknown singlet	37,373 (23,829–65,360)	25,998 (18,988–29,115)	0.72	1.32	0.020 *
_416_C	Acetaminophen	122,276 (98,341–146,314)	91,822 (84,232–97,395)	0.71	1.29	0.023 *
_333_C		23558 (21,121–26,910)	20,066 (14,804–23,496)	0.70	1.30	0.150
_21_C	Unknown; diclofenac?	5046 (0–12,759)	0 (0–0)	0.69	1.25	0.010 *
_352_C	Unknown singlet; dimethylamine?	66,322 (56,259–74,161)	51,341 (45,414–62,591)	0.68	1.25	0.051
_546_C	Pregabalin?	23,466 (20,505–49,519)	17,954 (15,269–19,301)	0.67	1.21	0.003 *
_396_C	Unknown singlet; acetylsalicylate?	17,326 (14,477–23,720)	13,263 (12,062–14,112)	0.67	1.21	0.007 *
_28_C	Acetaminophen	5756 (0–18,558)	0 (0–0)	0.67	1.24	0.010 *
_322_C		23,721 (21,822–25,907)	21,357 (13,720–22,045)	0.66	1.24	0.086
_502_C	Unknown singlet	19,648 (16,848–30,175)	15,496 (5388–17,337)	0.66	1.20	0.023 *
_543_C	Pregabalin?	20,593 (16,462–42,854)	15,809 (14,127–20,877)	0.65	1.17	0.014 *
_339_C	Unknown singlet; N,N-dimethylglycine?	12,799 (10,537–15,528)	0 (0–5595)	0.64	1.16	0.007 *
_35_C	Unknown; diclofenac?	5230 (0–12,274)	0 (0–0)	0.63	1.18	0.010 *
tyr_33_C	Tyrosine	35,814 (30,869–39,163)	32,743 (28,207–33,807)	0.62	1.13	0.114
_545_C	Pregabalin?	20,732 (14,992–50,151)	16,375 (15,239–18,050)	0.62	1.12	0.041 *
_548_C	Pregabalin?	20,748 (18,226–47,331)	18,624 (15,957–22,198)	0.61	1.10	0.063
ala + fructose_205_C	ALANINE + fructose	248,350 (214,837–268,264)	199,950 (190,866–223,795)	0.60	1.22	0.020 *

The metabolites are listed in descending order of absolute p(corr). A positive p(corr) indicates higher levels in patients than in healthy controls, while a negative p(corr) indicates the opposite. Intensity is expressed as median (IQR). * denotes significance at the 0.05 level; all remained significant at a false discovery rate (FDR) of 10%. The suffix C denotes cerebrospinal fluid.

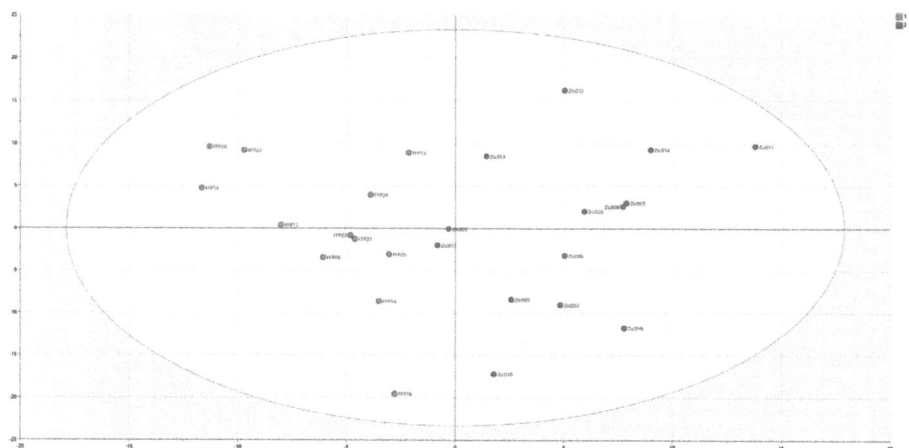

Figure 1. Score plot of OPLS-DA model, showing group separation between patients and controls along the first predictive component (x-axis). Each patient is a blue dot, each healthy control is a green.

The top 10 features of Table 2 were then analyzed in more depth, focusing on patients (n = 14). A bivariate correlation matrix for the top 10 features is presented in Table 3, showing that 8 of the features demonstrated a high degree of intercorrelation (the exceptions being 450_C and 503_C). This pattern was confirmed by the loading plot of the OPLS-DA model, part of which is depicted in Supplementary Materials S3. Going back to Table 3 and looking specifically at the six features absent in healthy controls, all bivariate correlation coefficients except for 36_C ranged 0.789–0.995, i.e., there was (in patients) a very high degree of intercorrelation between five features that were absent in healthy controls.

Table 3. Correlation matrix in *patients* (n = 14) by Spearman's rho for the top 10 features separating patients from healthy controls.

		_43_C	_26_C	_44_C	_41_C	_40_C	_29_C	_30_C	_450_C	_36_C	_503_C
_43_C	Rho	1.000	0.856 **	0.842 **	0.867 **	0.881 **	0.872 **	0.777 **	0.284	0.540 *	0.424
	p-value		<0.001	<0.001	<0.001	<0.001	<0.001	0.001	0.326	0.046	0.131
_26_C	Rho		1.000	0.960 **	0.978 **	0.973 **	0.983 **	0.823 **	0.290	0.571 *	0.254
	p-value			<0.001	<0.001	<0.001	<0.001	<0.001	0.315	0.033	0.381
_44_C	Rho			1.000	0.947 **	0.956 **	0.956 **	0.819 **	0.270	0.641 *	0.160
	p-value				<0.001	<0.001	<0.001	<0.001	0.350	0.014	0.584
_41_C	Rho				1.000	0.981 **	0.995 **	0.779 **	0.204	0.581 *	0.190
	p-value					<0.001	<0.001	0.001	0.485	0.029	0.516
_40_C	Rho					1.000	0.990 **	0.828 **	0.213	0.562 *	0.199
	p-value						<0.001	<0.001	0.465	0.037	0.495
_29_C	Rho						1.000	0.789 **	0.194	0.557 *	0.199
	p-value							0.001	0.505	0.038	0.495
_30_C	Rho							1.000	0.406	0.574 *	0.289
	p-value								0.150	0.032	0.317
_450_C	Rho								1.000	0.384	0.486
	p-value									0.175	0.078
_36_C	Rho									1.000	0.318
	p-value										0.268
_503_C	Rho										1.000
	p-value										

Correlation coefficients in bold. * denotes significance at the 0.05 level and ** denotes significance at the 0.001 level. The feature id suffix C denotes cerebrospinal fluid.

Then, the features tabulated in Table 2 were tentatively annotated, revealing that most of them were related to medication, mainly acetaminophen (paracetamol), see Table 2. When the features related to medication were removed from the above-mentioned OPLS-DA model, it was no longer significant (n = 26, 1 component, 197 X-variables, R^2 = 0.29, Q^2 = 0.18, p = 0.10 by CV-ANOVA).

3.4. OPLS Models in Patients

In patients (n = 14), it was not possible to regress VAS by OPLS using the 444 features as in the OPLS-DA model above as X-variables. Likewise, a non-significant model resulted when regressing pain duration by OPLS (n = 14, 2 components, R^2 = 0.85 and Q^2 = 0.21, p = 0.68 by CV-ANOVA) with the same 444 features.

Additionally, to investigate a potential confounding effect of age (which different significantly between groups) on the main OPLS-DA results as per the above, an OPLS model with age as outcome variable (Y-variable) was computed using the 215 features of the final OPLS-DA model as X-variables. The initial model had n = 14, R^2 = 0.87, Q^2 = 0.40 and p = 0.28 by CV-ANOVA. After the backward elimination procedure, the final model had 174 X-variables, n = 14, R^2 = 0.82, Q^2 = 0.44 and p = 0.21 by CV-ANOVA. Notwithstanding the fact that the OPLS model was not significant, we still scrutinized the absolute p(corr) values for the 12 features listed in Table 2 that remained in the OPLS model after the backward elimination procedure; none of them showed any indication of being correlated to age (all had absolute p(corr) $\leq$ 0.45). Moreover, using bivariate statistics, none of the features listed in Table 2 had any significant correlation to age. Hence, we found no indication that our findings in Table 2 were primarily related to age rather than to belonging to a specific group.

Finally, in a manner similar to age, we also investigated a potential confounding effect of sex on the main OPLS-DA results. After the backward elimination procedure, the final model with sex as Y variable had 175 X-variables, n = 14, R^2 = 0.37, Q^2 = 0.20 and p = 0.29 by CV-ANOVA. Notwithstanding the fact that the model was statistically non-significant, we still scrutinized the absolute p(corr) values for the eight features listed in Table 2 that remained in the model after the backward elimination procedure; only one of them, namely ala + fructose_205_C, showed an indication of being correlated to sex (absolute p(corr) = 0.78). We therefore compared ala + fructose_205_C in men vs. women, finding a statistically non-significant tendency towards higher levels of ala + fructose_205_C in men (p = 0.125, see Supplementary Materials S4).

4. Discussion

Unexpectedly, the main finding of the study was that CSF metabolomics was a sensitive method to detect ongoing analgesic medication, especially acetaminophen (also known as paracetamol), in chronic pain patients. We wish to highlight three aspects of this "negative" result.

First, our findings are a reminder of the importance of collecting information about concomitant medication when conducting pain biomarker studies in general, and perhaps in particular when studying CSF. In correlative studies such as this one, several confounding factors may be at work simultaneously. Ideally, controls should be age-, BMI- and sex-matched. However, this is especially difficult in CSF studies, given the difficulty in obtaining CSF in contrast to blood or saliva. Other possible confounders could be concomitant diseases or concomitant medication—and the latter seems to be the case in the present study.

Second, although in a sense disappointing, our results clearly demonstrate the power of CSF metabolomics combined with MVDA in identifying real and relevant group differences for central nervous system processes. Given that modern omics studies can generate a vast amount of data (meaning that the number of variables can by far exceed the number of participants), the omics field actualizes the multiple testing problem—hence, the potential accusation of being on a fishing expedition, also known as data dredging or p-hacking.

Indeed, the phenomenon of alpha inflation means that if two groups are compared two times, the risk of getting at least one significant result due to chance is not 5%, but almost 10%. If instead 20 comparisons are made, the probability increases to 64%; this phenomenon is captured by the formula $1 - 0.95^k$, where k is the number of comparisons [27,28]. If 100 comparisons are made, the probability hence rises to 99%. While we do understand and concur with such concerns, we also think that explorative studies such as this one are important to conduct, and that this can be sensibly achieved. One crucial aspect is the possibility of using not only traditional univariate statistics but MVDA, thereby taking the whole correlation structure of the material into consideration, hence better separating the valuable information from the noise [21]. MVDA is of course no panacea, but it is an important tool [20]. If we go back to the present study, it is notable that the combination of omics (in this case, metabolomics) and MVDA was able to detect a difference between the groups that we indeed know to be true (i.e., patients were on medication). We think that this should give researchers in the field some level of confidence that similar proteomics or proteomics-related studies using this statistical methodology can generate true results.

Third, our results are in line with the view that acetaminophen acts in the CNS. Until quite recently, at least in Sweden, the standard textbook teaching was that acetaminophen is a *peripherally* acting analgesic [29]. After more than 100 years of use, the exact mechanism of action of paracetamol remains to be determined [30]. In the CNS, acetaminophen has been said to have effects on cyclooxygenase, on serotonergic descending neuronal pathways, on L-arginine/NO pathways and on the endocannabinoid system [31]. Alternatively, acetaminophen analgesia could be mediated by the formation of its bioactive AM404 metabolite in the central nervous system [32]. Even if our findings do not prove that acetaminophen is centrally acting (it could be an epiphenomenon), they are nonetheless highly congruent with that view.

There are few NMR metabolomics studies on neuropathic pain in general, and on CSF in particular. We have previously reported interesting NMR metabolomic findings in blood from the same patients with chronic neuropathic pain [16]. In that study, 50 out of 326 features in blood significantly contributed to group separation between patients and healthy controls, the significant metabolites being involved in inflammation, CNS functioning and neural signaling [16]. In the present CSF study, the "metabolomic trace" of the treatment given to patients had a much higher magnitude than differences due to chronic pain pathophysiology. Therefore, should patients taking analgesics be excluded in future CSF metabolomic studies? The difficulty in obtaining CSF would be an argument in that direction, i.e., given the low number of patients included in CSF studies, group homogeneity is all the more important when studying CSF as opposed to blood or saliva (which are more easily collected).

5. Limitations

The low number of participants in this observational study is an obvious limitation. However, it is important to understand that studies such as the present one are not intended to generate *clinical* biomarker candidates. If that had been our purpose, dozens or perhaps hundreds of samples would have been necessary. Instead, using the terminology proposed by Pavlou et al., this was an early discovery phase, pre-clinical exploratory study [33]. For such studies, in which the aim is to strive towards a better understanding of pathophysiological mechanisms in humans, the study design requirements are different from clinical biomarker studies [34]. Another limitation pertains to the fact that, as already mentioned, it would have been better to have age-matched controls. Also, given the small sample size, a narrower age range would have been preferable (the age range of all participants was 21–75 years).

6. Conclusions

We have shown that the combination of CSF metabolomics and MVDA is a powerful tool to detect ongoing molecular events in the central nervous system. We were unable to detect a disease signal in patients with chronic neuropathic pain vs. healthy controls, centrally acting medication overshadowing the putative pathophysiologically interesting findings. These negative results notwithstanding, CSF metabolomics still have a role to play when investigating the mechanisms of chronic pain; however, our study shows that the power of an investigative method can also be its problem.

Supplementary Materials: The following supporting information can be downloaded at: https://www.mdpi.com/article/10.3390/biomedicines11092525/s1.

Author Contributions: Conceptualization, B.G. (Bijar Ghafouri), B.G. (Björn Gerdle) and E.B.; methodology, B.G. (Bijar Ghafouri), B.G. (Björn Gerdle), and E.B.; investigation, B.G. (Bijar Ghafouri) and K.T.; data curation, B.G. (Bijar Ghafouri) and K.T.; formal analysis, B.G. (Björn Gerdle) and E.B.; writing—original draft preparation, E.B.; writing—review and editing, B.G. (Bijar Ghafouri), B.G. (Björn Gerdle), E.B. and K.T.; visualization, E.B.; supervision, B.G. (Bijar Ghafouri); funding acquisition, E.B.; project administration, E.B. All authors have read and agreed to the published version of the manuscript.

Funding: This research was funded by NEURO Sweden (E.B.), and ALF Grants, Region Östergötland (E.B.).

Institutional Review Board Statement: The regional ethics committee in Linköping approved the study (Dnr M136-06 and Dnr 2012/94-32). The study was conducted in accordance with the Helsinki Declaration.

Informed Consent Statement: Informed consent was obtained from all subjects involved in the study.

Data Availability Statement: Data are not publicly available.

Acknowledgments: The support of Swedish NMR Centre at the University of Gothenburg, Gothenburg, Sweden, is hereby acknowledged.

Conflicts of Interest: The authors declare no conflict of interest. The funders NEURO Sweden and ALF Grants, Region Östergötland, had no role in the design, execution, interpretation, or writing of the study.

References

1. Sommer, C. Exploring pain pathophysiology in patients. *Science* **2016**, *354*, 588–592. [CrossRef] [PubMed]
2. Ji, R.R.; Nackley, A.; Huh, Y.; Terrando, N.; Maixner, W. Neuroinflammation and Central Sensitization in Chronic and Widespread Pain. *Anesthesiology* **2018**, *129*, 343–366. [CrossRef] [PubMed]
3. Yezierski, R.P.; Hansson, P. Inflammatory and Neuropathic Pain from Bench to Bedside: What Went Wrong? *J. Pain* **2018**, *19*, 571–588. [CrossRef] [PubMed]
4. Bäckryd, E.; Tanum, L.; Lind, A.L.; Larsson, A.; Gordh, T. Evidence of both systemic inflammation and neuroinflammation in fibromyalgia patients, as assessed by a multiplex protein panel applied to the cerebrospinal fluid and to plasma. *J. Pain Res.* **2017**, *10*, 515–525. [CrossRef]
5. Bäckryd, E.; Lind, A.L.; Thulin, M.; Larsson, A.; Gerdle, B.; Gordh, T. High levels of cerebrospinal fluid chemokines point to the presence of neuroinflammation in peripheral neuropathic pain: A cross-sectional study of 2 cohorts of patients compared with healthy controls. *Pain* **2017**, *158*, 2487–2495. [CrossRef]
6. Gonçalves Dos Santos, G.; Delay, L.; Yaksh, T.L.; Corr, M. Neuraxial Cytokines in Pain States. *Front. Immunol.* **2019**, *10*, 3061. [CrossRef]
7. Sommer, C.; Leinders, M.; Uceyler, N. Inflammation in the pathophysiology of neuropathic pain. *Pain* **2018**, *159*, 595–602. [CrossRef]
8. Bäckryd, E.; Ghafouri, B.; Carlsson, A.K.; Olausson, P.; Gerdle, B. Multivariate proteomic analysis of the cerebrospinal fluid of patients with peripheral neuropathic pain and healthy controls—A hypothesis-generating pilot study. *J. Pain Res.* **2015**, *8*, 321–333. [CrossRef]
9. Balogh, M.; Aguilar, C.; Nguyen, N.T.; Shepherd, A.J. Angiotensin receptors and neuropathic pain. *Pain Rep.* **2021**, *6*, e869. [CrossRef]
10. Rice, A.S.; Dworkin, R.H.; McCarthy, T.D.; Anand, P.; Bountra, C.; McCloud, P.I.; Hill, J.; Cutter, G.; Kitson, G.; Desem, N.; et al. EMA401, an orally administered highly selective angiotensin II type 2 receptor antagonist, as a novel treatment for postherpetic neuralgia: A randomised, double-blind, placebo-controlled phase 2 clinical trial. *Lancet* **2014**, *383*, 1637–1647. [CrossRef]
11. Jensen, T.S.; Baron, R.; Haanpaa, M.; Kalso, E.; Loeser, J.D.; Rice, A.S.; Treede, R.D. A new definition of neuropathic pain. *Pain* **2011**, *152*, 2204–2205. [CrossRef] [PubMed]
12. Baron, R.; Binder, A.; Wasner, G. Neuropathic pain: Diagnosis, pathophysiological mechanisms, and treatment. *Lancet Neurol.* **2010**, *9*, 807–819. [CrossRef] [PubMed]

13. Finnerup, N.B.; Attal, N.; Haroutounian, S.; McNicol, E.; Baron, R.; Dworkin, R.H.; Gilron, I.; Haanpaa, M.; Hansson, P.; Jensen, T.S.; et al. Pharmacotherapy for neuropathic pain in adults: A systematic review and meta-analysis. *Lancet Neurol.* **2015**, *14*, 162–173. [CrossRef] [PubMed]
14. Gerdle, B.; Ghafouri, B. Proteomic studies of common chronic pain conditions—A systematic review and associated network analyses. *Expert Rev. Proteom.* **2020**, *17*, 483–505. [CrossRef] [PubMed]
15. Teckchandani, S.; Nagana Gowda, G.A.; Raftery, D.; Curatolo, M. Metabolomics in chronic pain research. *Eur. J. Pain* **2021**, *25*, 313–326. [CrossRef] [PubMed]
16. Ghafouri, B.; Thordeman, K.; Hadjikani, R.; Bay Nord, A.; Gerdle, B.; Bäckryd, E. An investigation of metabolome in blood in patients with chronic peripheral, posttraumatic/postsurgical neuropathic pain. *Sci. Rep.* **2022**, *12*, 21714. [CrossRef]
17. Malatji, B.G.; Meyer, H.; Mason, S.; Engelke, U.F.H.; Wevers, R.A.; van Reenen, M.; Reinecke, C.J. A diagnostic biomarker profile for fibromyalgia syndrome based on an NMR metabolomics study of selected patients and controls. *BMC Neurol.* **2017**, *17*, 88. [CrossRef]
18. Chang, L.; Munsaka, S.M.; Kraft-Terry, S.; Ernst, T. Magnetic resonance spectroscopy to assess neuroinflammation and neuropathic pain. *J. Neuroimmune Pharmacol. Off. J. Soc. NeuroImmune Pharmacol.* **2013**, *8*, 576–593. [CrossRef]
19. Zabek, A.; Swierkot, J.; Malak, A.; Zawadzka, I.; Deja, S.; Bogunia-Kubik, K.; Mlynarz, P. Application of (1)H NMR-based serum metabolomic studies for monitoring female patients with rheumatoid arthritis. *J. Pharm. Biomed. Anal.* **2016**, *117*, 544–550. [CrossRef]
20. Wheelock, A.M.; Wheelock, C.E. Trials and tribulations of 'omics data analysis: Assessing quality of SIMCA-based multivariate models using examples from pulmonary medicine. *Mol. Biosyst.* **2013**, *9*, 2589–2596. [CrossRef]
21. Eriksson, L.; Byrne, T.; Johansson, E.; Trygg, J.; Vikström, C. *Multi- and Megavariate Data Analysis: Basic Principles and Applications*, 3rd ed.; MKS Umetrics AB: Malmo, Sweden, 2013.
22. Bäckryd, E.; Sorensen, J.; Gerdle, B. Ziconotide Trialing by Intrathecal Bolus Injections: An Open-Label Non-Randomized Clinical Trial in Postoperative/Posttraumatic Neuropathic Pain Patients Refractory to Conventional Treatment. *Neuromodulation* **2015**, *18*, 404–413. [CrossRef]
23. Jönsson, M.; Bäckryd, E.; Jonasson, L.; Gerdle, B.; Ghafouri, B. Differences in plasma lipoprotein profiles between patients with chronic peripheral neuropathic pain and healthy controls: An exploratory pilot study. *Pain Rep.* **2022**, *7*, e1036. [CrossRef] [PubMed]
24. Wishart, D.S.; Guo, A.; Oler, E.; Wang, F.; Anjum, A.; Peters, H.; Dizon, R.; Sayeeda, Z.; Tian, S.; Lee, B.L.; et al. HMDB 5.0: The Human Metabolome Database for 2022. *Nucleic Acids Res.* **2022**, *50*, D622–D631. [CrossRef] [PubMed]
25. Glickman, M.E.; Rao, S.R.; Schultz, M.R. False discovery rate control is a recommended alternative to Bonferroni-type adjustments in health studies. *J. Clin. Epidemiol.* **2014**, *67*, 850–857. [CrossRef] [PubMed]
26. Mehmood, T.; Sæbø, S.; Liland, K.H. Comparison of variable selection methods in partial least squares regression. *J. Chemom.* **2020**, *34*, e3226. [CrossRef]
27. Ranganathan, P.; Pramesh, C.S.; Buyse, M. Common pitfalls in statistical analysis: The perils of multiple testing. *Perspect. Clin. Res.* **2016**, *7*, 106–107. [CrossRef]
28. M.G. Why is multiple testing a problem? 2008. Available online: http://www.stat.berkeley.edu/~mgoldman/Section0402.pdf (accessed on 16 April 2023).
29. Hasselstrom, J.; Olsson, G.L. Smärtbehandling. In *Läkemedelsboken*; Bogentoft, S., Ed.; Apoteket AB: Stockholm, Sweden, 2001; pp. 675–698.
30. Sharma, C.V.; Mehta, V. Paracetamol: Mechanisms and updates. *Contin. Educ. Anaesth. Crit. Care Pain* **2014**, *14*, 153–158. [CrossRef]
31. Jóźwiak-Bebenista, M.; Nowak, J.Z. Paracetamol: Mechanism of action, applications and safety concern. *Acta Pol. Pharm.* **2014**, *71*, 11–23.
32. Mallet, C.; Desmeules, J.; Pegahi, R.; Eschalier, A. An Updated Review on the Metabolite (AM404)-Mediated Central Mechanism of Action of Paracetamol (Acetaminophen): Experimental Evidence and Potential Clinical Impact. *J. Pain Res.* **2023**, *16*, 1081–1094. [CrossRef]
33. Pavlou, M.P.; Diamandis, E.P.; Blasutig, I.M. The long journey of cancer biomarkers from the bench to the clinic. *Clin. Chem.* **2013**, *59*, 147–157. [CrossRef]
34. Mischak, H.; Vlahou, A.; Righetti, P.G.; Calvete, J.J. Putting value in biomarker research and reporting. *J. Proteom.* **2014**, *96*, A1–A3. [CrossRef] [PubMed]

Disclaimer/Publisher's Note: The statements, opinions and data contained in all publications are solely those of the individual author(s) and contributor(s) and not of MDPI and/or the editor(s). MDPI and/or the editor(s) disclaim responsibility for any injury to people or property resulting from any ideas, methods, instructions or products referred to in the content.

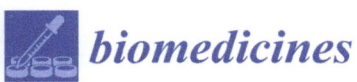

Article

Platelet Membrane Proteins as Pain Biomarkers in Patients with Severe Dementia

Hugo Ribeiro [1,2,3,4,5,6,*], Raquel Alves [3,4,5,6], Joana Jorge [3,4,5,6], Ana Cristina Gonçalves [3,4,5,6], Ana Bela Sarmento-Ribeiro [3,4,5,6,7], Manuel Teixeira-Veríssimo [3,7], Marília Dourado [3,4,6] and José Paulo Andrade [8,9]

[1] Community Support Team in Palliative Care—Group of Health Centers Gaia, 4430-999 Vila Nova de Gaia, Portugal
[2] Faculty of Medicine, University of Porto, 4200-319 Porto, Portugal
[3] Faculty of Medicine, University of Coimbra, 3000-548 Coimbra, Portugal
[4] Coimbra Institute for Clinical and Biomedical Research (iCBR)—Group of Environment, Genetics and Oncobiology (CIMAGO), University of Coimbra (FMUC), 3000-548 Coimbra, Portugal
[5] University Clinics of Hematology and Oncology and Laboratory of Oncobiology and Hematology (LOH), Faculty of Medicine, University of Coimbra (FMUC), 3000-548 Coimbra, Portugal
[6] Center for Innovative Biomedicine and Biotechnology (CIBB), 3000-548 Coimbra, Portugal
[7] Hematology Service, Centro Hospitalar e Universitário de Coimbra (CHUC), 3000-548 Coimbra, Portugal
[8] CINTESIS@RISE, Faculty of Medicine, University of Porto, 4200-319 Porto, Portugal
[9] Unit of Anatomy, Department of Biomedicine, Faculty of Medicine, University of Porto, 4200-319 Porto, Portugal
* Correspondence: hribeiroff@gmail.com

Abstract: Pain is one of the most frequent health problems, and its evaluation and therapeutic approach largely depend on patient self-report. When it is not possible to obtain a self-report, the therapeutic decision becomes more difficult and limited. This study aims to evaluate whether some membrane platelet proteins could be of value in pain characterization. To achieve this goal, we used 53 blood samples obtained from palliative patients, 44 with non-oncological pain and nine without pain. We observed in patients with pain a decrease in the percentage of platelets expressing CD36, CD49f, and CD61 and in the expression levels of CD49f and CD61 when compared with patients without pain. Besides that, an increase in the percentage of platelets expressing CD62p was observed in patients with pain. These results suggest that the levels of these platelet cluster differentiations (CDs) could have some value as pain biomarkers objectively since they are not dependent on the patient's participation. Likewise, CD40 seems to have some importance as a biomarker of moderate and/or severe pain. The identification of pain biomarkers such as CD40, CD49f, CD62p and CD61 can lead to an adjustment of the therapeutic strategy, contributing to a faster and more adequate control of pain and reduction in patient-associated suffering.

Keywords: chronic pain; pharmacology; platelets; biomarkers; palliative care

1. Introduction

The International Association for the Study of Pain (IASP) defines pain as an "unpleasant sensory and emotional experience associated with, or resembling that associated with, actual or potential tissue damage" [1]. Pain is multifactorial, with multiple pathways involved [2], which explains why it is a multidimensional experience that can significantly impair an individual's quality of life [3]. Pain can be classified according to tissue damage (nociceptive pain), nerve damage (neuropathic pain), and altered pain modulation (nociplastic pain) [3].

Pain characterization is essential for the correct approach for patients with chronic pain, starting with the assessment of pain intensity [4]. The proper characterization is dependent on patient self-report; pain multidimensional hetero-assessment scales can be used as an alternative, especially for dementia patients with and/or patients that cannot characterize their pain [5–7]. However, as pain is a sensory and emotional experience, it is subjective, and its expression is primarily determined by the perceived intensity of the painful sensation [5].

Preclinical and clinical studies have investigated the hypothesis that biomarkers may also be used to identify and quantify pain. Findings from a preclinical study show that inflammatory pain and neuropathic pain have different biomarkers [8], but most studies do not correlate with pain duration or intensity. Further studies are needed to gain insights into pain biomarkers to enhance pain management practices improving patient care, especially for those who suffer from severe cognitive decline or dementia and are unable to express themselves.

Platelet heterogeneity and subpopulations may suggest distinct biological roles for different platelet subpopulations and may be useful in evaluating inherited or acquired platelet disorders and platelet function in health and disease [9]. Besides their role in hemostasis, thrombosis, and wound healing, platelets are now known to play major effector activities in several additional functions, including inflammatory reactions and innate immune responses [9]. Further, platelets are the closest and most accessible peripheral neuronal-like cellular system likely to provide a wealth of information about neuronal functioning [10].

Since discovered by Giulio Bizzozero in 1882 [11], platelets have been exploited for their clinical value. Platelet surface receptors, such as CD62p (P-selectin) and CD41 (GPIIb-IIIa), have also been quantified as markers of the activation state of platelets [12]. The extravascular activation of platelets may contribute to nociceptor excitation and pain since platelets store and, upon stimulation, release potential allogenic substances such as serotonin, histamine, and precursor molecules of bradykinin [13,14].

Identifying blood and platelet pain biomarkers has been advanced as the next great tool for pain identification and characterization, allowing tailored treatments [15,16].

Few studies relate pain with platelet activation, as pain inhibition occurs with platelet antiaggregants [17–20]. However, there are other studies on specific situations, for instance, knee osteoarthritis or post-teeth extraction pain, where platelet-rich plasma (PRP) or fibrin-rich platelets (PRF) may have a significant analgesic effect [21–24]. However, the role of peripheral blood platelets membrane proteins as markers for pain evaluation and characterization is not yet clarified [25,26].

Here, we evaluated the levels of membrane proteins, namely receptors related to several recognized functions of platelets, such as recognition, adhesion, aggregation, activation, inflammation, and immune modulation. In this context, the levels of the glycoprotein IV (CD36), the adhesion molecules, integrin α6 (CD49f), integrin β3 (CD61) and p-selectin (CD62p), the complement activation inhibitor protein (CD59) and the TNFα family receptor CD40 were evaluated in palliative patients platelets.

The main aim of this study is to evaluate whether some known platelet membrane proteins could be of value in pain characterization and can be used as non-invasive pain biomarkers in patients where we cannot rely on their self-report, particularly patients with advanced dementia.

2. Materials and Methods

For this study, we collected individual and clinical data and peripheral blood samples from 53 palliative patients with non-oncological diseases, followed by a specialized palliative care team between 1 September and 31 December 2021.

This is an observational, analytic, transversal, non-interventional study using medical and nursing records on chronic pain patients.

The Ethics Committees of the Faculty of Medicine of the University of Porto and the North Regional Health Administration of Portugal approved the research procedures, and the study was conducted following the Declaration of Helsinki. Before enrollment, participants or their legal representatives provided informed consent for participation. The international ethical guidelines of confidentiality, the anonymity of personal data, and the abandonment option were followed.

For the collection of individual and clinical data, we consulted the records in the individual clinical files, after which they were registered in a protected Microsoft Excel sheet. To identify each patient, an alphanumeric code was used, thus keeping the identity confidential since only the researcher knows it. Following the European General Data Protection Regulation (GDPR), these electronic files will be deleted after the end of the study and the publication of the results. Data were collected regarding the following variables: age, sex, type and intensity of pain, opioid and other analgesics, such as nonsteroidal anti-inflammatory drugs (NSAIDs) and acetaminophen, and doses in use. We also noted whether the patient had pain control at the moment of blood sample collection.

We also collected information regarding the presence of a diagnosis of dementia and its type. For patients that had severe dementia, we used the Pain Assessment in Advanced Dementia Scale (PAINAD) [27] to identify and distinguish those who probably have uncontrolled pain, and we separated PAINAD values (under 5, between 5 and 7 and 8 to 10), to evaluate a possible clinical correlation of these PAINAD values and mild, moderate or severe pain, respectively. For patients who could self-report their pain, we used the pain numeric scale [28].

For the purpose of analyzing the expression of the platelet biomarkers, we selected the following: glycoprotein IV (CD36), integrin α6 (CD49f), integrin β3 (CD61), and p-selectin (CD62p), the complement activation inhibitor protein (CD59) and TNFα family receptor CD40, that we analyzed in absolute and relative concentration.

We proceeded to the ROC curve analysis to evaluate the significance of the area under the curve and if we have a cut-off point for CD40.

2.1. Platelets Membrane Proteins Evaluation by Flow Cytometry

The platelet phenotyping was performed in freshly prepared platelet suspensions. None of the participants were recently transfused. Briefly, platelets were separated by centrifuging citrated blood specimens at $120\times g$ for 20 min at room temperature (RT). Then, the platelet-rich plasma was collected into a tube, and the platelets were washed using 2 mL of wash buffer (BD cell wash). Next, 1×10^6 platelets were incubated with the monoclonal antibodies anti-CD36 conjugated with FITC (BD Pharmingen, BD Biosystems, San Diego, CA, USA), anti-CD49f conjugated with PE conjugate (BD Pharmingen, BD Biosystems), anti-CD61 conjugated with PerCP-Cy5.5 (BD Pharmingen, BD Biosystems), anti-CD62 conjugated with APC (BD Pharmingen, BD Biosystems), anti-CD59 conjugated with BV421(BD Horizon, BD Biosystems), and anti-CD40 conjugated with BV510 (BD Horizon, BD Biosystems) for 15 min at RT in the dark, according to manufacture instructions. Then, cells were washed twice with FACS flow (BD Biosystems) by centrifugation at $300\times g$ for 5 min and immediately analyzed in a FACS Canto II flow cytometer (BD Biosystems). At least 50,000 events were collected using FACS DIVA software (BD Biosystems), and the results were analyzed through Infinicyte software (Cytognos, Salamanca, Spain). The results are expressed in the percentage of cells expressing each protein marker and as mean fluorescence intensity (MIF).

2.2. Statistical Analysis

Statistical analysis was performed using the SPSS software (Statistical Package for the Social Sciences, version 28.0 for Windows, IBM Corp., Armonk, NY, USA). For the statistical analysis of data, we used measures of descriptive statistics (absolute and relative frequencies, means, and respective standard deviations) and inferential statistics. The significance level for rejecting the null hypothesis was set at $(\alpha) \leq 0.05$. We used the Pearson correlation coefficient, Fisher's test, Chi-squared test of independence, Student's t-test for independent samples, Mann–Whitney U test, and Kruskal–Wallis test. The normality of distribution was analyzed with the Shapiro-Wilk test, and the homogeneity of variances was analyzed with Levene's test. We analyzed the Chi-squared assumption that there should not be more than 20% of cells with expected frequencies inferior to 5. In those situations where this assumption could not be satisfied, we used the Chi-squared test with the Monte Carlo simulation.

The following variables were included: age, sex, type of pain, the intensity of pain, opioid and dose used, and other analgesics, such as nonsteroidal anti-inflammatory drugs (NSAIDs) and paracetamol, and absolute (MIF) and relative concentration levels of CD36, CD49f, CD61, CD62p, CD59, and CD40. We also included the type of dementia (because most of the patients had this condition) and controlled pain time for patients diagnosed with chronic pain, but their pain is controlled at the moment of blood collection. For patients that had severe dementia, we used the Pain Assessment in Advanced Dementia Scale (PAINAD) [27] to identify uncontrolled pain. Other variables that could have a relationship with our findings were also included, such as renal function (using the Cockcroft–Gault formula [29], body mass index (BMI), functionality (using the Karnovsky scale [30]), and nutritional status (using Mini-Nutritional Assessment scale [31]).

2.3. Inclusion Criteria

All patients under clinical follow-up from a palliative care specialized team from the North region of Portugal with non-oncological diseases.

All patients or their legal representatives provided informed consent for participation.

3. Results

We selected 95 patients. However, five patients or their legal representatives refused to participate in this study and 20 of them were in their last days of life, and it was decided not to conduct a blood collection in this clinical condition. We could not collect blood samples from 17 patients, as they were too fragile, with hypovolemia and bad venous accesses.

So, we collected samples from a total of 53 patients with an average age of 74.8 years old, a minimum of 29 and a maximum of 98 years old; most were female [n = 39 (73.6%)]. Forty-four patients suffered from pain, and nine had no pain. We had no patients with known autoimmune diseases (inflammatory bowel disease, multiple sclerosis, psoriasis, or other of these conditions).

Among the 44 patients with chronic pain, 38 had severe dementia. We could not evaluate the type of pain and intensity in these patients. Therefore, we used PAINAD to distinguish those who probably have uncontrolled pain (PAINAD $\geq$ 5, present in 32 patients), and we separated PAINAD values (under 5, between 5 and 7 and 8 to 10) because in the clinical evaluation, there was a correlation between these PAINAD values and the possibility of having mild, moderate or severe pain, respectively. Among the 44 patients with pain, 19 were under opioid treatment (15 with dementia and four without dementia).

We had six patients with pain and without dementia and nine without pain and without dementia (controls), as shown in Table 1.

Table 1. Characterization of the Study Population.

Total of Patients: 53		Patients with Pain and Dementia (n = 38)	Patients with Pain and without Dementia (n = 6)	Patients without Pain and without Dementia (Controls) (n = 9)
Gender	Male	29% (n = 11)	50% (n = 3)	0
	Female	71% (n = 27)	50% (n = 3)	100%
Average age (years)		84.1	62.5	44.7
PAINAD	<5	15.8% (n = 6)	NA	NA *
	5–7	73.7% (n = 28)	NA	NA
	8–10	10.5% (n = 4)	NA	NA
Average numeric pain scale		NA	4.3	0

Table 1. Cont.

Total of Patients: 53		Patients with Pain and Dementia (n = 38)	Patients with Pain and without Dementia (n = 6)	Patients without Pain and without Dementia (Controls) (n = 9)
Type of Pain	Nociceptive	39.5% (n = 15)	50% (n = 3)	NA
	Neuropathic	2.6% (n = 1)	16.7% (n = 1)	NA
	Mixed	57.9% (n = 22)	33.3% (n = 2)	NA
Type of Dementia	Vascular	36.8% (n = 14)	NA	NA
	Alzheimer	36.8% (n = 14)	NA	NA
	Mixed	7.9% (n = 3)	NA	NA
	Other	18.4% (n = 7)	NA	NA
Under opioid treatment		39.5% (n = 15)	66.7% (n = 4)	NA

* NA: Not Applicable.

In the platelets of patients with chronic pain, we observe a statistically significant decrease in the percentage of platelets expressing CD36, CD49f, and CD61, but the decrease in the expression levels of these biomarkers was only observed for CD49f and CD61, compared with those patients without pain (Table 2). An increase in the percentage of platelets expressing CD62p was detected when compared with patients without pain ($p = 0.002$) (Table 2).

Table 2. Platelets Membrane Proteins in Patients with and without Chronic Pain.

	Patients without Pain and without Dementia Controls (n = 9)	Patients with Pain (n = 44)	
	M ± SD	M ± SD	p
CD36 (%)	98.04 ±1.97	91.54 ± 12.30	0.004 **
CD36 (MIF)	6475.64 ± 2081.58	5506.31 ± 2168.98	0.228
CD49f (%)	99.16 ± 0.35	95.31 ± 10.79	0.037 *
CD49f (MIF)	5385.83 ± 855.09	4540.24 ± 969.50	0.021 *
CD61 (%)	99.37 ± 0.18	95.28 ± 10.76	0.026 *
CD61 (MIF)	16561.81 ± 1404.83	13571.25 ± 4064.78	0.009 **
CD62P (%)	8.47 ± 4.87	22.62 ± 23.65	0.002 **
CD62P (MIF)	760.75 ± 114.10	1357.76 ± 2606.10	0.499
CD59 (%)	4.76 ± 3.03	3.45 ± 5.67	0.507
MIF CD59 (MIF)	1556.62 ± 509.90	1771.15 ± 858.56	0.478
CD40 (%)	0.15 ± 0.09	0.09 ± 0.17	0.289
CD40 (MIF)	1476.08 ± 352.14	1456.12 ± 501.07	0.911

MIF—Mean Fluoresce intensity; * $p \leq 0.05$, ** $p \leq 0.01$. F: median intensity fluorescence; M: mean; SD: standard deviation; p: significance.

While the differences observed in CD36, CD49f and CD61 are age and sex independent, the difference observed in CD62p were more accentuated in men (about three times higher) comparatively with the observed in women (Table 3). When we compared the platelets phenotype between patients with dementia with those without dementia, we did not observe any statistically significant difference. Further, the relationship between the type of pain and the type of dementia is also not statistically significant (Table 3).

Table 3. Gender And Membrane Protein Platelets.

	Female (*n* = 39)	Male (*n* = 14)	
	M ± SD	M ± SD	*p*
% CD36	92.89 ± 10.89	92.58 ± 13.25	0.899
MIF CD36	5392.26 ± 2050.79	6662.28 ± 2330.91	0.090
% CD49f	96.35 ± 8.80	95.18 ± 12.86	0.445
MIF CD49f	4617.57 ± 978.43	4986.02 ± 1057.26	0.291
% CD61	96.38 ± 8.80	95.13 ± 12.83	0.272
MIF CD61	14465.44 ± 3481.59	13172.91 ± 4992.24	0.525
% CD62P	**13.76 ± 17.43**	**39.24 ± 24.50**	**0.006 *****
MIF CD62P	829.68 ± 261.73	2549.57 ± 4691.50	0.251
% CD59	3.74 ± 5.35	3.59 ± 5.20	0.839
MIF CD59	1643.84 ± 790.28	2000.70 ± 815.41	0.130
% CD40	0.09 ± 0.10	0.14 ± 0.28	0.939
MIF CD40	1471.59 ± 505.76	1423.23 ± 362.89	0.899

*** $p \leq 0.001$; MIF: median intensity fluorescence; M: mean; SD: standard deviation; *p*: significance; bold: values statistically significant.

As we can observe in Table 4, patients under opioids, when compared with patients that did not receive opioids, present a statistically significant decrease in the percentage of platelets expressing CD36 (88.52% vs. 95.58, $p = 0.026$) and in the expression levels of CD49f (4254.22 vs. 4995.90, $p = 0.012$), CD61 (12643.79 vs. 15128.72, $p = 0.029$) and CD59 (1345.35 vs. 1975.92, $p = 0.008$).

Table 4. Comparative Analysis Of Membrane Platelets Proteins Between Patients Receiving And Not Receiving Opioids Medication.

	No Opioids (*n* = 25)	Opioids (*n* = 19)	
	M ± SD	M ± SD	*p*
% pos CD36	95.58 ± 8.38	88.52 ± 14.02	0.026 *
MIF CD36	6007.26 ± 2091.56	5211.73 ± 2246.28	0.228
% pos CD49f	98.82 ± 2.39	91.78 ± 14.55	0.070
MIF CD49f	**4995.90 ± 850.84**	**4254.22 ± 1065.23**	**0.012 ***
% pos CD61	98.87 ± 2.40	91.73 ± 14.51	0.077
MIF CD61	**15128.72 ± 3014.28**	**12643.79 ± 4616.87**	**0.029 ***
% pos CD62P	21.08 ± 22.70	17.93 ± 21.35	0.290
MIF CD62P	1483.69 ± 2983.98	863.37 ± 388.08	0.242
% pos CD59	2.94 ± 3.33	4.90 ± 7.28	0.597
MIF CD59	**1975.92 ± 886.94**	**1345.35 ± 444.10**	**0.008 ****
% pos CD40	0.07 ± 0.08	0.15 ± 0.23	0.742
MIF CD40	1485.36 ± 467.55	1420.60 ± 490.21	0.458

* $p \leq 0.05$, ** $p \leq 0.01$; MIF: median intensity fluorescence; M: mean; SD: standard deviation; *p*: significance; bold: values statistically significant.

Regarding the type of pain and its relationship with biomarkers under study, we found statistically significant differences, as shown in Table 5. A decrease in the expression levels of CD62p in the platelets of patients with nociceptive pain was observed compared with patients presenting mixed pain (723.52 vs. 1953.63, $p = 0.002$) (Table 5).

Table 5. Membrane Proteins Platelets In Patients Suffering From Nociceptive Pain Or Mixed Pain.

	Nociceptive (n = 18)	Mixed (n = 26)	
	M ± SD	M ± SD	p
% pos CD36	91.17 ± 11.90	92.52 ± 10.84	0.762
MIF CD36	4751.72 ± 1640.23	5952.76 ± 2468.46	0.118
% pos CD49f	94.47 ± 12.16	97.46 ± 5.19	0.789
MIF CD49f	4206.69 ± 995.35	4859.81 ± 890.59	0.056
% pos CD61	94.37 ± 12.13	97.45 ± 5.15	0.762
MIF CD61	12507.53 ± 5215.25	14025.16 ± 3190.66	0.682
% pos CD62P	13.89 ± 14.69	31.73 ± 28.35	0.117
MIF CD62P	**723.55 ± 184.49**	**1953.63 ± 3679.90**	**0.002 ****
% pos CD59	4.49 ± 6.59	3.05 ± 5.46	0.789
MIF CD59	1570.69 ± 826.36	1963.51 ± 937.17	0.274
% pos CD40	0.16 ± 0.25	0.04 ± 0.02	0.145
MIF CD40	1530.59 ± 601.99	1466.89 ± 448.98	0.986

** $p \leq 0.01$, MIF: median intensity fluorescence; M: mean; SD: standard deviation; p: significance; bold: values statistically significant.

The clinical history (other diseases) of the patients does not seem to interfere with platelet biomarkers.

With regard to pain intensity, we observed a significant relationship with the percentage of platelets expressing CD40. In fact, the percentage of platelets expressing CD40 is significantly higher in patients with moderate-severe pain (considering PAINAD ≥5) compared with those with mild pain (0.18% vs. 0.02%, $p = 0.047$), as it is shown in Table 6.

Table 6. Membrane Proteins Platelets In Patients Suffering From Mild Pain And With Moderate Or Severe Pain.

	Mild Pain (PAINAD < 5)	Moderate or Severe Pain (PAINAD 5-10)	
	M	M	p
% pos CD36	90.34 ± 18.24	92.88 ± 9.64	0.563
MIF CD36	5635.97 ± 2538.02	5424.41 ± 2158.15	0.859
% pos CD49f	99.19 ± 0.66	95.94 ± 9.29	0.625
MIF CD49f	4310.17 ± 1200.38	4549.61 ± 949.86	0.723
% pos CD61	99.16 ± 0.66	95.90 ± 9.27	0.625
MIF CD61	10900.50 ± 4611.48	13915.31 ± 3929.31	0.059
% pos CD62P	16.62 ± 21.39	23.77 ± 24.53	0.690
MIF CD62P	3966.84 ± 7066.90	918.62 ± 383.06	0.533
% pos CD59	1.25 ± 1.49	3.90 ± 6.08	0.282
MIF CD59	1699.58 ± 1043.69	1793.88 ± 856.69	0.533
% pos CD40	**0.02 ± 0.02**	**0.10 ± 0.18**	**0.047 ***
MIF CD40	1202.00 ± 232.79	1509.31 ± 524.97	0.207

* $p \leq 0.05$, MIF: median intensity fluorescence; M: mean; SD: standard deviation; p: significance; bold: values statistically significant.

We used receiver operating characteristic curve (ROC) analysis to verify if CD40 could be a peripheral biomarker of pain intensity. We proceed to the ROC curve analysis to evaluate the significance of the area under the curve and if we have a cut-off point for this biomarker. The area under the curve is statistically significant, 0.777, with $p = 0.049$, as shown in Figure 1 and Table 7.

The ideal cut-off point corresponds to 0.025 (sensitivity 74.2%, specificity 80%, positive predictive value = 95.8%, negative predictive value = 33.3%).

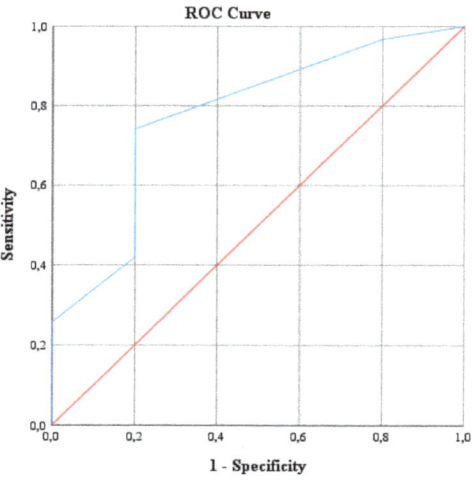

Figure 1. ROC curve of CD 40 as a biomarker of moderate or severe pain.

Table 7. ROC Analysis Data for CD40.

Area	SE [a]	Asymptotic p [b]	Asymptotic 95% Confidence Interval	
			Lower Bound	Upper Bound
0.777	0.114	0.049	0.555	1.000

[a]: Standard Error; [b]: Significance.

4. Discussion

In patients with severe dementia, we cannot rely on self-report, and the characterization of the pain is difficult. The identification of biomarkers could be a valuable solution to enable targeted medical treatment. In this study, we find that CD36, CD49f, percentage of CD49f, CD61, percentage of CD61, and CD62p can be considered as platelet biomarkers of pain, CD62p as a platelet biomarker for nociceptive pain and CD40 as a platelet biomarker for moderate-severe pain.

The hypothesis that biomarkers may be used to identify and quantify pain was investigated in several preclinical and clinical studies. A preclinical study showed that inflammatory and neuropathic pain have different biomarkers [8]. Further investigations provided mixed results. For example, cystatin C levels in the cerebrospinal fluid appear to be a predictive marker for postherpetic neuralgia in patients with varicella-zoster virus and a pain marker in women experiencing labor pain. However, it is not correlated with pain duration or intensity. Investigations into potential biomarkers for chest pain showed that cardiac markers used to aid in the diagnosis and prognosis of cardiac disease correlate with tissue damage rather than with pain [8]. Further studies are needed to gain insights into biomarkers for pain to enhance pain management practices.

Platelet receptors are important for their normal functioning as they either activate platelets or act as adhesion molecules interacting with the damaged endothelium, other platelets, and leukocytes. Besides the platelet role in hemostasis, they also have a role in inflammation, antimicrobial activity, angiogenesis, tumor growth, and metastasis. In the absence of their receptors, platelets are unable to perform these functions. Some of the well-recognized platelet receptors are integrins, leucine-rich repeats receptors, selectins, tetraspanins, transmembrane receptors, prostaglandin receptors, lipid receptors, immunoglobulin superfamily receptors, tyrosine kinase receptors, and other platelet receptors [32]. The present study focused on membrane glycoproteins, such as CD36, CD49f, CD61, CD62p, CD59, and CD40.

CD36 or Glycoprotein IV is a member of the class B scavenger receptor family of cell surface proteins, a multiligand pattern recognition receptor that interacts with a large number of structurally dissimilar ligands, including long chain fatty acid (LCFA), advanced glycation end products (AGE), thrombospondin-1, oxidized low-density lipoproteins (oxLDLs), high density lipoprotein (HDL), phosphatidylserine, apoptotic cells, beta-amyloid fibrils (fAβ), collagens I and IV, and Plasmodium falciparum-infected erythrocytes [33].

CD49f is an adhesion molecule, namely α6-integrin 1, associated with inflammation towards the regulation of differentiation, adhesion, and migration of human mesenchymal stem cells [34]. CD61 is the integrin β3, a glycoprotein that plays a role in platelet aggregation and also as a receptor for fibrinogen, fibronectin, von Willebrand factor and vitronectrin [35]. CD62p or P-selectin is a membrane protein that redistributes to the plasma membrane during platelet activation and degranulation and mediates the interaction of activated endothelial cells or platelets with leukocytes [36]. CD59 is the complement activation inhibitor protein that binds to complement components C5 and C9 and prevents the polymerization of C9, which is required for the formation of the membrane attack complex (MAC) [37]. CD40 is a receptor of the TNFα family, being a cytokine produced by many cells, and was originally identified by its cytotoxic effects. In addition to inducing cell death in some types of cells, it also elicits a wide range of physiological responses, such as inflammation, cell proliferation, and differentiation [38]. Further, circulating biomarkers of platelet activation, including soluble CD40 and CD62p, have also been studied as a strategy to monitor the efficacy of combination antiretroviral therapy (cART) in patients infected with HIV [39].

Platelet surface receptors have also been quantified as markers of the activation state of platelets, and platelet activation is increased in dementia [40]. Both platelet CD62p (P-selectin) expression and CD41 (GPIIb-IIIa) complex activation are significantly elevated in Alzheimer's Dementia (AD) patients [41]. CD41 is a platelet activation marker in dementia, and the increase in CD41 complex expression in platelets was associated with faster cognitive decline in AD [41]. However, there is an overwhelming lack of additional clinical studies. Another platelet receptor, CD62p, is present on activated platelet membranes [42] and promotes platelet adhesion and thrombin formation [43]. Increased levels of CD62p were found in circulation in AD patients, but there was no significant change in the membrane-bound [12,38]. The soluble form of CD62p was also significantly elevated in HIV patients not under cART, compared with those cART-treated and with healthy control groups, suggesting its role in monitoring combination antiretroviral therapy [39].

We already know that there is platelet activation in pain, especially inflammatory pain (Barkai et al., 2019; Beurling-Harbury and Schade, 1989), but we are still unaware of all the pathophysiology and molecular biology involved [19]. The identification of CD36, CD49f, percentage of CD49f, CD61, percentage of CD61, and CD62p as platelet biomarkers of pain was statistically significant. These new markers must be considered in the process of obtaining pain biomarkers in peripheral blood.

For patients with well-controlled pain, in comparison with those with non-controlled pain, we did not find statistically significant differences regarding laboratory data, including patients with well-controlled pain for seven or more days. These data are relevant because we could expect a reduction in platelet activation with pain control, considering that the half-life of platelets is seven days. However, it may mean that some underlying mechanisms and causes of pain may be equally active, and there is only pain desensitization.

In opioid-treated patients presenting a better control of pain, there is less expression of biomarkers such as CD36, CD49f, CD61, and CD59. These data are in agreement with the literature on the effect of opioids on platelets, particularly in reducing their activity [44–46].

The sample was too small to assess more types of pain in addition to nociceptive and mixed pain. However, CD62p has been shown to be a reliable marker of nociceptive pain. Although it has not yet been specifically studied in this regard, the role of p-selectin is already known and has been linked to inflammatory pain [47,48].

CD40 (TNFα receptor family) was identified as a potential biomarker of moderate or severe pain intensity. The association of a biomarker with pain severity has not yet been established, although there are several references to platelet markers and disease severity [49–51]. In addition to the biomarkers of the existence or not of pain, which can be a powerful aid in the therapeutic approach of patients, the identification of biomarkers that allow the characterization of pain, in this case by intensity, can allow the therapeutic adjustment as quickly as possible, reducing suffering and minimizing the adverse effects of drugs.

Further, and besides the involvement of platelets in several diseases the presented markers, such as CD40, in autoimmune diseases such as inflammatory bowel disease, multiple sclerosis, psoriasis, or other autoimmune diseases, we had no patients with these diseases. Other diseases from the known medical history of these patients (such as hypertension) did not influence the platelet markers, according to what we found in the literature [9,10,12,17,26].

This is one of the largest studies on pain biomarkers that we know of, and it is the only study comparing patients with non-oncological pain with specific platelet biomarkers. However, the sample is small, and further studies are needed considering these markers to confirm their viability as pain markers and CD40 as a marker of moderate-severe pain.

In vulnerable and dependent patients, in whom we cannot rely on self-report, the identification of pain biomarkers such as CD40 can lead to an adjustment of the therapeutic strategy, according to the WHO ladder [4], contributing to a faster and more adequate control of pain and reduction in associated suffering.

Author Contributions: Conceptualization, H.R., M.D., A.B.S.-R. and J.P.A.; methodology, H.R., R.A., J.J. and A.C.G.; software, H.R.; validation, A.B.S.-R., J.P.A., M.D., M.T.-V.; formal analysis, H.R. and A.B.S.-R.; investigation, H.R., R.A., J.J. and A.C.G.; resources, H.R. and A.C.G.; data curation, H.R., R.A., J.J. and A.B.S.-R.; writing—original draft preparation, H.R.; writing—review and editing, all authors; visualization, H.R., A.B.S.-R., J.P.A., M.T.-V. and M.D.; supervision, J.P.A., M.T.-V. and M.D.; project administration, H.R.; funding acquisition, H.R., A.B.S.-R., J.P.A. and M.D. All authors have read and agreed to the published version of the manuscript.

Funding: This article was supported by National Funds through FCT—Fundação para a Ciência e a Tecnologia, I.P., within CINTESIS, R&D Unit (reference UIDB/4255/2020) and within the scope of the project RISE, Associated Laboratory (reference LA/P/0053/2020).

Institutional Review Board Statement: The study was conducted in accordance with the Declaration of Helsinki, and approved by the Ethics Committees of the Faculty of Medicine of the University of Porto and the North Regional Health Administration of Portugal (PI 20210013, 27 Januray 2022).

Informed Consent Statement: Informed consent was obtained from all subjects involved in the study or their legal representatives.

Data Availability Statement: The data presented in this study are available on request from the corresponding author.

Acknowledgments: Júlia Magalhães, Elisabete Costa, Tatiana Cardoso, Patrícia Rocha, Luísa Lopes, Isabel Chaves-Castro, Carla Lopes-Mota, Ângela Bouça, Cristina Pereira, Foco Saúde Gaia, LAPI Norte Gaia, Health Care Centers Group Gaia.

Conflicts of Interest: The authors declare no conflict of interest.

References

1. Raja, S.N.; Carr, D.B.; Cohen, M.; Finnerup, N.B.; Flor, H.; Gibson, S.; Keefe, F.J.; Mogil, J.S.; Ringkamp, M.; Sluka, K.A.; et al. The revised International Association for the Study of Pain definition of pain: Concepts, challenges, and compromises. *Pain* **2020**, *161*, 1976–1982. [CrossRef]
2. Garcia-Larrea, L.; Peyron, R. Pain matrices and neuropathic pain matrices: A review. *Pain* **2013**, *154* (Suppl. 1), S29–S43. [CrossRef] [PubMed]
3. Orr, P.M.; Shank, B.C.; Black, A.C. The Role of Pain Classification Systems in Pain Management. *Crit. Care Nurs. Clin. N. Am.* **2017**, *29*, 407–418. [CrossRef] [PubMed]
4. World Health Organization. *WHO's Pain Relief Ladder*; WHO: Geneva, Switzerland, 2009.
5. Ribeiro, H.; Moutinho, R.; Dourado, M. *Particularidades da Avaliação e Tratamento da dor no Idoso: Contributo Para a Validação da Pain Quality Assessment Scale© e Abordagem Terapêutica na População Idosa*; Universidade de Coimbra: Coimbra, Portugal, 2017.
6. World Health Organization. *Normative Guidelines on Pain Management*; WHO: Geneva, Switzerland, 2007.
7. Ali, A.; Arif, A.W.; Bhan, C.; Kumar, D.; Malik, M.B.; Sayyed, Z.; Akhtar, K.H.; Ahmad, M.Q. Managing Chronic Pain in the Elderly: An Overview of the Recent Therapeutic Advancements. *Cureus* **2018**, *10*, e3293. [CrossRef]
8. Marchi, A.; Vellucci, R.; Mameli, S.; Piredda, A.R.; Finco, G. Pain Biomarkers. *Clin. Drug Investig.* **2009**, *29* (Suppl. 1), 41–46. [CrossRef]
9. Chen, Y.; Zhong, H.; Zhao, Y.; Luo, X.; Gao, W. Role of platelet biomarkers in inflammatory response. *Biomark. Res.* **2020**, *8*, 28. [CrossRef] [PubMed]
10. Kopeikina, E.; Ponomarev, E.D. The Role of Platelets in the Stimulation of Neuronal Synaptic Plasticity, Electric Activity, and Oxidative Phosphorylation: Possibilities for New Therapy of Neurodegenerative Diseases. *Front. Cell. Neurosci.* **2021**, *15*, 269. [CrossRef] [PubMed]
11. Ribatti, D.; Crivellato, E. Giulio Bizzozero and the discovery of platelets. *Leuk. Res.* **2007**, *31*, 1339–1341. [CrossRef]
12. Akingbade, O.E.; Gibson, C.; Kalaria, R.N.; Mukaetova-Ladinska, E.B. Platelets: Peripheral Biomarkers of Dementia? *J. Alzheimer's Dis.* **2018**, *63*, 1235–1259. [CrossRef]
13. Arman, M.; Payne, H.; Ponomaryov, T.; Brill, A. Role of Platelets in Inflammation. *InTech* **2015**. [CrossRef]
14. Ringkamp, M.; Schmelz, M.; Kress, M.; Allwang, M.; Ogilvie, A.; Reeh, P. Activated human platelets in plasma excite nociceptors in rat skin, in vitro. *Neurosci. Lett.* **1994**, *170*, 103–106. [CrossRef] [PubMed]
15. Osman, Y.; Vatte, C.B. Study of platelet activation markers and plasma cytokines in sickle cell disease patients during vaso-occlusive pain crises. *J. Hematop.* **2018**, *11*, 37–44. [CrossRef]
16. Niculescu, A.B.; Le-Niculescu, H.; Levey, D.F.; Roseberry, K.; Soe, K.C.; Rogers, J.; Khan, F.; Jones, T.; Judd, S.; Mc-Cormick, M.A.; et al. Towards precision medicine for pain: Diagnostic biomarkers and repurposed drugs. *Mol. Psychiatry* **2019**, *24*, 501–522. [CrossRef]
17. Salem, H.H. Leg Pain and Platelet Aggregates in Thrombocythemic Myeloproliferative Disease. *JAMA* **1980**, *244*, 1122. [CrossRef] [PubMed]
18. Kwon, Y.-J.; Koh, I.; Chung, K.; Lee, Y.-J.; Kim, H.-S. Association between platelet count and osteoarthritis in women older than 50 years. *Ther. Adv. Musculoskelet. Dis.* **2020**, *12*. [CrossRef] [PubMed]
19. Barkai, O.; Puig, S.; Lev, S.; Title, B.; Katz, B.; Eli-Berchoer, L.; Gutstein, H.B.; Binshtok, A.M. Platelet-derived growth factor activates nociceptive neurons by inhibiting M-current and contributes to inflammatory pain. *Pain* **2019**, *160*, 1281–1296. [CrossRef]
20. Weth, D.; Benetti, C.; Rauch, C.; Gstraunthaler, G.; Schmidt, H.; Geisslinger, G.; Sabbadini, R.; Proia, R.; Kress, M. Activated platelets release sphingosine 1-phosphate and induce hypersensitivity to noxious heat stimuli in vivo. *Front. Neurosci.* **2015**, *9*, 140. [CrossRef]
21. Jankovic, S.; Aleksic, Z.; Klokkevold, P.; Lekovic, V.; Dimitrijevic, B.; Kenney, E.B.; Camargo, P. Use of platelet-rich fibrin membrane following treatment of gingival recession: A randomized clinical trial. *Int. J. Periodontics Restor. Dent.* **2012**, *32*, e41-50.
22. Chignon-Sicard, B.; Georgiou, C.A.; Fontas, E.; David, S.; Dumas, P.; Ihrai, T.; Lebreton, E. Efficacy of Leukocyte- and Platelet-Rich Fibrin in Wound Healing. *Plast. Reconstr. Surg.* **2012**, *130*, 819e–829e. [CrossRef]
23. Kumar, N.; Prasad, K.; Ramanujam, L.; Ranganath, K.; Dexith, J.; Chauhan, A. Evaluation of Treatment Outcome After Impacted Mandibular Third Molar Surgery With the Use of Autologous Platelet-Rich Fibrin: A Randomized Controlled Clinical Study. *J. Oral Maxillofac. Surg.* **2015**, *73*, 1042–1049. [CrossRef]
24. Ozgul, O.; Senses, F.; Er, N.; Tekin, U.; Tuz, H.H.; Alkan, A.; Kocyigit, I.D.; Atil, F. Efficacy of platelet rich fibrin in the reduction of the pain and swelling after impacted third molar surgery: Randomized multicenter split-mouth clinical trial. *Head Face Med.* **2015**, *11*, 37. [CrossRef] [PubMed]
25. Ludwig, N.; Hilger, A.; Zarbock, A.; Rossaint, J. Platelets at the Crossroads of Pro-Inflammatory and Resolution Pathways during Inflammation. *Cells* **2022**, *11*, 1957. [CrossRef] [PubMed]
26. Gianazza, E.; Brioschi, M.; Baetta, R.; Mallia, A.; Banfi, C.; Tremoli, E. Platelets in Healthy and Disease States: From Biomarkers Discovery to Drug Targets Identification by Proteomics. *Int. J. Mol. Sci.* **2020**, *21*, 4541. [CrossRef] [PubMed]
27. Warden, V.; Hurley, A.C.; Volicer, L. Development and Psychometric Evaluation of the Pain Assessment in Advanced Dementia (PAINAD) Scale. *J. Am. Med. Dir. Assoc.* **2003**, *4*, 9–15. [CrossRef] [PubMed]
28. Rodriguez, C.S. Pain measurement in the elderly: A review. *Pain Manag. Nurs.* **2001**, *2*, 38–46. [CrossRef] [PubMed]

29. Michels, W.M.; Grootendorst, D.C.; Verduijn, M.; Elliott, E.G.; Dekker, F.W.; Krediet, R.T. Performance of the Cockcroft-Gault, MDRD, and New CKD-EPI Formulas in Relation to GFR, Age, and Body Size. *Clin. J. Am. Soc. Nephrol.* **2010**, *5*, 1003–1009. [CrossRef]
30. Mor, V.; Ms, L.L.; Morris, J.N.; Wiemann, M. The Karnofsky performance status scale: An examination of its reliability and validity in a research setting. *Cancer* **1984**, *53*, 2002–2007. [CrossRef]
31. Soysal, P.; Isik, A.T.; Arik, F.; Kalan, U.; Eyvaz, A.; Veronese, N. Validity of the Mini-Nutritional Assessment Scale for Evaluating Frailty Status in Older Adults. *J. Am. Med. Dir. Assoc.* **2019**, *20*, 183–187. [CrossRef]
32. Saboor, M.; Ayub, Q.; Ilyas, S. Moinuddin Platelet receptors; an instrumental of platelet physiology. *Pak. J. Med. Sci.* **2013**, *29*, 891–896. [CrossRef]
33. Silverstein, R.L.; Febbraio, M. CD36, a Scavenger Receptor Involved in Immunity, Metabolism, Angiogenesis, and Behavior. *Sci. Signal.* **2009**, *2*, re3. [CrossRef]
34. Yang, Z.; Dong, P.; Fu, X.; Li, Q.; Ma, S.; Wu, D.; Kang, N.; Liu, X.; Yan, L.; Xiao, R. CD49f Acts as an Inflammation Sensor to Regulate Differentiation, Adhesion, and Migration of Human Mesenchymal Stem Cells. *Stem Cells* **2015**, *33*, 2798–2810. [CrossRef]
35. Barbar, L.; Jain, T.; Zimmer, M.; Kruglikov, I.; Sadick, J.S.; Wang, M.; Kalpana, K.; Rose, I.V.; Burstein, S.R.; Rusielewicz, T.; et al. CD49f Is a Novel Marker of Functional and Reactive Human iPSC-Derived Astrocytes. *Neuron* **2020**, *107*, 436–453.e12. [CrossRef] [PubMed]
36. Antibody Engineering & Therapeutics, Human P Selectin CD62P. Available online: https://www.creative-biolabs.com/magic-antibody-discovery-human-p-selectin-cd62p-42-771-membrane-protein-partial-higg1-fc-tag-4597.htm?gclid=CjwKCAiA9qKbBhAzEiwAS4yeDb2xogl7NOfoyX_wAeIwqYZ7Uvy2cbPeaGyuErgcsu-zrgV7CMsuIRoC2boQAvD_BwE (accessed on 10 October 2022).
37. Weinstock, C.; Anliker, M.; Von Zabern, I. CD59: A long-known complement inhibitor has advanced to a blood group system. *Immunohematology* **2015**, *31*, 145–151. [CrossRef]
38. Dostert, C.; Grusdat, M.; Letellier, E.; Brenner, D. The TNF Family of Ligands and Receptors: Communication Modules in the Immune System and Beyond. *Physiol. Rev.* **2019**, *99*, 115–160. [CrossRef]
39. Steel, H.C.; Venter, W.D.F.; Theron, A.J.; Anderson, R.; Feldman, C.; Arulappan, N.; Rossouw, T.M. Differential Responsiveness of the Platelet Biomarkers, Systemic CD40 Ligand, CD62P, and Platelet-Derived Growth Factor-BB, to Virally-Suppressive Antiretroviral Therapy. *Front. Immunol.* **2021**, *11*, 594110. [CrossRef]
40. Ramos-Cejudo, J.; Johnson, A.D.; Beiser, A.; Seshadri, S.; Salinas, J.; Berger, J.S.; Fillmore, N.R.; Do, N.; Zheng, C.; Kovbasyuk, Z.; et al. Platelet Function Is Associated With Dementia Risk in the Framingham Heart Study. *J. Am. Heart Assoc.* **2022**, *11*, e023918. [CrossRef]
41. Sevush, S.; Jy, W.; Horstman, L.L.; Mao, W.-H.; Kolodny, L.; Ahn, Y.S. Platelet Activation in Alzheimer Disease. *Arch. Neurol.* **1998**, *55*, 530–536. [CrossRef]
42. Green, S.A.; Smith, M.; Hasley, R.B.; Stephany, D.; Harned, A.; Nagashima, K.; Abdullah, S.; Pittaluga, S.; Imamichi, T.; Qin, J.; et al. Activated platelet–T-cell conjugates in peripheral blood of patients with HIV infection. *Aids* **2015**, *29*, 1297–1308. [CrossRef]
43. Valkonen, S.; Mallas, B.; Impola, U.; Valkeajärvi, A.; Eronen, J.; Javela, K.; Siljander, P.R.-M.; Laitinen, S. Assessment of Time-Dependent Platelet Activation Using Extracellular Vesicles, CD62P Exposure, and Soluble Glycoprotein V Content of Platelet Concentrates with Two Different Platelet Additive Solutions. *Transfus. Med. Hemotherapy* **2019**, *46*, 267–275. [CrossRef]
44. Reches, A.; Eldor, A.; Vogel, Z.; Salomon, Y. Do human platelets have opiate receptors? *Nature* **1980**, *288*, 382–383. [CrossRef]
45. Gruba, S.M.; Francis, D.H.; Meyer, A.F.; Spanolios, E.; He, J.; Meyer, B.M.; Kim, D.; Xiong-Hang, K.; Haynes, C.L. Characterization of the Presence and Function of Platelet Opioid Receptors. *ACS Meas. Sci. Au* **2021**, *2*, 4–13. [CrossRef]
46. Farag, M.; Srinivasan, M.; A Gorog, D. 28 Impact of Opiate Analgesia on Platelet Reactivity in Patients Presenting for Primary Percutaneous Coronary Intervention. *Heart* **2016**, *102* (Suppl. 6), A19. [CrossRef]
47. Schedel, A.; Thornton, S.; Klüter, H.; Bugert, P. The Effect of Psychoactive Drugs on in vitro Platelet Function. *Transfus. Med. Hemotherapy* **2010**, *37*, 9. [CrossRef]
48. Bekő, K.; Koványi, B.; Gölöncsér, F.; Horváth, G.; Denes, A.; Környei, Z.; Botz, B.; Helyes, Z.; Müller, C.E.; Sperlágh, B. Contribution of platelet $P2Y_{12}$ receptors to chronic Complete Freund's adjuvant-induced inflammatory pain. *J. Thromb. Haemost.* **2017**, *15*, 1223–1235. [CrossRef]
49. Altintoprak, F.; Arslan, Y.; Yalkin, O.; Uzunoglu, Y.; Ozkan, O.V. Mean platelet volume as a potential prognostic marker in patients with acute mesenteric ischemia–retrospective study. *World J. Emerg. Surg.* **2013**, *8*, 49. [CrossRef] [PubMed]
50. Levi, M.; Toh, C.H.; Thachil, J.; Watson, H.G. Guidelines for the diagnosis and management of disseminated intravascular coagulation. *Br. J. Haematol.* **2009**, *145*, 24–33. [CrossRef] [PubMed]
51. Avcioğlu, S.N.; Altinkaya, S.; Küçük, M.; Demircan-Sezer, S.; Yüksel, H. Can Platelet Indices Be New Biomarkers for Severe Endometriosis? *ISRN Obstet. Gynecol.* **2014**, *2014*, 1–6. [CrossRef] [PubMed]

Disclaimer/Publisher's Note: The statements, opinions and data contained in all publications are solely those of the individual author(s) and contributor(s) and not of MDPI and/or the editor(s). MDPI and/or the editor(s) disclaim responsibility for any injury to people or property resulting from any ideas, methods, instructions or products referred to in the content.

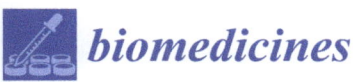

Article

Central Sensitization and Psychological State Distinguishing Complex Regional Pain Syndrome from Other Chronic Limb Pain Conditions: A Cluster Analysis Model

Hana Karpin [1,2], Jean-Jacques Vatine [2,3], Yishai Bachar Kirshenboim [2,4], Aurelia Markezana [5] and Irit Weissman-Fogel [1,*]

1. Physical Therapy Department, Faculty of Social Welfare and Health Sciences, University of Haifa, Haifa 3498838, Israel
2. Reuth Rehabilitation Hospital, Tel Aviv 6772829, Israel
3. Physical Medicine and Rehabilitation Department, Sackler Faculty of Medicine, Tel Aviv University, Tel Aviv 6997801, Israel
4. Department of Occupational Therapy, School of Health Professions, Sackler Faculty of Medicine, Tel Aviv University, Tel Aviv 6997801, Israel
5. Goldyne Savad Institute of Gene Therapy, Hadassah Hebrew University Medical Center, Jerusalem 91120, Israel
* Correspondence: ifogel@univ.haifa.ac.il

Abstract: Complex regional pain syndrome (CRPS) taxonomy has been updated with reported subtypes and is defined as primary pain alongside other chronic limb pain (CLP) conditions. We aimed at identifying CRPS clinical phenotypes that distinguish CRPS from other CLP conditions. Cluster analysis was carried out to classify 61 chronic CRPS and 31 CLP patients based on evoked pain (intensity of hyperalgesia and dynamic allodynia, allodynia area, and after-sensation) and psychological (depression, kinesiophobia, mental distress, and depersonalization) measures. Pro-inflammatory cytokine IL-6 and TNF-α serum levels were measured. Three cluster groups were created: 'CRPS' (78.7% CRPS; 6.5% CLP); 'CLP' (64.5% CLP; 4.9% CRPS), and 'Mixed' (16.4% CRPS; 29% CLP). The groups differed in all measures, predominantly in allodynia and hyperalgesia ($p < 0.001$, $\eta^2 > 0.58$). 'CRPS' demonstrated higher psychological and evoked pain measures vs. 'CLP'. 'Mixed' exhibited similarities to 'CRPS' in psychological profile and to 'CLP' in evoked pain measures. The serum level of TNF-α was higher in the 'CRPS' vs. 'CLP' ($p < 0.001$) groups. In conclusion, pain hypersensitivity reflecting nociplastic pain mechanisms and psychological state measures created different clinical phenotypes of CRPS and possible CRPS subtypes, which distinguishes them from other CLP conditions, with the pro-inflammatory TNF-α cytokine as an additional potential biomarker.

Keywords: complex regional pain syndrome; chronic limb pain; nociplastic pain; psychological state; cluster analysis; CRPS clinical phenotypes

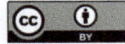

1. Introduction

Complex regional pain syndrome (CRPS) is a multifaceted pain disorder that mainly emerges after limb trauma or a lesion in the peripheral nervous system. The syndrome is comprised of CRPS-Type I (without nerve damage) and CRPS-Type II (with major nerve damage) subtypes, although their clinical presentation is similar [1]. Typical features include continuing pain (disproportionate to any inciting event or underlying pathology), and sensory, vasomotor, sudomotor, motor, and trophic changes [2,3]. The syndrome is diagnosed according to the Budapest Criteria, a decision rules method based on objective clinical signs and reported self-subjective symptoms [4]. Epidemiologically, the syndrome's incidence rates range between 5.6 [5], 26.2 [6], and 29 [7] per 10,000 person-years in the USA, Europe, and Korea, respectively.

The severity of the syndrome may be determined by the CRPS Severity Score (CSS), which reflects features of CRPS included in the Budapest Criteria [4] CRPS was recently defined as a Chronic Primary Pain (CPP) disorder, a pain condition in its own right which is not better accounted for by another disease. The pain persists for over three months and is associated with significant emotional distress and/or functional disability [8]. Mechanistically, CPP is viewed as nociplastic pain that is maintained by abnormal central processes, i.e., hypersensitivity of pain transmitting pathways (i.e., central sensitization) and/or an inefficient endogenous pain inhibition process. These are manifested as hyperpathia, hyperalgesia, and allodynia in response to evoked pain [9]. Nociplastic pain was accepted by the IASP as a third mechanistic pain descriptor in addition to neuropathic and nociceptive pain [9].

The literature suggests that CRPS is a heterogeneous syndrome based on different pathophysiological mechanisms [10,11] including central sensitization, inflammation, immune alterations, brain changes, genetic predisposition, and psychological state [12,13]. Cluster analysis procedures that were performed to detect different CRPS subtypes have yielded various classifications: 'warm' (inflammatory) vs. 'cold' (chronic) [11] and 'central' (maladaptive sensory-motor processing) vs. 'peripheral' (inflammatory signs) subtypes [10]. Additional classification is based on the serum level of TNF-α; in the high-level TNF-α group, levels of TNF-α were shown to be correlated with greater disease severity and longer disease duration [14]. Other classifications were focused on the syndrome's cognitive, perceptual, or emotional features. For example, different subtypes of neuropsychological function in CRPS patients (i.e., normal performance, executive difficulties, and global cognitive impairment) [15] or 'motor' vs. 'cognitive' neglect reflecting different phenotypes of body perception disturbances [16]. However, research aimed at subgrouping CRPS based on clinical features has failed to support the traditional sequential staging of CRPS mainly because the pain duration was similar across the subgroups [1,14].

Recently, the CRPS taxonomy was updated [17] with newly reported subtypes and a clarified diagnosis procedure. Specifically, the updated taxonomy includes two CRPS subtypes: (1) 'CRPS Not Otherwise Specified' meaning patients who display insufficient features of CRPS that are required for formal diagnosis (based on the Budapest Criteria) with no other diagnosis to better explain their clinical state, and (2) 'CRPS with Remission of Some Features' (CRPS RoSF) meaning patients that were previously diagnosed with CRPS but then display insufficient signs and symptoms to fully meet the diagnostic criteria [17]. However, it is still unclear whether these subtypes are distinct subtypes with unique clinical features or are part of the sequential stages of the syndrome reflecting recovery processes [17]. Moreover, to improve the therapeutic outcome of CRPS patients, it is essential not only to identify subgroups within CRPS that probably reflect different mechanisms but also to differentiate CRPS from other chronic limb pain (CLP) conditions.

The diagnostical definition of CLP has been changed recently, including the differentiation between primary chronic limb pain (which is considered a disease on its own [18,19] and secondary chronic limb pain when the pain is defined as a symptom [19,20]. Although these clarifications give more precision to the diagnostic process, many chronic pain conditions involve a combination of pain mechanisms [9,21], which makes this process harder and accordingly requires more clinical clarifications.

A previous study that explored measures that differentiate CRPS patients from CLP patients found that spontaneous pain, pinprick hyperalgesia, and dynamic allodynia were more prominent in CRPS patients. This suggests that augmented pain in CRPS [3] can be attributed at least in part to central sensitization. In another study, CRPS and CLP patients were compared based on a broad clinical but limited psychological battery. Two discriminating factors were identified: (i) clinical pain based on self-reporting and evoked pain (i.e., pinprick and pressure pain sensitivity), and (ii) psychological measures (i.e., anxiety and depression). CRPS demonstrated higher intensity in both factors [22]. Additional psychological factors including catastrophization [23,24], kinesiophobia [25,26], and somatization characterize CRPS and other CLP conditions [24]. Interestingly, depersonalization is the only measure that distinguishes CRPS from other chronic pain groups (i.e., CLP and migraine) [24].

An interesting potential phenotype of CRPS, namely Body Perception Disturbances (BPD), which is measured by limb neglect, was compared between CRPS and CLP patients. Results showed that neglect scores were higher in CRPS patients and that they were correlated with psychological factors. Nonetheless, the neglect scores were associated with clinical pain intensity only in CLP patients, indicating a different role for BPD in various CLP disorders [24].

Taken together, the evidence suggests a combination of factors, specifically those reflecting pain hypersensitivity and psychological distress distinguishes CRPS from CLP. Therefore, the current study's aims were: (1) to identify phenotypes that distinguish CRPS from other CLP based on comprehensive evoked pain and psychological measures, and (2) to explore the validity of these measures and their usage as a novel, clinically oriented classification method. The main findings show that nociplastic pain and the level of psychological distress can distinguish between CLP conditions; the CRPS group has a unique psychological and pain profile derived from central sensitization and central neuro-inflammation processes.

2. Materials and Methods

2.1. Patients

This was a cross-sectional observational study comprised of two patient groups: a research group and a control group. The inclusion criteria for the research group were: (1) subjects aged > 18; (2) diagnosed with CRPS type 1 or 2 in the upper or lower limb, according to a medical evaluation of a pain specialist physician and based on the Budapest clinical criteria; and (3) pain that has persisted > 4 months since the primary injury. The exclusion criteria were: (1) bilateral CRPS; (2) primary psychiatric diagnosis of depression, anxiety, or post-traumatic stress disorder; (3) a different pain syndrome causing a major pain; (4) disorders of the central nervous system (epilepsy, intracranial injury, stroke, Parkinson's disease, multiple sclerosis), or other diseases with sensory or inflammatory components; (5) pregnant or nursing women; (6) severe visual deficiency; (7) intellectual disability; and (8) insufficient proficiency in spoken Hebrew.

The control group was comprised of subjects aged > 18 who were diagnosed with chronic secondary musculoskeletal pain [20] according to a medical evaluation by a pain specialist physician. The pain in this group was from a nociceptive origin and associated with traumatic structural changes in the musculoskeletal system and some of the subjects in this group also had a nerve injury. All subjects in this group did not reach the CRPS criteria [27]. Both patient groups were referred to the pain rehabilitation units at Reuth Rehabilitation Hospital (Tel-Aviv, Israel) and were voluntarily recruited during their rehabilitation course from June 2018 to January 2021. The study was approved by the Institutional Review Board (IRB) of Reuth Rehabilitation Center (2017-14) and by the IRB of the University of Haifa (Haifa, Israel, 135/18; File 1822). Participants signed written informed consent forms before inclusion in the study.

2.2. Disease Severity Measures

2.2.1. CRPS Severity Score

The CSS [4,27] is an index consisting of 16 signs and symptoms, including sensory, vasomotor, sudomotor/edema, and motor/trophic criteria. The index is scored based on the presence/absence (coded 1/0) of signs and symptoms. A higher CSS score indicates a greater extent of CRPS symptoms.

2.2.2. Short-Form McGill Pain Questionnaire (MPQ-SF)

The MPQ-SF [28] is a self-report questionnaire that assesses the multi-dimensional aspects of current clinical pain. The questionnaire includes 11 sensory descriptions and four emotional descriptions (on a 0–3 scale; no, mild, moderate, and strong, respectively).

The total score ranges from 0 to 45 points; a higher score represents a more intense pain experience. The MPQ includes two measures of pain intensity: The Visual Analogue Scale (VAS) with the two ends denoting 'no pain' and 'maximal pain imaginable', and a verbal pain bar ranging from 0 'no pain at all' to 5 'very strong pain'. We used the validated Hebrew version of the SF-MPQ [29].

2.3. Psychophysical Measures

The psychophysical tests were performed on the dorsal aspect of the involved hand or foot, in the area defined as having 'secondary hyperalgesia' (i.e., increased pain sensitivity in non-injured skin surrounding a site of tissue damage [30]. The rationale was to explore and quantify central processes and to prevent a ceiling effect (i.e., unbearable pain) in case the stimulus was placed in the center of the primary hyperalgesia area. In cases where allodynia or hyperalgesia was not identified, the tests were taken adjacent to the injury site. If this area was scarred, the tests were performed on the nearest intact skin area.

2.3.1. Thermal and Pain Thresholds

This set of tests was performed by an occupational therapist according to the standardized DFNS (German Research Network on Neuropathic Pain) protocol [31]. The threshold tests included cold detection threshold (CDT), warm detection threshold (WDT), cold pain threshold (CPT), and heat pain threshold (HPT) that were performed on the dorsal aspects of the hand or the feet of both sides of the body, depending on the affected extremity [22], with the unaffected side tested first. The thermal tests were applied before the pain threshold tests. The threshold tests were performed by the Thermal Sensory Analyzer (TSA) system (Medoc, Ltd., Ramat Yishai, Israel) using the 3×3 cm contact thermode that warms and cools using a temperature range from $0\ °C$ to a safety limit of $50\ °C$. The baseline temperature was $32\ °C$ and the thermode heat and cool rate was $1\ °C/s$. For the WDT and CDT, the participant was asked to press a computer mouse button when warm and cold sensations were felt. For the HPT and CPT, they were asked to detect the moment that warm and cold sensations became painful and to press the button. Each test was performed three times and averaged. The mean value of each test was Z transformed, based on the following equation, according to the standardized and published instructions [31].

Z score = (patient mean value) − (mean value of the published reference) ÷ SD of the published reference.

The z scores were adjusted as follows: z score > 0 indicated high sensitivity and z score < 0 indicated low sensitivity; z score > +1 indicated somatosensory gain and z score < −1 indicated somatosensory loss; z score > ±1.96 indicated pathologic changes in somato-sensory function [10].

2.3.2. Mechanical Hyperalgesia Intensity

The intensity of supra-threshold mechanical stimuli was assessed using a pinprick stimulator at 256 mN (MRC Systems Pin Prick Stimulator, Heidelberg, Germany). The participant was asked to rate the pain intensity using the 0–10 Numerical Rating Scale (NRS; 0 denoted 'no pain' and 10 denoted 'maximal pain imaginable').

2.3.3. Static Mechanical Allodynia Intensity

The intensity of static allodynia was assessed using a cotton stick. The stimulus was applied once perpendicular to the skin, for two seconds, with a pressure force that was less than 15 gr [32]. The participants were asked to rate the pain intensity using the 0–10 NRS.

2.3.4. Dynamic Mechanical Allodynia Intensity

The intensity of dynamic allodynia was assessed using a cotton stick. The stimulus was applied once perpendicular to the skin, while the tester moved over a five cm skin area for two seconds with a pressure force that was less than 15 gr [32]. The participants were asked to rate the pain intensity using the 0–10 NRS.

2.3.5. Dynamic Allodynia Area

We used a novel method developed for the current study to quantify the allodynia area [33]. The method protocol consisted of (i) identification and marking of the allodynia area using a cotton swab and makeup pencil; (ii) measurement of this area length with a cm tape; and (iii) calculation of the allodynia area by using the Lund and Browder chart for estimation of burned areas as a percentage of the total skin area (i.e., % fragment) [33,34], according to the following equation:

Allodynia area (%) = Length of allodynia area ÷ Length of body fragment × % fragment.

The calculated score represents the percentage of allodynia area relative to body surface.

2.3.6. Aftersensation Intensity

Continued pain beyond the noxious stimulus presentation was recorded using the VAS immediately after the completion of the dynamic allodynia area test.

2.4. Psychological Self-Reported Measures

2.4.1. Pain Catastrophizing Scale (PCS) [35]

The PCS is a questionnaire that was developed to test an exaggerated negative mental set during actual or anticipated painful experiences [35]. The PCS includes 13 items on a scale ranging from 0 'not at all' to 4 'all the time' that represent three aspects of catastrophic thoughts related to pain: rumination (4 items), magnification (3 items), and helplessness (6 items). The overall score ranges from 0 to 52. The higher the score, the more negative the attitude toward the pain. We used the validated Hebrew version of the PCS [36].

2.4.2. Tampa Scale of Kinesiophobia (TSK) [37]

The TSK is a questionnaire that was developed to test fear of movement, fear of physical activity, and fear avoidance. The TSK includes 17 items ranging from 1 ('I do not agree') to 4 ('completely agree'). The overall score ranges from 17 to 68. The higher the score, the higher the level of kinesiophobia. We used the standard Hebrew version of the TSK [38].

2.4.3. Beck Depression Inventory (BDI-II) [39]

This rating inventory measures characteristic attitudes and symptoms of depression. The BDI-II includes 21 items (on a scale of 0–3). The overall score ranges from 0 to 63. Higher scores suggest a greater severity of depression. We used the validated Hebrew version of the BDI-II [40].

2.4.4. Brief Symptom Inventory (BSI) [41]

The BSI evaluates mental distress expressed in nine dimensions: obsessive-compulsive, interpersonal sensitivity, depression, anxiety, hostility, somatization, phobic-anxiety, paranoid ideation, and psychoticism. The BSI consists of 53 items on a scale ranging from 0 ('not at all') to 4 ('extremely'). It can be summed up based on an overall score (General Severity Index) calculated using the sum of the nine symptom dimension scores and dividing by the total number of items. The higher the score the higher the level of mental distress. We used the validated Hebrew version of the BSI [42].

2.4.5. Cambridge Depersonalization Scale (CDS) [43]

The CDS measures the frequency and duration of depersonalization symptoms during the past six months. The CDC includes 29 items coded by two scales—a frequency scale ranging from 0 (never) to 4 (always) and a duration scale ranging from 1 (seconds) to 6 (over a week). The final score ranges from 0 to 290 points; a score above 70 was determined to be clinically significant depersonalization. The CDS was Hebrew translated for the benefit of the study using the back translation method [44] by four stages: (i) the CDS was translated to Hebrew by a bilingual occupational therapist; (ii) the Hebrew version was retranslated to English by a different bilingual occupational therapist; (iii) the two versions were compared for concept equivalence; and (iv) the final version was synthesizing after a discussion between the two translators. The internal consistency of the Hebrew scale was high (Cronbach's alpha= 0.94).

2.4.6. The Bath Body Perception Disturbances Questionnaire (Bath-BPD) [45]

The Bath-BPD is comprised of seven items covering different aspects related to the affected limb: a sense of ownership, limb position awareness, attention to the painful limb, feelings toward the limb, perceptual disparities in size, temperature, pressure, and weight, limb amputation desire, and a mental representation of the affected limb. The total score is calculated by summing the individual scores of the seven items ranging from 0 to 57 points. The higher the score, the greater the degree of disturbance [44]. We used the Hebrew version of the Bath-BPD that was translated using the Vallerand method [45]. The internal consistency of the Hebrew-translated questionnaire was similar to the original English version (Cronbach's alpha = 0.63 and 0.66, respectively) [46].

2.5. Biological Measures

Pro-Inflammatory Cytokines

The blood samples were drawn using standardized venipuncture on the participants' non-affected arm; 2 mL plasma was extracted from each patient and collected into EDTA-coated (purple top) vacutainers. After clotting, the plasma was separated by centrifugation (1500 rpm, 10 min, at 4 °C), the serum was extracted and then centrifuged again (3000 rpm, 10 min at 4 °C), split into two 250 microliter aliquots and stored at −20 °C until assayed.

The serum levels of Tumor Necrosis Factor- α (TNF-α) and Interluekin-6 (IL-6) were measured by a human TNF-α immuno-assay (Quantikine HS ELISA HSTA00E, R&D Systems, Minneapolis, Minnesota) and a human IL-6 immuno-assay (Quantikine ELISA D6050 R&D Systems, Minneapolis, Minnesota), respectively. The kits were used according to the manufacturer's instructions by a trained laboratory technician.

All samples were tested in duplicate and data were obtained by the standard curve that was created using the recombinant standards and expressed as the average protein levels in pg/mL for each group. Measurements were performed on the Infinite F50 ELISA microplate reader (TECAN Ltd., Männedorf, Switzerland) together with the Magellan^{TM} reader control and data analysis software (TECAN Ltd. Switzerland).

2.6. Statistical Analysis

The required sample size was estimated a priori for the ANOVA procedure that tested the cluster model sensitivity. Using the G*power program [47], α = 0.05, statistical power of 85%, and effect size of 0.35, the calculation yielded a total sample size of N = 93 participants. The final sample comprised 92 participants (61 CRPS and 31 CLP patients).

All statistical analyses were performed using SPSS version 27.0 for Windows. Data are presented as mean ± SD or as median (in the case of non-parametric analysis) for continuous variables and as count and percentage for categorical variables. Effect sizes are presented by partial eta squared [48]. The statistical significance was defined as a value of $p \leq 0.05$.

A repeated measures ANOVA was performed to compare the effect of group membership (CRPS/CLP) and the tested side (affected vs. not affected) on the thermal and pain thresholds.

A cluster analysis was performed to classify the sample based on evoked pain and psychological measures, aiming to identify different clinical phenotypes within the study sample. Eight measures were selected for the final model (four evoked pain measures: dynamic allodynia intensity, mechanical hyperalgesia intensity, dynamic allodynia area, and after-sensation intensity; and four psychological measures: depression, mental distress, kinesiophobia, and de-personalization). Two measures: the intensity of static mechanical allodynia and the PCS questionnaire were excluded due to their strong positive correlation with dynamic mechanical allodynia intensity and kinesiophobia, respectively ($r > 0.57$, $p < 0.001$).

A statistical procedure of Two-Step Cluster Analysis was chosen due to its ability to ensure that one variable does not dominate the cluster solution. Furthermore, it enables the user to identify the importance of each item in the cluster solution [49]. The classification variables were z transformed and the cluster analysis was performed using a predetermined fixed number of clusters (k = 3), aiming to uncover a pattern in the data set, i.e., a latent group within the CRPS-CLP spectrum.

The model fit was assessed by Schwarz's Bayesian Information Criterion [50] and evaluated by the average silhouette coefficient, an internal validity index representing cluster cohesion and separation quality, ranging between 0 and 1; the closer to 1, the better the model [51].

A crosstab analysis was performed to test the association ($\chi 2$) and its strength (Cramer's V-rc) between the derived clusters and the participants' original diagnosis, and a MANOVA to detect differences in the classification variables based on cluster groups.

The cluster sensitivity was measured using ANOVA and Kruskal–Wallis tests to explore differences in the CSS score, MPQ-SF, Bath-BPD, and pro-inflammatory plasma cytokines levels depending on the three cluster groups.

Lastly, a spearman correlation was conducted to test the correlations between the pro-inflammatory cytokines and the pain measures -evoked and clinical pair (MPQ-SF). Bonferroni/Mann–Whitney analyses were used to detect significant mean differences using a pairwise comparison method. The Bonferroni correction was conducted in cases of multiple comparisons.

Missing Variables

The thermal and pain threshold tests were added as an additional descriptive measure of the cohort and were tested on a subsample of CRPS (n = 33) and CLP (n = 25) subjects. Twenty-eight CRPS and six CLP patients were enrolled before the protocol was established and therefore were not examined by these measures. The pro-inflammatory cytokine samples were collected from a subsample of CRPS (n = 20) and CLP (n = 13) subjects. Only measures with less than 10% missing values were included in the cluster model; the completion of the data, if required, was based on mean imputation [52].

2.7. The Study Protocol

All subjects were diagnosed according to the clinical Budapest Criteria and underwent the CSS evaluation by a pain specialist physician. Each participant completed four or five one-hour research sessions in a quiet room. The sessions included (1) blood samples performed during daylight hours between 8:00 AM to 2:00 PM, conducted by a paramedic or a physician; (2) psychophysical tests including thermal and pain thresholds, evoked pain measures, and allodynia area in percentages; and (3) self-administered questionnaires including demographic, psychological, and clinical pain, performed by a trained occupational therapist. The research sessions were conducted in random order, except for the first meeting, which was dedicated to acquainting the participants with the research team and completing the demographic questionnaires.

3. Results

3.1. Patients

The socio-demographics, pain characteristics, and comorbid medical diagnostic data of the CRPS and CLP participants are shown in Table 1. There were no significant differences between the groups regarding age, years of education, and disease duration ($p > 0.05$). In the CRPS group, the female/male ratio was 32/29 (52.5/47.5%). In the CLP group, the ratio was 23/8 (74.2/25.8%), with significantly more females than males ($p = 0.044$,

Φ = 0.210). The average 24-h pain level and the current pain level based on the CSS index were significantly higher in the CRPS group ($p < 0.001$).

Table 1. Demographic data in CRPS and CLP patients.

Variables	CRPS	CLP	p
Patients, n	61	31	
Age (years), mean (SD)	34.69 (11.52)	39.0 (15.09)	0.164
Sex (female/male), n (%)	32/29 (52.5/47.5)	23/8 (74.2/25.8)	0.044
Education (years), mean (SD)	12.93 (2.14)	13.71 (2.25)	0.111
Disease duration (days), mean (SD)	728.62 (903.96)	775.81 (843.25)	0.809
Work status, n (%)			
Working	15 (24.59)	13 (41.93)	
Not working	43 (70.49)	14 (45.16)	
Soldier	3 (4.91)	4 (12.90)	
Type of injury, n (%):			
Fracture	31 (50.81)	14 (45.16)	
Trauma	27 (44.26)	15 (48.38)	
Other	3 (4.91)	2 (6.45)	
Limb involved, n (%):Hand	24 (39.35)	12 (38.7)	
Leg	37 (60.65)	19 (61.29)	
Side involved, n (%):			
Rt.	31 (50.81)	12 (38.71)	
Lt.	30 (49.19)	19 (61.29)	
Nerve injury, n (%)	38 (62.35)	16 (51.61)	
Pain characteristics, mean (SD):			
NRPS—Current	7.15 (1.5)	4.29 (2.59)	<0.001
NRPS—24 H	7.42 (1.38)	5.11 (2.57)	<0.001
Comorbid diagnosis n (%):			
Cardiovascular/Hematology	5 (8.19)	3 (9.66)	
Endocrine diseases	5 (8.19)	1 (3.22)	
Enzyme deficiency/Allergies	4 (6.55)	1 (3.22)	
Neurodevelopmental disorder	3 (4.91)	2 (6.45)	
Missing	1 (1.63)	6 (19.35)	

Note. CRPS—Complex Regional Pain Syndrome; CLP—Chronic Limb Pain; Other—inflammation, acute disease, spontaneous onset. The presence of nerve injury was determined by a pain specialist physician based on clinical tests and/or EMG findings.

Medications and drug usage: the medical pain therapy included opiates, antiepileptics, anti-depressives, sleep drugs, analgesics, and B-phosphonate medications. Six participants suffered from hypertension, and two from hypothyroidism and used relevant medications. In addition, 16 participants had a medical license for cannabis. During the research period, the participants did not report substantial adverse drug reactions [53]; however, a complete medical follow-up regarding this issue was impossible as most of the participants were not fully hospitalized.

3.2. Thermal and Pain Thresholds Profile

Statistically significant effects of the tested side were found in all the thermal tests ($p < 0.05$), except for HPT ($p > 0.05$). Specifically, the involved limb showed more sensitivity to painful stimuli (gain of function) and less sensitivity to non-painful stimuli (loss of function). Although the differences between the groups were insignificant, the CLP group showed more loss of function for CDT and WDT and the CRPS showed more gain of function for CPT and HPT. The differences between the affected and non-affected sides were more prominent in the CLP than in the CRPS group. The data are shown in Table 2 and in Figure 1.

Table 2. The differences in thermal and pain threshold between limbs in CRPS and CLP groups.

Variables, Mean (SD)	CRPS (n = 33)		CLP (n = 25)		$F_{(1, 56)}$	p	η^2
	Involved	Not involved	Involved	Not involved			
CDT	−1.74 (1.87)	−1.39 (1.45)	−2.21 (1.26)	−1.61 (1.19)	4.08	0.048	0.068
WDT	−1.26 (1.82)	−0.82 (1.55)	−1.82 (1.18)	−0.96 (1.35)	7.27	0.009	0.115
CPT	1.19 (1.16)	0.33 (1.21)	0.68 (1.18)	0.29 (1.19)	10.74	0.002	0.161
HPT	1.15 (2.11)	0.43 (1.61)	−0.02 (1.60)	0−.03 (1.30)	1.55	ns	

Note. CRPS—Complex Regional Pain Syndrome; CLP—Chronic Limb Pain; CDT—Cold Detection Threshold; WDT—Warm Detection Threshold; CPT—Cold Pain Threshold; HPT—Heat Pain Threshold.

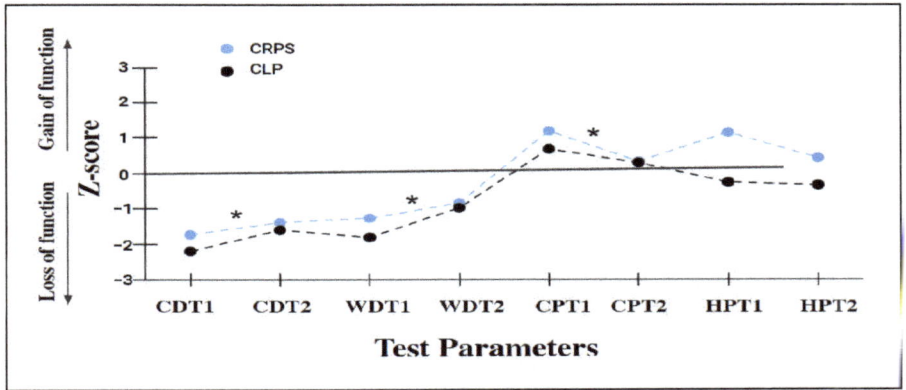

Figure 1. The thermal and pain threshold profile. Note. CRPS—Complex Regional Pain Syndrome; CLP—Chronic Limb Pain; CDT1—Cold Detection Threshold in the involved limb; CDT2—Cold Detection Threshold in the non-involved limb; WDT1—Warm Detection Threshold in the involved limb; WDT2—Warm Detection Threshold in the non-involved limb. CPT1—Cold Pain Threshold in the involved limb; CPT2—Cold Pain Threshold in the non-involved limb; HPT1—Heat Pain Threshold in the involved limb; HPT2—Heat Pain Threshold in the non-involved limb. Gain of function ($z > 1$); 'loss of function' ($z < -1$). Pathologic gain of function ($z > 1.96$) pathologic loss of function ($z < -1.96$). * $p < 0.05$- significant differences between the affected and non-affected sides in each group.

3.3. The Cluster Analysis Model

The derived model yielded three clusters group (CRPS, CLP, and Mixed), The 'CRPS' group included 78.7% CRPS patients and 6.5% CLP patients; the 'CLP' group included 64.5% CLP patients and 4.9% CRPS patients; and the 'Mixed' included 16.4% CRPS and 29% CLP patients. Each cluster group comprised both pain-evoked and psychological measures and therefore the cluster was named CRPSycho-noci. χ^2 analysis showed a significant correlation between the cluster and the original diagnosis ($\Phi = 0.741$, $p < 0.001$).

The cluster quality was fair (silhouette = 0.4); a silhouette coefficient equal to or above 0.50 indicates a good model fit [45]. The cluster cohesion indexes were good, with all measures having a silhouette value range between 0.4 and 1. The most important predictors were hyperalgesia and mechanical allodynia indicating a perfect model fit (silhouette = 1). The silhouette value of each measure (i.e., predictive importance) is shown in Figure 2.

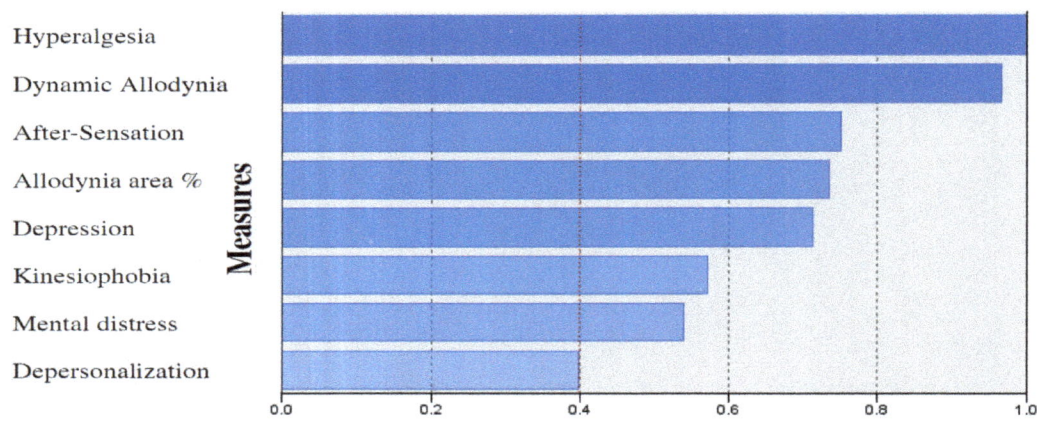

Figure 2. The measures' predictive importance. Note: Two-step cluster analysis predictive importance measures. All measures are within the cutoff level of 0.4 silhouette index.

The differences in the intensity of the measures between the cluster groups are shown in Table 3. The MANOVA model was significant ($F_{(16, 164)} = 18.94$, $p<0.001$; Wilk's $\Lambda = 0.12$, $\eta^2 = 0.64$), dynamic allodynia and hyperalgesia demonstrated the largest effect size ($\eta^2 > 0.58$). A post-hoc analysis revealed significant differences between the CRPS and CLP groups in all measures: the 'CRPS' demonstrated higher scores for psychological and evoked pain vs. the 'CLP'. The 'Mixed' group exhibited similarities to CRPS in psychological measures and to CLP in evoked pain measures. The data are presented in Figure 3.

Table 3. Differences in the intensities of the measures between the cluster groups.

Variables, Mean (SD)	Cluster 'CRPS' ($n = 50$)	Cluster 'Mixed' ($n = 19$)	Cluster 'CLP' ($n = 23$)	$F (2, 89)$	Multiple pairwise comparisons	η^2
Dynamic allodynia	7.32 (1.53)	2.11 (2.92)	1.94 (2.78)	64.96 *	CLP = Mixed < CRPS	0.59
Hyperalgesia	7.72 (2.58)	2.86 (2.99)	2.63 (2.38)	61.67 *	CLP = Mixed < CRPS	0.58
After-sensation	7.66 (1.39)	5.11 (3.47)	2.23 (2.85)	42.97 *	CRPS > Mixed > CLP	0.49
Allodynia area %	5.84 (3.03)	0.97 (1.54)	0.87 (2.11)	41.64 *	CLP = Mixed < CRPS	0.48
Depression	28.55 (10.06)	23.63 (7.11)	9.29 (5.42)	40.01 *	CRPS = Mixed > CLP	0.47
Kinesiophobia	42.89 (6.08)	41.79 (6.62)	30.43 (7.44)	29.89 *	CRPS = Mixed > CLP	0.40
Mental distress	2.64 (0.57)	2.62 (0.45)	1.72 (0.39)	27.81 *	CRPS = Mixed > CLP	0.38
De-personalization	76.61 (47.29)	68.31 (45.51)	12.66 (18.09)	19.21 *	CRPS = Mixed > CLP	0.30

Note. CRPS—Complex Regional Pain Syndrome; CLP—Chronic Limb Pain; Mixed—a mixed cluster group.
* $p < 0.001$.

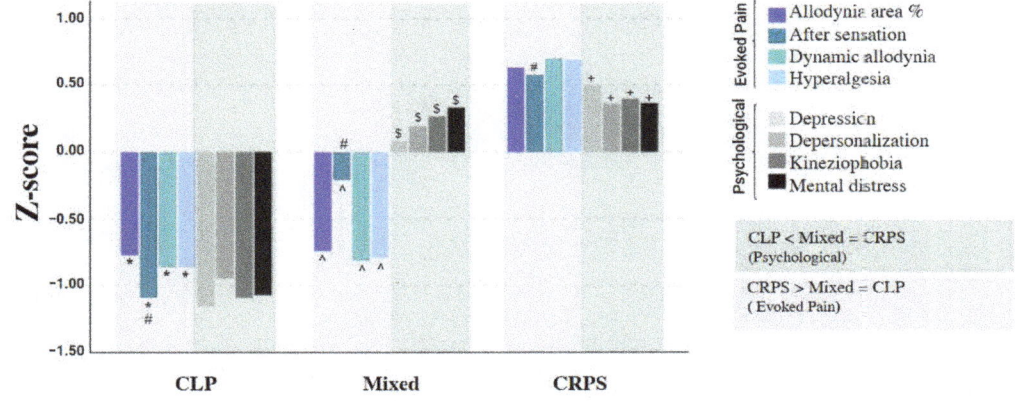

Figure 3. The three groups of the CRPSyco-noci cluster. Note. CRPS—Complex Regional Pain Syndrome; CLP—chronic limb pain; evoked pain and psychological measures distinguish between CLP, Mixed, and CRPS groups. All measures were z transformed. CLP showed lower values than CRPS in evoked pain measures (* CLP vs. CRPS) and CRPS showed higher values than CLP in psychological measures (+ CRPS vs. CLP). The Mixed group showed lower scores than CRPS in evoked pain measures (^ Mixed vs. CRPS) and higher scores than CLP in psychological measures ($ Mixed vs. CLP). After-sensation significantly differed in all groups (#).

3.4. The Model Sensitivity

The secondary analysis aimed to test the model's sensitivity in detecting differences between the cluster groups regarding the CSS score, clinical pain (MPQ-SF), Bath-BPD, and pro-inflammatory cytokines. The results are shown in Table 4. The analysis revealed significant differences in CSS scores between all the cluster groups ($p < 0.001$). The post-hoc analysis revealed that the CRPS, Mixed, and CLP cluster groups demonstrated the highest, moderate, and lowest scores, respectively. In addition, the CRPS group showed significantly higher clinical pain intensity, Bath-BPD scores, and TNF-α serum levels vs. the CLP group. However, the Mixed group did not differ significantly from the CRPS group. IL-6 serum levels did not differ significantly between the cluster groups.

Table 4. Cluster group differences in CSS, MPQ-SF, Bath-BPD scores and pro-inflammatory cytokines.

Variables, Mean (SD)	Cluster 'CRPS' ($n = 50$)	Cluster 'Mixed' ($n = 19$)	Cluster 'CLP' ($n = 23$)	$F (2, 89)$	Multiple pairwise comparisons	η^2
CSS Score	12.08 (2.54)	8.93 (2.83)	6.16 (3.28)	36.74 **	CRPS > Mixed > CLP	0.45
MPQ-SF	27.22 (9.01)	22.21 (9.63)	10.61 (7.41)	28.2 **	CRPS = Mixed > CLP	0.38
Bath-BPD	25.61 (10.07)	21.36 (7.17)	12.93 (10.54)	13.49 **	CRPS = Mixed > CLP	0.23
Variables, Median (Interquartile range)	Cluster CRPS ($n = 17$)	Cluster Mixed ($n = 7$)	Cluster CLP ($n = 9$)	$H (2)$	Multiple pairwise comparisons	r
TNF-α (pg/mL)	1.27 (0.50)	1.77 (1.28)	0.61 (0.42)	6.28 *	CRPS = Mixed > CLP	−0.53
IL-6 (pg/mL)	1.97 (2.48)	1.39 (0.85)	3.73 (1.63)	4.15	rs	−0.30

Note. CRPS—Complex Regional Pain Syndrome; CLP—Chronic Limb Pain; Mixed—a mixed cluster group; CSS—CRPS Severity Score; MPQ-SF—McGill Pain Questionnaire Short Form; BATH-BPD—Bath Body Perception Disturbances questionnaire; ** $p < 0.001$; * $p < 0.05$.

3.5. Correlation between the Pro-Inflammatory Cytokines and the Pain Measures

The correlations of TNF-α and IL-6 serum levels with the evoked and clinical pain measures of hyperalgesia, dynamic allodynia, allodynia area, after-sensation, and MPQ-SF were tested by Spearman correlations, separately for each cytokine. After a Bonferroni correction, the adjusted alpha level was 0.01 (α = 0.05/5). The correlations that remained significant were between TNF-α and MPQ-SF (rs = 0.51, p = 0.002, n = 33) and between TNF-α and allodynia area (rs = 0.44, p = 0.001, n = 33).

4. Discussion

The study aimed to identify the clinical phenotypes of subgroups along the CLP-CRPS spectrum.

We used a unique classification method based on evoked pain and psychological measures that revealed a cluster solution based on a combination of these two realms (named the CRPSyco-noci cluster). The cluster comprised three groups: CRPS, CLP, and Mixed, which highly correlated with the original diagnoses and differed significantly in their CSS means. The most predictive factors, which shaped the cluster cohesion and separation, were mechanical sensitivity and pain after-sensation, with the CRPS group showing a higher pain hypersensitivity and psychological distress.

Interestingly, the Mixed group, as named, showed a mixed pattern; it was similar to the CRPS group in the psychological measures and to the CLP group in evoked pain measures. Further testing of the cluster sensitivity revealed that the CSS score was significantly different between CRPS, Mixed, and CLP cluster groups demonstrating high, moderate, and lowest scores, respectively. Likewise, the CRPS group demonstrated significantly higher clinical pain, TNF-α serum level, and Bath-BPD score than the CLP, with no differences in IL-6 serum level. Nonetheless, these parameters did not differentiate CRPS from the Mixed group. On the contrary, the CRPS group showed a combination of gain and loss of thermal sensory function, and the CLP showed a more dominant loss of sensory function but these differences were insignificant. These findings further emphasize the role of central sensitization as a mechanism that differentiates between the chronic limb pain disorders tested here.

4.1. Central Sensitization Processes That Differ between the Cluster Groups

The study results show that the most discriminating between-group measures were mechanical hyperalgesia and dynamic allodynia. Both are clinical manifestations of the central sensitization process that occurs due to increased excitability and synaptic efficacy of neurons in the ascending transmitting pathways [54]. Furthermore, in the cases where the tests were undergone in the secondary hyperalgesia area, these serve as an additional indication of central sensitization [55]. The results indicate that the CRPS participants were more influenced than the CLP subjects by these central processes, demonstrating possible nociplastic pain. As we did not collect data regarding the participants' comorbidity, such as cognitive problems, sleep disturbances, fatigue, or other senses hypersensitivity, we use the term 'possible' as recommended by the IASP clinical criteria of nociplastic pain [21,56], which is characterized as a pro-nociceptive profile [57]. This profile may be derived from a neural hyper-responsiveness in the ascending transmitting pathways that causes enhanced facilitatory processes at the spinal and supra-spinal levels, and/or reduced neural activity in the inhibitory pathways interrupting the endogenous analgesia. In both situations, this results in pain amplification [57,58].

A few potential mechanisms may explain the pro-nociceptive profile in CRPS: (i) Higher post-injury pain level (i.e., in the week after the trauma) [59,60]; the CRPS group showed higher clinical and evoked pain levels than the CLP group, although it is unknown whether their pain levels shortly after the trauma were also higher. Yet, this group was diagnosed with CRPS due to continuous and disproportionate pain levels, which is one of the CRPS diagnosis criteria [1,4,61]. Moreover, ongoing nociceptive pain is a risk factor for developing nociplastic pain [21] and continuous high pain intensity can exhaust the capacity of participants' ability to inhibit pain due to their need to cope with the ongoing pain in the long-term [57,58]. (ii) Another potential mechanism is the inflammatory process, which is derived from and interacts with central sensitization processes [13,62]. Inflammatory processes are suggested to play a substantial role in the pathogenesis of CRPS, both in acute and chronic stages, producing sensitization via secretion of pro-inflammatory cytokines, e.g., TNF-α and IL-6 [13,62,63]. Indeed, the CRPS group showed a higher TNF-α serum level, implying its role in the inflammatory process at the chronic CRPS stages. (iii) Predisposing genetic factors causing heightened pain sensitivity and reduced efficiency of pain inhibition processes can contribute to the pro-nociceptive profile [55,57,64]. This possibility was supported by a previous study that suggested a pre-existing inter-individual difference in the pain modulatory network activity among CRPS patients [55]. This could not be tested here because this was a cross-sectional study. On the contrary, we found no group differences in thermal thresholds, which is in line with another previous study that demonstrated no differences in thermal sensitivity between CRPS and CLP patients when comparing both body sides [22]. The thermal thresholds evaluate the function of the peripheral nervous system, namely C and Aδ fibers [65], which may be similar in the CRPS and CLP groups in our cohort. This further supports central mechanisms as a diagnostic marker.

Mechanical pain sensitivity measures were found to differentiate the CRPS from the CLP group [3,22], but interestingly, pain after-sensation was the only measure that differed significantly between the three cluster groups. After-sensation is an index of central sensitization [54,66] reflecting sensitization of second-order neurons. Namely, wide dynamic range pain transmission neurons that produce prolonged pain after discharge, which outlasts the period of stimulation [67]. In a case where hyperalgesia is identified, this response can also occur after a non-painful sensory stimulus, as was seen in the current study [68]. These results align with a previous study that demonstrated after-sensation and secondary hyperalgesia, both manifestations of central sensitization, as a dominant underlying mechanism in nociplastic pain and specifically in chronic CRPS [69].

4.2. Psychological State Differences between the Cluster Groups

The most important discriminative measure was depression, which is mutually associated with chronic pain via shared brain mechanisms [70]. For example, the nigra-subthalamic circuit is involved in the maintenance of both hyperalgesia and depression and is modulated by the impairment of substantia nigra reticulata-subthalamic nucleus GABAergic projection [71]. In CRPS, depression is a measure associated with pain severity [26,72,73] and disability [26], reflecting these prominent aspects of the disease burden [74]. Kinesiophobia was the second most important measure among the psychological measures. Kinesiophobia reflects a fear of movement and (re)injury [75], manifested as pain-related fear and avoidance behavior [76]. A systematic review among chronic musculoskeletal pain patients revealed that a greater degree of kinesiophobia is associated with greater levels of pain intensity, pain severity, disability, and a lower quality of life [77]. In CRPS, fear of pain is a predictor of pain intensity [26] and disability [75]. Furthermore, kinesiophobia is correlated with longer symptom durations and a lower illness perception [78]. These may lead to the adoption of poor coping strategies including immobilization, protecting, and neglecting the limb [78], which themselves aggravate the severity of the syndrome. Accordingly, this implies that there is a link between kinesiophobia and other psychological measures that establishes a vicious cycle of pain, emotional distress, and functional limitation in CRPS.

4.3. The Mutual Association between Pain Hypersensitivity and Psychological State

The cluster classification, with each group characterized by various degrees of pain hypersensitivity and psychological distress, suggests a mutual association between pain and emotional suffering [79]. The suggested underlying central processes are brain circuits that are involved in pain chronicity, e.g., the cortico-limbic pain circuit including the prefrontal cortex, anterior cingulate cortex, amygdala, and nucleus accumbens. All these brain areas are involved in the emotional and affective processing of pain as well as in its modulation, amplification, and chronicity [80,81]. fMRI assessment of CRPS patients has shown that hyperalgesia and allodynia stimulation in the affected side produced an increase and widespread brain activation in somatosensory regions, prefrontal cortex, bilateral insula, and anterior cingulate cortex compared to the non-involved side [82,83]. The two latter brain areas are involved in interoception, inherently integrated pain, emotion, and body awareness [84]. Thus, the mutual association between pain and psychological distress in CRPS and CLP represents their bidirectional influence at the chronic pain stages yet, with a different relative contribution depending on the magnitude of the central sensitization [85–88].

The Mixed group showed similarity to the CRPS group in their psychological profile along with low evoked-pain intensity, like the CLP group. This pattern implies that although the Mixed group displayed a relatively minor clinical presentation of CRPS signs and symptoms, there was substantial psychological distress, specifically a high intensity of kinesiophobia and somatization. Moreover, the CSS scores demonstrated significant differences between groups with severe, moderate, and mild scores in the CRPS, Mixed, and CLP groups, respectively. These findings further validate CSS as an outcome measure [4] and support the cluster sensitivity in detecting different clinical phenotypes reflecting different chronic pain states. Examining the Mixed group distribution revealed that it comprised 29% of the CLP and 16.4% of the CRPS group, suggesting that this group can fit CRPS not otherwise specified, CRPS with remission of some features subtypes [17], or mild CRPS patients.

4.4. TNF-α and Central Neuro-Inflammation Processes

Our cluster model was further tested for TNF-α and IL-6 serum levels. TNF-α was found to be higher in the CRPS and Mixed groups compared to CLP, while the differences in IL-6 levels between the cluster groups were insignificant. TNF-α is a pro-algesic cytokine released by microglia and astrocytes, is involved in the central neuro-inflammation process [89], and serves as a neuromodulator in the spinal cord dorsal horn. It enhances synaptic plasticity after peripheral injury through the excitation of synaptic transmission. In CRPS, central sensitization processes are more prominent due to ongoing pain and continuous nociceptive input [63,90]. This process leads to the ongoing activation of glial cells in the dorsal horn and the brain [91], which in turn increases the release of pro-inflammatory cytokines and enhances central sensitization [62]. As a result, these central processes contribute to pain persistency in CRPS [13,92]. The CRPS literature regarding the role of IL-6 and TNF-α in the chronic stages is controversial and based on substantial variability in patient characteristics (i.e., acute vs. chronic), testing methods (i.e., CSF, blister fluid, mRNA, and blood), and type of control group (healthy vs. limb pain or the contralateral noninvolved limb) [93]. Thus, it is difficult to draw clear conclusions. However, a systematic meta-analysis has demonstrated an elevated level of TNF-α in a serum sample of chronic CRPS, while IL-6 was found to be elevated in a blister fluid only [94]. In the current study, positive correlations were found between TNF-α, clinical pain intensity, and allodynia area but not IL-6. This further confirms the potential involvement of TNF-α as a marker of centralized pain and neuro-inflammation processes in chronic CRPS.

4.5. BPD in CRPS

Testing the cluster sensitivity in detecting differences in the Bath-BPD score revealed a significantly higher Bath-BPD score in CRPS compared to CLP, with no differences between the Mixed and CRPS groups. BPD is a well-known phenomenon reported in CRPS [59] and CLP [95], yet to a lesser extent in the latter [96,97]. BPD is proposed to be a consequence of learned nonuse processes derived from pain, movement suppression, and fear avoidance in CRPS patients [98]. Although learned nonuse processes can also result from movement avoidance as a pain preventive strategy in the CLP group, we can postulate that this process was amplified in the CRPS group due to mechanical hypersensitivity (i.e., allodynia and hyperalgesia), leading to touch avoidance as well.

Kuttikat et al. [99], suggested two potential neurocognitive mechanisms for somatosensory misperception that leads to BPD in CRPS. The first mechanism is derived from a disruption in the quality of ascending sensory input arising from the involved limb. This disruption is due to neuro-inflammatory processes leading to greater weight on brain prediction processes without online sensory precision, resulting in limb misperception and BPD. The second mechanism is derived from decreased attention to the involved limb, which may be due to psychological distress (e.g., fear of pain, depression) leading to 'cognitive neglect' and limb depersonalization. Our results suggest that these mechanisms probably exist to a greater extent in CRPS compared to CLP since we found significantly greater BPD in the CRPS group.

4.6. Limitations

The study has a few limitations: (i) Although we used the thermal tests as bilateral measures, the evoked pain measures (i.e., the intensity of allodynia, hyperalgesia, and allodynia area) were not tested bilaterally; hence, we could not evaluate the central sensitization process in the contralateral side by using these measures. (ii) The study did not include the conditioned pain modulation test. This test could have gained further understanding of the differences in the pain inhibition modulation function between groups. (iii) The pro-inflammatory samples were taken from a sub-sample that included 33 subjects, thus limiting the strength of the results, which will need further validation in future studies. (iv) A few subjects used cannabis which has possible anti-inflammatory effects on TNF-α levels. However, as the IL-6 levels did not differ between groups, we do not think it was an influential factor.

5. Conclusions

The research findings show that central processes underlying nociplastic pain can distinguish between different CLP conditions. CRPS and its possible subtypes have a unique combination of psychological and pain phenotypes derived from central sensitization and central neuro-inflammation processes. These processes possibly lead to changes in the perception of nociceptive stimuli resulting in pain amplification and mechanical hypersensitivity, along with changes in cognitive and affective brain areas, which may lead to psychological distress and BPD. Future studies can use the described classification method to identify specific markers in other chronic primary pain syndromes, and therefore promote the planning of multimodal, personalized pain medicine interventions.

Author Contributions: H.K. and I.W.-F. developed the study design and wrote the original draft preparation. J.-J.V. clinical and psychophysical supervision and writing—review and editing, A.M. and Y.B.K. participated in data collection and data analysis. All authors have read and agreed to the published version of the manuscript.

Funding: This research was funded by the Reuth Rehabilitation Hospital Internal Research Grant Program, Research grant No. 2017-14.

Institutional Review Board Statement: The study was conducted in accordance with the Declaration of Helsinki, and approved by the Institutional Review Board (IRB) of Reuth Rehabilitation Hospital (2017/14-1, 22/11/2017) and by the IRB of the University of Haifa (Haifa, Israel, 135/18; File 1822).

Informed Consent Statement: Informed consent was obtained from all subjects involved in the study.

Data Availability Statement: The data presented in this study are available on request from the corresponding author.

Acknowledgments: The authors thank Eithan Galun and Sagit Arbel-Alon for their supervision and support in the analysis of the biological measures, Sandra Zukerman for her statistical advisory, and Ruth Moont for reviewing and editing the manuscript.

Conflicts of Interest: The authors declare no conflict of interest.

References

1. Harden, N.; McCabe, C.S.; Goebel, A.; Massey, M.; Suvar, T.; Grieve, S.; Bruehl, S. Complex Regional Pain Syndrome: Practical Diagnostic and Treatment Guidelines, 5th Edition. *Pain Med.* 2022, 23, S1–S53. [CrossRef] [PubMed]
2. Chang, C.; McDonnell, P.; Gershwin, M.E. Complex regional pain syndrome—Autoimmune or functional neurologic syndrome. *J. Transl. Autoimmun.* 2021, 4, 100080. [CrossRef] [PubMed]
3. Ott, S.; Maihöfner, C. Signs and Symptoms in 1,043 Patients with Complex Regional Pain Syndrome. *J. Pain* 2018, 19, 599–611. [CrossRef] [PubMed]
4. Harden, N.; Bruehl, S.; Perez, R.S.G.M.; Birklein, F.; Marinus, J.; Maihofner, C.; Lubenow, T.; Buvanendran, A.; Mackey, S.; Graciosa, J.; et al. Development of a severity score for CRPS. *Pain* 2010, 151, 870–876. [CrossRef] [PubMed]
5. Sandroni, P.; Benrud-Larson, L.M.; Mcclelland, R.L.; Low, P.A. Complex regional pain syndrome type I: Incidence and prevalence in Olmsted county, a population-based study. *Pain* 2003, 103, 199–207. [CrossRef]
6. De Mos, M.; de Bruijn, A.G.J.; Huygen, F.J.P.M.; Dieleman, J.P.; Stricker, B.H.C.; Sturkenboom, M.C.J.M. The incidence of complex regional pain syndrome: A population-based study. *Pain* 2007, 129, 12–20. [CrossRef]
7. Kim, H.; Lee, C.H.; Kim, S.H.; Kim, Y.D. Epidemiology of complex regional pain syndrome in Korea: An electronic population health data study. *PLoS ONE* 2018, 13, e0198147. [CrossRef]
8. Nicholas, M.; Vlaeyen, J.W.S.; Rief, W.; Barke, A.; Aziz, Q.; Benoliel, R.; Cohen, M.; Evers, S.; Giamberardino, M.A.; Goebel, A.; et al. The IASP classification of chronic pain for ICD-11: Chronic primary pain. *Pain* 2019, 160, 28–37. [CrossRef]
9. Fitzcharles, M.-A.; Cohen, S.P.; Clauw, D.J.; Littlejohn, G.; Usui, C.; Häuser, W. Nociplastic pain: Towards an understanding of prevalent pain conditions. *Lancet* 2021, 397, 2098–2110. [CrossRef]
10. Dimova, V.; Herrnberger, M.S.; Escolano-Lozano, F.; Rittner, H.L.; Vlckova, E.; Sommer, C.; Maihöfner, C.; Birklein, F. Clinical phenotypes and classification algorithm for complex regional pain syndrome. *Neurology* 2020, 94, e357–e367. [CrossRef]
11. Bruehl, S.; Maihöfner, C.; Stanton-Hicks, M.; Perez, R.S.G.M.; Vatine, J.J.; Brunner, F.; Birklein, F.; Schlereth, T.; Mackey, S.; Mailis-Gagnon, A.; et al. Complex regional pain syndrome: Evidence for warm and cold subtypes in a large prospective clinical sample. *Pain* 2016, 157, 1674–1681. [CrossRef] [PubMed]
12. Bruehl, S. Complex regional pain syndrome. *BMJ* 2015, 351, h2730. [CrossRef] [PubMed]
13. Mangnus, T.J.P.; Bharwani, K.D.; Dirckx, M.; Huygen, F.J.P.M. From a Symptom-Based to a Mechanism-Based Pharmacotherapeutic Treatment in Complex Regional Pain Syndrome. *Drugs* 2022, 82, 511–531. [CrossRef] [PubMed]
14. Alexander, G.M.; Peterlin, B.L.; Perreault, M.J.; Grothusen, J.R.; Schwartzman, R.J. Changes in plasma cytokines and their soluble receptors in complex regional pain syndrome. *J. Pain* 2012, 13, 10–20. [CrossRef] [PubMed]
15. Libon, D.J.; Schwartzman, R.J.; Eppig, J.; Wambach, D.; Brahin, E.; Peterlin, B.L.; Alexander, G.; Kalanuria, A. Neuropsychological deficits associated with Complex Regional Pain Syndrome. *J. Int. Neuropsychol. Soc.* 2010, 16, 566–573. [CrossRef]
16. Ten Brink, A.F.; Bultitude, J.H. Predictors of Self-Reported Neglect-like Symptoms and Involuntary Movements in Complex Regional Pain Syndrome Compared to Other Chronic Limb Pain Conditions. *Pain Med.* 2021, 22, 2337–2349. [CrossRef]
17. Goebel, A.; Birklein, F.; Brunner, F.; Clark, J.D.; Gierthmühlen, J.; Harden, N.; Huygen, F.; Knudsen, L.; McCabe, C.; Lewis, J.; et al. The Valencia consensus-based adaptation of the IASP complex regional pain syndrome diagnostic criteria. *Pain* 2021, 162, 2346–2348. [CrossRef]
18. Fitzcharles, M.A.; Cohen, S.P.; Clauw, D.J.; Littlejohn, G.; Usui, C.; Häuser, W. Chronic primary musculoskeletal pain: A new concept of nonstructural regional pain. *Pain Rep.* 2022, 7, e1024. [CrossRef]
19. Treede, R.D.; Rief, W.; Barke, A.; Aziz, Q.; Bennett, M.I.; Benoliel, R.; Cohen, M.; Evers, S.; Finnerup, N.B.; First, M.B.; et al. Chronic pain as a symptom or a disease: The IASP Classification of Chronic Pain for the International Classification of Diseases (ICD-11). *Pain* 2019, 160, 19–27. [CrossRef]
20. Perrot, S.; Cohen, M.; Barke, A.; Korwisi, B.; Rief, W.; Treede, R.-D.; IASP Taskforce for the Classification of Chronic Pain. The IASP classification of chronic pain for ICD-11: Chronic secondary musculoskeletal pain. *Pain* 2019, 160, 77–82. [CrossRef]
21. Kosek, E.; Clauw, D.; Nijs, J.; Baron, R.; Gilron, I.; Harris, R.E.; Mico, J.-A.; Rice, A.S.; Sterling, M. Chronic nociplastic pain affecting the musculoskeletal system: Clinical criteria and grading system. *Pain* 2021, 162, 2629–2634. [CrossRef] [PubMed]
22. Dietz, C.; Müller, M.; Reinhold, A.K.; Karch, L.; Schwab, B.; Forer, L.; Vlckova, E.; Brede, E.-M.; Jakubietz, R.; Üçeyler, N.; et al. What is normal trauma healing and what is complex regional pain syndrome I? An analysis of clinical and experimental biomarkers. *Pain* 2019, 160, 2278–2289. [CrossRef] [PubMed]
23. Alam, O.H.; Zaidi, B.; Pierce, J.; Moser, S.E.; Hilliard, P.E.; Golmirzaie, G.; Brummett, C.M. Phenotypic features of patients with complex regional pain syndrome compared with those with neuropathic pain. *Reg. Anesth. Pain Med.* 2019, 44, 881–885. [CrossRef] [PubMed]
24. Michal, M.; Adler, J.; Reiner, I.; Wermke, A.; Ackermann, T.; Schlereth, T.; Birklein, F. Association of Neglect-Like Symptoms with Anxiety, Somatization, and Depersonalization in Complex Regional Pain Syndrome. *Pain Med.* 2017, 18, 764–772. [CrossRef] [PubMed]
25. Farzad, M.; MacDermid, J.C.; Packham, T.; Khodabandeh, B.; Vahedi, M.; Shafiee, E. Factors associated with disability and pain intensity in patients with complex regional pain syndrome. *Disabil. Rehabil.* 2022, 44, 8243–8251. [CrossRef]
26. Bean, D.J.; Johnson, M.H.; Kydd, R.R. Relationships Between Psychological Factors, Pain, and Disability in Complex Regional Pain Syndrome and Low Back Pain. *Clin. J. Pain* 2014, 30, 647–653. [CrossRef]

27. Harden, N.; Maihofner, C.; Abousaad, E.; Vatine, J.J.; Kirsling, A.; Perez, R.S.G.M.; Kuroda, M.; Brunner, F.; Stanton-Hicks, M.; Marinus, J.; et al. A prospective, multisite, international validation of the Complex Regional Pain Syndrome Severity Score. *Pain* **2017**, *158*, 1430–1436. [CrossRef]
28. Melzack, R. The short-form McGill pain questionnaire. *Pain* **1987**, *30*, 191–197. [CrossRef]
29. Sloman, R.; Rosen, G.; Rom, M.; Shir, Y. Nurses' assessment of pain in surgical patients. *J. Adv. Nurs.* **2005**, *52*, 125–132. [CrossRef]
30. Treede, R.D.; Magerl, W. Multiple mechanisms of secondary hyperalgesia. *Prog. Brain Res.* **2000**, *129*, 331–341. [CrossRef]
31. Rolke, R.; Magerl, W.; Campbell, K.A.; Schalber, C.; Caspari, S.; Birklein, F.; Treede, R.-D. Quantitative sensory testing: A comprehensive protocol for clinical trials. *Eur. J. Pain* **2006**, *10*, 77. [CrossRef] [PubMed]
32. Packham, T.L.; Spicher, C.J.; MacDermid, J.C.; Michlovitz, S.; Buckley, D.N. Somatosensory rehabilitation for allodynia in complex regional pain syndrome of the upper limb: A retrospective cohort study. *J. Hand Ther.* **2018**, *31*, 10–19. [CrossRef] [PubMed]
33. Karpin, H.; Shmueli, S.; Turgeman, N.; Weissman-Fogel, I.; Vatin, J.J. A new allodynography quantification method for somatosensory rehabilitation in Complex Regional Pain Syndrome. In Proceedings of the 11th Congress of the European Pain Federation, Valencia, Spain, 4–7 September 2019.
34. Lund, C.C.; Browder, N.C. The estimation of areas of burns. *Surg. Gynecol. Obst.* **1944**, *79*, 352–358.
35. Sullivan, M.J.L.; Bishop, S.R.; Pivik, J. The Pain Catastrophizing Scale: Development and Validation. *Psychol. Assess.* **1995**, *7*, 524–532. [CrossRef]
36. Granot, M.; Ferber, S.G. The Roles of Pain Catastrophizing and Anxiety in the Prediction of Postoperative Pain Intensity—A Prospective Study. *Pain* **2005**, *21*, 439–445. [CrossRef]
37. Miller, R.P.; Kori, S.H.; Todd, D.D. Miller, R.P.; Kori, S.H.; Todd, D.D. The Tampa Scale—A measiure of kinesiophobia. *Clin. J. Pain* **1991**, *7*, 51. [CrossRef]
38. Sarig Bahat, H.; Weiss, P.L.T.; Sprecher, E.; Krasovsky, A.; Laufer, Y. Do neck kinematics correlate with pain intensity, neck disability or with fear of motion? *Man. Ther.* **2014**, *19*, 252–258. [CrossRef]
39. Beck, A.T.; Steer, R.A.; Brown, G. Beck Depression Inventory–II (BDI-II). *Psychol. Assess.* **1996**, *67*, 588–597.
40. *BDI-II Guide*, 2nd ed.; Psyctech: Jerusalem, Israel, 2010.
41. Derogatis, L.R.; Melisaratos, N. The brief symptom inventory: An introductory report. *Psychol. Med.* **1983**, *13*, 595–605. [CrossRef]
42. Canetti, L.; Kaplan De-Nour, A.; Shalev, A.Y. Israeli adolescents' norms of the Brief Symptom Inventory (BSI). *Isr. J. Psychiatry Relat. Sci.* **1994**, *31*, 13–18.
43. Sierra, M.; Berrios, G.E. The Cambridge Depersonalisation Scale: A new instrument for the measurement of depersonalisation. *Psychiatry Res.* **2000**, *93*, 153–164. [CrossRef] [PubMed]
44. Lewis, J.; McCabe, C. Body perception disturbance (BPD) in CRPS. *Pract. Pain Manag.* **2010**, 60–66.
45. Vallerand, R.J.; Pelletier, L.G.; Blais, M.R.; Briere, N.M.; Senecal, C.; Vallieres, E.F. The Academic Motivation Scale: A measure of intrinsic, extrinsic, and amotivation in education. *Educ. Psychol. Meas.* **1992**, *52*, 1003–1017. [CrossRef]
46. Lewis, J.S.; Schweinhardt, P. Perceptions of the painful body: The relationship between body perception disturbance, pain and tactile discrimination in complex regional pain syndrome. *Eur. J. Pain* **2012**, *16*, 1320–1330. [CrossRef]
47. Faul, F.; Erdfelder, E.; Buchner, A.; Lang, A.G. Statistical power analyses using G* Power 3.1: Tests for correlation and regression analyses. *Behav. Res. Methods* **2009**, *41*, 1149–1160. [CrossRef]
48. Richardson, J.T.E. Eta squared and partial eta squared as measures of effect size in educational research. *Educ. Res. Rev.* **2011**, *6*, 135–147. [CrossRef]
49. Tkaczynski, A. Segmentation using two-step cluster analysis. In *Segmentation in Social Marketing*; Springer: Singapore, 2017; pp. 109–125.
50. Schwarz, G. Estimating the Dimension of a Model. *Ann. Stat.* **1978**, *6*, 261–464. [CrossRef]
51. Rousseeuw, P.J. Silhouettes: A graphical aid to the interpretation and validation of cluster analysis. *J. Comput. Appl. Math.* **1987**, *20*, 53–65. [CrossRef]
52. Baraldi, A.N.; Enders, C.K. An introduction to modern missing data analyses. *J. Sch. Psychol.* **2010**, *48*, 5–37. [CrossRef] [PubMed]
53. Edwards, I.R.; Aronson, J.K. Adverse drug reactions: Definitions, diagnosis, and management. *Lancet* **2000**, *356*, 1255–1259. [CrossRef]
54. Woolf, C.J.; Warner, D.S.; Ch, B. Central Sensitization Uncovering the Relation between Pain and Plasticity. *Anesthesiology* **2007**, *106*, 864–867. [CrossRef]
55. Seifert, F.; Kiefer, G.; Decol, R.; Schmelz, M.; Maihöfner, C. Differential endogenous pain modulation in complex-regional pain syndrome. *Brain* **2009**, *132*, 788–800. [CrossRef]
56. Nijs, J.; Lahousse, A.; Kapreli, E.; Bilika, P.; Saraçoğlu, İ.; Malfliet, A.; Coppieters, I.; De Baets, L.; Leysen, L.; Roose, E.; et al. Nociplastic pain criteria or recognition of central sensitization? Pain phenotyping in the past, present and future. *J. Clin. Med.* **2021**, *10*, 3203. [CrossRef]
57. Yarnitsky, D. Role of endogenous pain modulation in chronic pain mechanisms and treatment. *Pain* **2015**, *156*, S24–S31. [CrossRef] [PubMed]
58. Yarnitsky, D.; Granot, M.; Granovsky, Y. Pain modulation profile and pain therapy: Between pro- and antinociception. *Pain* **2014**, *155*, 663–665. [CrossRef]
59. Birklein, F.; Ajit, S.K.; Goebel, A.; Perez, R.S.G.M.; Sommer, C. Complex regional pain syndrome-phenotypic characteristics and potential biomarkers. *Nat. Rev. Neurol.* **2018**, *14*, 272–284. [CrossRef]

60. Moseley, G.L.; Herbert, R.D.; Parsons, T.; Lucas, S.; van Hilten, J.J.; Marinus, J. Intense pain soon after wrist fracture strongly predicts who will develop complex regional pain syndrome: Prospective cohort study. *J. Pain* 2014, *15*, 16–23. [CrossRef]
61. Harden, R.N.; Oaklander, A.L.; Burton, A.W.; Perez, R.S.G.M.; Richardson, M.K.; Swan, O.M.; Barthel, M.J.; Costa, C.B.; Graciosa, B.J.R.; Bruehl, S. Complex Regional Pain Syndrome: Practical Diagnostic and Treatment Guidelines, 4th Edition. *Pain Med.* 2013, *14*, 180–229. [CrossRef]
62. Ji, R.-R.; Nackley, A.; Huh, Y.; Terrando, N.; Maixner, W. Neuroinflammation and central sensitization in chronic and widespread pain. *Anesthesiology* 2018, *129*, 343–366. [CrossRef]
63. Bharwani, K.D.; Dik, W.A.; Dirckx, M.; Huygen, F.J.P.M. Highlighting the Role of Biomarkers of Inflammation in the Diagnosis and Management of Complex Regional Pain Syndrome. *Mol. Diagn. Ther.* 2019, *23*, 615–626. [CrossRef]
64. Edwards, R.R. Medical Hypotheses Individual differences in endogenous pain modulation as a risk factor for chronic pain. *Neurology* 2005, *65*, 437–443. [CrossRef] [PubMed]
65. Zaslansky, R.; Yarnitsky, D. Clinical applications of quantitative sensory testing (QST). *J. Neurol. Sci.* 1998, *153*, 215–238. [CrossRef]
66. Gottrup, H.; Kristensen, A.D.; Bach, F.W.; Jensen, T.S. Aftersensations in experimental and clinical hypersensitivity. *Pain* 2003, *103*, 57–64. [CrossRef] [PubMed]
67. Morisset, V.; Nagy, F. Plateau potential-dependent windup of the response to primary afferent stimuli in rat dorsal horn neurons. *Eur. J. Neurosci.* 2000, *12*, 3087–3095. [CrossRef]
68. Monteiro, C.; Lima, D.; Galhardo, V. Switching-on and -off of bistable spontaneous discharges in rat spinal deep dorsal horn neurons. *Neurosci. Lett.* 2006, *398*, 258–263. [CrossRef]
69. Wolanin, M.W.; Schwartzman, R.J.; Alexander, G.; Grothusen, J. Loss of Surround Inhibition and After Sensation as Diagnostic Parameters of Complex Regional Pain Syndrome. *Neurosci. Med.* 2012, *03*, 344–353. [CrossRef]
70. Sheng, J.; Liu, S.; Wang, Y.; Cui, R.; Zhang, X. The Link between Depression and Chronic Pain: Neural Mechanisms in the Brain. *Neural. Plast.* 2017, *2017*, 9724371. [CrossRef]
71. Yin, C.; Jia, T.; Luan, Y.; Zhang, X.; Xiao, C.; Zhou, C. A nigra–subthalamic circuit is involved in acute and chronic pain states. *Pain* 2022, *163*, 1952–1966. [CrossRef]
72. Margalit, D.; ben Har, L.; Brill, S.; Vatine, J.J. Complex regional pain syndrome, alexithymia, and psychological distress. *J. Psychosom. Res.* 2014, *77*, 273–277. [CrossRef]
73. Park, H.Y.; Jang, Y.E.; Oh, S.; Lee, P.B. Psychological characteristics in patients with chronic complex regional pain syndrome: Comparisons with patients with major depressive disorder and other types of chronic pain. *J. Pain Res.* 2020, *13*, 389–398. [CrossRef]
74. Bean, D.J.; Johnson, M.H.; Heiss-Dunlop, W.; Kydd, R.R. Extent of recovery in the first 12 months of complex regional pain syndrome type-1: A prospective study. *Eur. J. Pain* 2016, *20*, 884–894. [CrossRef]
75. De Jong, J.R.; Vlaeyen, J.W.S.; de Gelder, J.M.; Patijn, J. Pain-related fear, perceived harmfulness of activities, and functional limitations in complex regional pain syndrome type I. *J. Pain* 2011, *12*, 1209–1218. [CrossRef]
76. Marinus, J.; Perez, R.S.; van Eijs, F.; van Gestel, M.A.; Geurts, J.J.; Huygen, F.J.; Bauer, M.C.; van Hilten, J.J. The Role of Pain Coping and Kinesiophobia in Patients with Complex Regional Pain Syndrome Type 1 of the Legs. *Clin. J. Pain* 2013, *29*, 563–569. [CrossRef]
77. Luque-Suarez, A.; Martinez-Calderon, J.; Falla, D. Role of kinesiophobia on pain, disability and quality of life in people suffering from chronic musculoskeletal pain: A systematic review. *Br. J. Sport. Med.* 2019, *53*, 554–559. [CrossRef]
78. Antunovich, D.R.; Horne, J.C.; Tuck, N.L.; Bean, D.J. Are Illness Perceptions Associated with Pain and Disability in Complex Regional Pain Syndrome? A Cross-Sectional Study. *Pain Med.* 2021, *22*, 100–111. [CrossRef]
79. Mansour, A.R.; Farmer, M.A.; Baliki, M.N.; Apkarian, A.V. Chronic pain: The role of learning and brain plasticity. *Restor. Neurol. Neurosci.* 2014, *32*, 129–139. [CrossRef]
80. Thompson, J.M.; Neugebauer, V. Amygdala Plasticity and Pain. *Pain Res. Manag.* 2017, *2017*, 8296501. [CrossRef]
81. Yang, S.; Chang, M.C. Chronic pain: Structural and functional changes in brain structures and associated negative affective states. *Int. J. Mol. Sci.* 2019, *20*, 3130. [CrossRef]
82. Maihöfner, C.; Handwerker, H.O.; Birklein, F. Functional imaging of allodynia in complex regional pain syndrome. *Neurology* 2006, *66*, 711–717. [CrossRef]
83. Maihfner, C.; Forster, C.; Birklein, F.; Neundörfer, B.; Handwerker, H.O. Brain processing during mechanical hyperalgesia in complex regional pain syndrome: A functional MRI study. *Pain* 2005, *114*, 93–103. [CrossRef]
84. Gilam, G.; Gross, J.J.; Wager, T.D.; Keefe, F.J.; Mackey, S.C. What Is the Relationship between Pain and Emotion? Bridging Constructs and Communities. *Neuron* 2020, *107*, 17–21. [CrossRef]
85. Woolf, C.J. Central sensitization: Implications for the diagnosis and treatment of pain. *Pain* 2011, *152*, S2–S15. [CrossRef]
86. Latremoliere, A.; Woolf, C.J. Central Sensitization: A Generator of Pain Hypersensitivity by Central Neural Plasticity. *J. Pain* 2009, *10*, 895–926. [CrossRef]
87. Harte, S.E.; Harris, R.E.; Clauw, D.J. The neurobiology of central sensitization. *J. Appl. Biobehav. Res.* 2018, *23*, e12137. [CrossRef]
88. Adams, L.M.; Turk, D.C. Central sensitization and the biopsychosocial approach to understanding pain. *J. Appl. Biobehav. Res.* 2018, *23*, e12125. [CrossRef]
89. Baral, P.; Udit, S.; Chiu, I.M. Pain and immunity: Implications for host defence. *Nat. Rev. Immunol.* 2019, *19*, 433–447. [CrossRef]

90. Reimer, M.; Rempe, T.; Diedrichs, C.; Baron, R.; Gierthmühlen, J. Sensitization of the nociceptive system in complex regional pain syndrome. *PLoS ONE* **2016**, *11*, e0154553. [CrossRef]
91. Li, W.W.; Guo, T.Z.; Shi, X.; Sun, Y.; Wei, T.; Clark, D.J.; Kingery, W. Substance P spinal signaling induces glial activation and nociceptive sensitization after fracture. *Neuroscience* **2015**, *310*, 73–90. [CrossRef]
92. Pohóczky, K.; Kun, J.; Szentes, N.; Aczél, T.; Urbán, P.; Gyenesei, A.; Bölcskei, K.; Szőke, É.; Sensi, S.; Dénes, Á.; et al. Discovery of novel targets in a complex regional pain syndrome mouse model by transcriptomics: TNF and JAK-STAT pathways. *Pharmacol. Res.* **2022**, *182*, 106347. [CrossRef]
93. Sommer, C.; Leinders, M.; Üçeyler, N. Inflammation in the pathophysiology of neuropathic pain. *Pain* **2018**, *159*, 595–602. [CrossRef]
94. Parkitny, L.; McAuley, J.H.; di Pietro, F.; Stanton, T.R.; O'Connell, N.E.; Marinus, J.; Van Hilten, J.J.; Moseley, G.L. Inflammation in complex regional pain syndrome A systematic review and meta-analysis. *Am. Acad. Neurol.* **2013**, *80*, 106–117. [CrossRef]
95. Hall, J.; Llewellyn, A.; Palmer, S.; Rowett-Harris, J.; Atkins, R.M.; McCabe, C.S. Sensorimotor dysfunction after limb fracture—An exploratory study. *Eur. J. Pain* **2016**, *20*, 1402–1412. [CrossRef]
96. Frettlöh, J.; Hüppe, M.; Maier, C. Severity and specificity of neglect-like symptoms in patients with complex regional pain syndrome (CRPS) compared to chronic limb pain of other origins. *Pain* **2006**, *124*, 184–189. [CrossRef]
97. Reinersmann, A.; Landwehrt, J.; Krumova, E.K.; Ocklenburg, S.; Güntürkün, O.; Maier, C. Impaired spatial body representation in complex regional pain syndrome type 1 (CRPS I). *Pain* **2012**, *153*, 2174–2181. [CrossRef]
98. Punt, T.D.; Cooper, L.; Hey, M.; Johnson, M.I. Neglect-like symptoms in complex regional pain syndrome: Learned nonuse by another name? *Pain* **2013**, *154*, 200–203. [CrossRef]
99. Kuttikat, A.; Noreika, V.; Shenker, N.; Chennu, S.; Bekinschtein, T.; Brown, C.A. Neurocognitive and neuroplastic mechanisms of novel clinical signs in CRPS. *Front. Hum. Neurosci.* **2016**, *10*, 16. [CrossRef]

Disclaimer/Publisher's Note: The statements, opinions and data contained in all publications are solely those of the individual author(s) and contributor(s) and not of MDPI and/or the editor(s). MDPI and/or the editor(s) disclaim responsibility for any injury to people or property resulting from any ideas, methods, instructions or products referred to in the content.

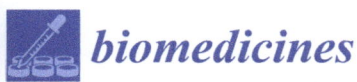

Article

FDG PET Imaging of the Pain Matrix in Neuropathic Pain Model Rats

Yilong Cui [1,*], Hiroyuki Neyama [1], Di Hu [1], Tianliang Huang [1], Emi Hayashinaka [2], Yasuhiro Wada [2] and Yasuyoshi Watanabe [2]

[1] Laboratory for Biofunction Dynamics Imaging, RIKEN Center for Biosystems Dynamics Research, Kobe 650-0047, Hyogo, Japan
[2] Laboratory for Pathophysiological and Health Science, RIKEN Center for Biosystems Dynamics Research, Kobe 650-0047, Hyogo, Japan
* Correspondence: cuiyl@riken.jp; Tel.: +81-78-304-7172

Abstract: Pain is an unpleasant subjective experience that is usually modified by complex multidimensional neuropsychological processes. Increasing numbers of neuroimaging studies in humans have characterized the hierarchical brain areas forming a pain matrix, which is involved in the different dimensions of pain components. Although mechanistic investigations have been performed extensively in rodents, the homologous brain regions involved in the multidimensional pain components have not been fully understood in the rodent brain. Herein, we successfully identified several brain regions activated in response to mechanical allodynia in neuropathic pain rat models using an alternative neuroimaging method based on 2-deoxy-2-[^{18}F]fluoro-D-glucose positron emission tomography (FDG PET) scanning. Regions such as the medial prefrontal cortex, primary somatosensory cortex hindlimb region, and the centrolateral thalamic nucleus were identified. Moreover, brain activity in these regions was positively correlated with mechanical allodynia-related behavioral changes. These results suggest that FDG PET imaging in neuropathic pain model rats enables the evaluation of regional brain activity encoding the multidimensional pain aspect. It could thus be a fascinating tool to bridge the gap between preclinical and clinical investigations.

Keywords: neuroimaging; FDG; neuropathic pain; objective biomarker; pain matrix; preclinic

Citation: Cui, Y.; Neyama, H.; Hu, D.; Huang, T.; Hayashinaka, E.; Wada, Y.; Watanabe, Y. FDG PET Imaging of the Pain Matrix in Neuropathic Pain Model Rats. *Biomedicines* **2023**, *11*, 63. https://doi.org/10.3390/biomedicines11010063

Academic Editors: Mats Eriksson and Anders O. Larsson

Received: 15 November 2022
Revised: 3 December 2022
Accepted: 23 December 2022
Published: 27 December 2022

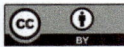

Copyright: © 2022 by the authors. Licensee MDPI, Basel, Switzerland. This article is an open access article distributed under the terms and conditions of the Creative Commons Attribution (CC BY) license (https://creativecommons.org/licenses/by/4.0/).

1. Introduction

Pain is an unpleasant subjective experience that interacts with multidimensional neuropsychological processes, including sensory discrimination, cognitive evaluation, and emotional affection [1]. Chronic pain is the most common cause for seeking medical care, affecting over 20% of adults worldwide [2]. Unfortunately, most patients with chronic pain are not satisfied with currently available analgesic therapy [3], suggesting that the development of more effective therapies for chronic pain is indispensable. Pain is a multidimensional neuropsychological process and is not linearly related to primary nociception, especially in chronic pain. Owing to such a subjective nature and complex interactions with conscious brain activity, non-invasive neuroimaging has received increasing attention as a potential biomarker for the objective assessment of pain and the comprehensive exploration of pharmacological targets of pain intervention [4–7]. Previously, neuroimaging studies in patients have attributed structural abnormalities and functional alterations to chronic pain [7–10]. In patients with chronic back pain, the gray matter density was decreased in the prefrontal cortex and thalamic region [11], whereas the functional connectivity between the prefrontal cortex and the nucleus accumbens was increased [9]. Functional neuroimaging studies have also characterized several regions of the brain that are thought to be involved in different dimensions of pain components. The lateral thalamus, sensory cortex, and posterior insular cortex are preferentially related to the sensory-discriminative dimension of pain [5,7,12]. The medial thalamus and anterior cingulate cortex seem to be associated with the emotional affective dimension of pain [1,13,14], whereas the prefrontal cortex is related to the cognitive evaluation dimension of pain [15,16].

Meanwhile, preclinical research employing diverse animal models that mimic certain forms of clinical pain has been extensively undertaken to explore the pathophysiology of pain and to identify effective therapeutic targets for pain treatment [17–20]. However, due to the lack of reliable coherent biomarkers for pain assessment throughout preclinical and clinical studies, the pathophysiology revealed in these preclinical studies has not been completely translated into clinical practice [21]. In general, reflex-based behavioral observations are often used for pain assessment in most preclinical studies [22]. However, self-reporting-based subjective evaluation has long been used as the gold standard in clinical endpoints [3,23,24]. Such inconsistencies between the biomarkers of pain assessment in preclinical and clinical research may also hinder our understanding of the pathophysiology of chronic pain.

Current advances in neuroimaging technologies provide a potential consistent biomarker for pain assessment throughout preclinical and clinical research. A growing number of neuroimaging studies, involving methods such as functional magnetic resonance imaging (fMRI) and positron emission tomography (PET), have been performed in rodent pain models and have highlighted that functional and structural changes in several brain regions may underlie the pathophysiology of chronic pain [25,26]. However, most neuroimaging studies in rodents require the immobilization of the animal with anesthesia or a specific head-fix system, which may interfere with normal neuropsychological processes and cause a reduction of neuronal activity [25,27,28]. Compared with the conscious condition, the cerebral glucose metabolic rate in the cerebral cortex of mice was decreased by 66% under isoflurane, one of the most frequently used anesthetics in animal neuroimaging studies [28]. Recently, an alternative 2-deoxy-2-[^{18}F]fluoro-D-glucose (FDG) PET imaging, which does not require immobilization, has been increasingly used for analyzing brain activity in rodents [29–32]. FDG is taken up by active regions of the brain and remains within the regions for at least an hour [33]; therefore, brain activity free from immobilization can be obtained by subsequent FDG PET scans performed under anesthesia, in which most FDG is taken up under a conscious condition prior to the PET scan. Using the FDG PET imaging and subsequent voxel-based statistical analysis, we investigated chronic pain-related brain activity in the spinal nerve ligated (SNL) neuropathic pain rat model.

2. Materials and Methods

All experimental protocols of our study were approved by the Animal Care and Use Committee of RIKEN, Kobe Branch, and were performed in accordance with the Principles of Laboratory Animal Care (NIH publication No. 85–23, revised 2011). This study was conducted in accordance with the Animal Research: Reporting in Vivo Experiments (ARRIVE) guidelines. All recommended means were followed to minimize animal suffering.

2.1. Neuropathic Pain Animal Model Preparation

Twenty-two male Wistar rats (SLC, Hamamatsu, Shizuoka, Japan) of approximately 8 weeks of age were used for the FDG PET scan. The rats were housed in a 12-h light/dark cycle at a temperature of 22 ± 1 °C and received food and water *ad libitum*. As shown in Figure 1, the neuropathic pain model was generated by tight ligation of the left L5 and L6 spinal nerves 1-week before the FDG PET scan [19]. The rats were anesthetized with a mixture of 1.5% isoflurane and nitrous oxide/oxygen (7:3). A dorsal midline incision was made at the back from L3 to S2. The left L5 and L6 spinal nerves were isolated adjacent to the vertebral column and tightly ligated with 3-0 silk sutures. In contrast, the sham-operated control rats underwent the same surgical procedure; however, the L5/L6 spinal nerves were not ligated. The incision was then closed in two layers. The rats in the SNL group underwent a PET scan only when the paw withdrawal threshold (PWT) was less than 6.0 g in response to von Frey filaments stimulation.

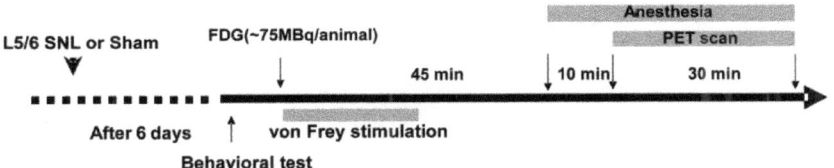

Figure 1. Experimental paradigm. The left L5 and L6 spinal nerve ligation (SNL) was performed one week before the FDG PET scan. Mechanical allodynia was examined using the von Frey test one day before the FDG PET scan in all SNL and sham-operated rats. FDG was intravenously injected into the tail vein via an indwelling catheter under free-moving conditions. Immediately after the FDG injection, mechanical stimulation with von Frey filaments lower than PWT in the sham-operated rats to evoke allodynia was initiated in SNL rats.

2.2. Behavior Test

Mechanical allodynia was tested using a series of von Frey filaments applied to the plantar of the left hind paw in a blinded fashion, as described previously [34]. The rats were placed in a plastic cage with a wire mesh bottom which allowed easy access to the paws. The center-plantar surface of the left hind paw was stimulated with a series of calibrated von Frey filaments with ascending stiffness (4, 6, 8, 10, 15, and 26 g) in an incremental order starting with the lowest filament weight (4 g) after a sufficient acclimation period. Stimuli were presented at intervals of at least 30 s. A positive response was noted if the paw was removed from the wire mesh bottom. The cut-off of 26 g filament (approximately 10% of the body weight of the rats) was selected as the upper limit for testing. When the hind paw was withdrawn from a certain filament in more than two of three applications, the value of that filament in grams was considered as the PWT.

2.3. PET Scanning

All PET scans were performed using microPET Focus220 (Siemens Co., Ltd., Knoxville, TN, USA), which was designed for the high-resolution imaging of laboratory small animals, as previously described [35]. As shown in Figure 1, seven days after the SNL surgery, each rat underwent tail vein cannulation under anesthesia with a mixture of 1.5% isoflurane and nitrous oxide/oxygen (7:3) before the PET scan. After more than an hour of recovery, the free-moving rat received an intravenous injection of ^{18}F-FDG (ca. 75 MBq/0.4 mL) in the home cage. Immediately after the FDG injection, the SNL rats were placed in the plastic cage and the left hind paw was stimulated every 30 s for 20 min with the von Frey filaments two levels higher than the corresponding PWT. The paw withdrawal rate was calculated as a percentage of positive response to total von Frey stimulations. The sham-operated control rats were kept in the home cage after the FDG injection. After a 45-min uptake period, the rats were anesthetized with a mixture of 1.5% isoflurane and nitrous oxide/oxygen (7:3), and positioned in the gantry of a PET scanner. Fifty-five minutes after receiving the ^{18}F-FDG injection, a 30-min emission scan was performed with 400–650 keV as the energy window and 6 nsec as the coincidence time window. A thermocouple probe was inserted into the rectum to monitor the rectal temperature. The body temperature was maintained at approximately 37 °C with a heating blanket during the PET scan. The emission data were acquired in the list mode. The acquired data were sorted into a single sinogram. The data were reconstructed by standard 2D filtered back projection (FBP) with a Ramp filter and cutoff frequency of 0.5 cycles per pixel, or by a statistical maximum a posteriori probability algorithm (MAP), 12 iterations with point spread function (PSF) effect.

2.4. Image Analysis

For voxel-based statistical analysis, individual MAP-reconstructed FDG images were coregistered to an FDG template image using a mutual information algorithm with Powell's convergence optimization method implemented with PMOD software package (version

3.2, PMOD Technologies, Ltd., Zurich, Switzerland). Subsequently, the FDG template was transformed into the space of an MRI reference template, which was placed in the Paxinos and Watson stereotactic space. The transformation parameters obtained from individual MAP-reconstructed FDG images were applied to each FBP image. For matching the default setting in SPM, the voxel size of the template was scaled by a factor of 10. Since the Paxinos stereotactic space had a slice thickness of 0.12 mm, the final voxel size was resampled at $1.2 \times 1.2 \times 1.2$ mm. To enhance the statistical power, each FBP image was spatially smoothed with an isotropic Gaussian kernel (6-mm full width at half of the maximum [FWHM]).

The voxel-based statistical analysis was assessed using SPM8 software (Welcome Department of Imaging Neuroscience, London, UK). Proportional scaling was used for global normalization. A two-sample t-test was used to detect statistical differences between the treatment groups. The statistical threshold was set at $p < 0.002$ (uncorrected) with an extent threshold of 100 contiguous voxels. T-value maps of results were overlaid on the MRI template to define the voxels with significance.

2.5. Data Analyses

Statistical analysis of the behavioral test was performed using GraphPad Prism 5.0 (GraphPad, San Diego, CA, USA). The statistical difference between the SNL and sham-operated rats was estimated using two-tailed unpaired t-tests. $p < 0.05$ was considered statistically significant. Data in the text is expressed as the mean $\pm$ standard deviation of the mean (SD).

3. Results

3.1. Mechanical Allodynia in SNL Rats

SNL is one of the popular neuropathic pain models in rodents that evoked mechanical allodynia restricted to the ipsilateral hind paw for at least 2 weeks [19]. To examine mechanical allodynia, the von Frey behavior test was performed in the SNL ($n = 10$) and sham-operated groups ($n = 12$) one day before the PET scan. As shown in Figure 2, the PWT in the ipsilateral hind paw (left hind paw) was significantly decreased in the SNL group compared with that in the sham-operated group ($p < 0.05$, two-tail unpaired t-test). In contrast, the PWT in the contralateral hind paw of SNL rats did not show any significant change. These results indicate that mechanical allodynia was developed in the ipsilateral hind paw but not in the contralateral hind paw of SNL rats approximately one week after SNL treatment.

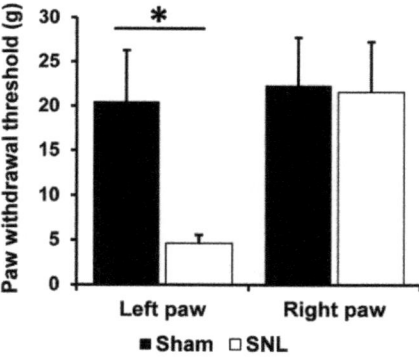

Figure 2. Behavior test for the assessment of mechanical allodynia one day before the FDG PET scan. Bilateral hind paw withdrawal thresholds (PWT) for von Frey filaments stimulation were assessed in the sham-operated (closed bar, $n = 12$) and SNL (open bar, $n = 10$) rats. The data are presented as mean $\pm$ standard deviation of the mean (SD). *, $p < 0.05$, two-tail unpaired t-tests.

3.2. Regional Brain Activity in Response to Mechanical Stimulation

To identify mechanical allodynia-related brain activity, we performed an FDG PET scan in SNL rats, wherein the rats underwent stimulation with von Frey filaments two levels higher than their own PWT (Figure 1). All von Frey filaments used for mechanical stimulation were lower than the mean value of PWT (20.5 ± 5.7 g) in the sham-operated group, indicating that von Frey stimulation was innocuous under normal conditions. Subsequently, the FDG uptake in the entire brain of these rats ($n = 10$) was compared with that of the sham-operated rats ($n = 12$) using voxel-based statistical analysis. As shown in Figure 3 and Table 1, significant activation was observed in response to mechanical allodynia in widespread regions of the brain. The regional brain activity was increased in the contralateral medial prefrontal cortex (mPFC), the primary motor cortex (M1), and the primary somatosensory cortex hindlimb region (S1HL). In the thalamus, brain activity was increased in the contralateral intralaminar nuclei, which are reported to be involved in the emotional affective component of pain, such as the centrolateral thalamic nucleus (CL) and central medial thalamic nucleus (CM). Bilateral posterior thalamic nuclei (Po) also showed significant activation, although predominant activation was observed in the contralateral hemisphere. Moreover, a vast area of the cerebellum was also activated by mechanical allodynia in SNL rats.

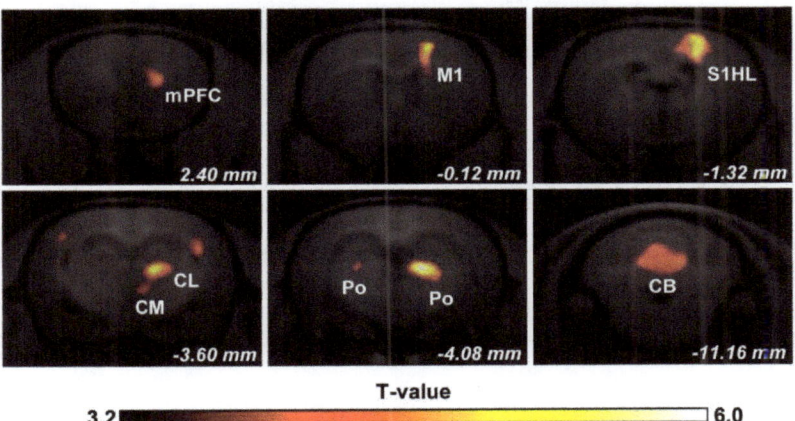

Figure 3. Regions of the brain activated in response to mechanical allodynia superimposed upon MRI coronal images. The images were obtained via a voxel-based statistical comparison between the FDG uptake of the SNL ($n = 10$) and sham-operated rats ($n = 12$). The T-value of 3.2 used as the threshold in the figure corresponds to the $p < 0.002$ (uncorrected) threshold. The right side of the images corresponds to the right hemisphere. The numbers in white indicate the anterior-posterior level of the coronal slices according to the rat brain atlas (Paxinos and Watson). Abbreviations: mPFC, medial prefrontal cortex; M1, primary motor cortex; S1HL, primary somatosensory cortex, hindlimb region; CL, centrolateral thalamic nucleus; CM, central medial thalamic nucleus. Po, posterior thalamic nuclei; CB, cerebellum.

3.3. Regional Brain Activity and Behavior Correlation

Finally, we further analyzed the correlation between mechanical allodynia-induced behavioral change and regional brain activity in SNL rats ($n = 10$) The calculated paw withdrawal rate in response to von Frey filaments stimulation during FDG uptake ranged from 55–100%. In these rats, the mean value of FDG uptake in the mPFC, S1HL, and CL showed a weak positive correlation with the paw withdrawal rate measured during the FDG uptake period (Figure 4). However, the mean value of FDG uptake in the M1 did not show an apparent correlation with the paw withdrawal rate.

Table 1. Regions of the brain activated in response to mechanical allodynia in a neuropathic pain rat model.

Brain Regions	Laterality	T-Value (Peak)	Volume (mm³)
Anterior olfactory nucleus lateral part (AOL)	R	3.97	0.32
Medial prefrontal cortex (mPFC)	R	4.45	1.49
Cluster 1			15.44
Primary motor cortex (M1)	R	5.3	
Primary somatosensory cortex hindlimb region (S1HL)	R	5.39	
Primary somatosensory cortex barrel field (S1BF)/ Primary somatosensory cortex dysgranular zone (S1DZ)	L	3.89	0.85
Cluster 2			7.54
Centrolateral thalamic nucleus (CL)	R	5.35	
Central medial thalamic nucleus (CM)	R	3.81	
Posterior thalamic nucleus (Po)	R	6.55	
Posterior thalamic nucleus (Po)	L	3.98	0.34
Cerebellum (CB)	R/L	5.92	30.06

SNL + stimuli (n = 10) vs. sham-operated (n = 12). Height threshold: T = 3.25, p < 0.002 (uncorrected). R and L indicate right and left side hemispheres, respectively.

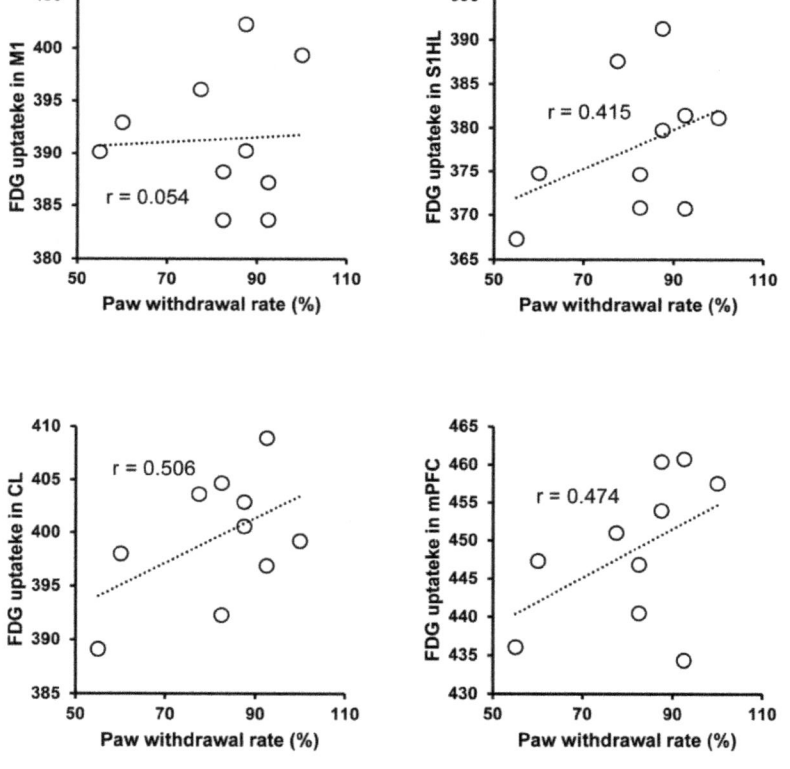

Figure 4. Correlation between mechanical allodynia-related behavioral changes and regional brain activity in neuropathic pain rats. The mean value of FDG uptake in the M1, S1HL CL, and mPFC were plotted against mechanical allodynia-related behavioral changes in SNL rats (n = 10). The Pearson coefficient value (r) is shown for each relation. Abbreviations: M1, primary motor cortex; S1HL, primary somatosensory cortex, hindlimb region; CL, centrolateral thalamic nucleus; mPFC, medial prefrontal cortex.

4. Discussion

In the present study, we successfully identified mechanical allodynia-related brain activity in the neuropathic pain model of rats using FDG PET imaging-based small animal neuroimaging. We found that the brain activity in the pain-related regions, such as the mPFC, S1HL, CL, Po, etc. was increased in response to mechanical allodynia (Figure 3 and Table 1). Moreover, the brain activity in the high-order prefrontal cortex (mPFC), the primary somatosensory cortex (S1HL), and the intralaminar thalamic nucleus (CL) were positively correlated with mechanical allodynia-related behavioral changes, which indicated that the brain activity in these areas may encode multidimensional pain aspects. These results suggest that FDG PET imaging in conscious neuropathic pain model rats acts as a reliable biomarker for the objective assessment of pain in the preclinical study, which may bridge the inconsistencies between preclinical and clinical investigations.

Neuroimaging has been used extensively to understand the neuronal basis of pain processing and perception, including the characterization of brain activity underlying the different dimensions of pain. The sensory-discriminative dimension of pain is thought to involve the lateral pain system, such as the lateral thalamus, sensory cortex, and posterior insular cortex [5,7,12]. Neuroimaging studies in humans and animal models have reported that the primary somatosensory cortex was activated in response to peripheral nociceptive stimulation [36]. Consistently, we demonstrated that brain activity in the contralateral S1HL, a primary somatosensory field of the hind limb, was significantly increased and positively correlated with mechanical allodynia-related behavior changes in SNL rats. Our results demonstrate that the brain activity in the S1HL could encode pain intensity and localization following neuropathic injury (Figures 3 and 4). In contrast, the medial pain system is known to be involved in the emotional affective dimension of pain, such as the medial thalamus and anterior cingulate cortex [1,13,14]. In the present study, we also found significant activation in the intralaminar thalamic nuclei, such as the CL, indicating that the brain activity in the CL may be used for assessing the affective aspect of pain in neuropathic injury. Indeed, a previous lesion study further supports the engagement of the intralaminar nuclei in the pathophysiology of neuropathic pain [37]. In the present study, we also found that brain activity in the mPFC was increased and correlated with mechanical allodynia-related pain behavior. The involvement of the prefrontal cortex in different types of neuropathic pain has been reported in several clinical neuroimaging studies [8,38]. Traditionally, activation of the prefrontal cortex is thought to be related to a more cognitive evaluation dimension of pain [15,16]. Meanwhile, the frontal cortex may also be engaged in pain modulation by innervating the descending pain modulation system in the diencephalon or brainstem [39,40]. Recently, our FDG PET imaging study in neuropathic pain model rats showed that the mPFC critically contributes to pharmacological conditioning-induced placebo analgesia by interacting with the ventrolateral periaqueductal gray matter [32]. The aberrant activation of the parvalbumin interneuron in the mPFC has been found in the neuropathic animal model, and optogenetic suppression of the parvalbumin interneuron activity alleviates mechanical allodynia of neuropathic pain [39,41]. Interestingly, in brachial plexus avulsion injury model rats, the metabolic connectivity between the mPFC and several regions of the brain, such as the frontal association cortex, medial hypothalamus, diagonal band, anterodorsal hippocampus, and caudate putamen, was increased [42]. However, the pathophysiology of brachial plexus avulsion injury is complicated and involves diverse symptoms. Therefore, the pathophysiological role of the mPFC in brachial plexus avulsion injury needs to be confirmed via neurophysiological experiments in the future. Taken together, these observations suggest that the regional brain activity identified by the present FDG PET imaging study in conscious rats could be a reliable biomarker for the objective assessment of neuropathic pain in preclinical investigations.

In the present study, mechanical allodynia-related brain activity was also observed in the contralateral M1 region. Altered M1 functions have been reported in diverse pain conditions. The corticospinal output from the M1 was decreased in acute muscle pain, which may represent adaptive protection against further injury [43], whereas increased excitability of the M1 was observed in sustained muscle pain [44]. Changes in the structure, organization, and function of the M1 have been reported heterogeneously in chronic neuropathic pain [45]. M1 activation was increased in postherpetic neuralgia pain [46], and M1 cortical thickness was increased in trigeminal neuralgia pain [47]. The absence of changes in M1 activation/connectivity [48] and decreased functional connectivity in the M1 and supplementary motor cortex [49] were also reported in lower back pain. These observations suggest that the pathophysiological role of the M1 in neuropathic pain is complex and may depend largely on the pain mechanism, severity, and duration from the onset. In the present study, the regional brain activity in the M1 increased but was not correlated with paw withdrawal behavior (Figures 3 and 4), indicating that the brain activity in the M1 may not encode pain intensity, at least in the current experimental setting. On the other hand, paw withdrawal behavior is a simple avoidance reflex thought to be innervated by the spinal cord, and not by the high-order motor cortex, including the M1 [22]. Therefore, the precise measurement of leg movements, such as velocity, distance, and coordinated movement, may be needed for the assessment of the functional change of the M1 of the SNL rats in the future.

The pathophysiology underlying chronic pain has been widely investigated in preclinical studies using various animal models, since mechanistic exploration using molecular, cellular, and genetic manipulation is feasible in these animal studies [17–20]. In drug development, the pharmacological efficacy of any candidate analgesic drug is primary proofed in preclinical animal models mimicking certain forms of chronic pain. However, most candidate compounds with promising efficacy in preclinical studies have failed to translate into clinical therapies [50]. This could be due to the lack of consistent biomarkers for the objective assessment of pain throughout preclinical studies to clinical application. Since pain is a subjective experience, a self-reporting-based subjective assessment is generally used as the gold standard for clinical diagnosis [3,23,24]. Whereas reflex-based behavior tests have been used widely in preclinical studies for the objective assessment of pain, such as paw withdrawal or tail-flick behavior, which are considered to measure the functional alteration in the spinal cord and brainstem but do not estimate the high-order neuropsychological processing [22]. As a potential consistent biomarker between preclinical and clinical investigations, neuroimaging has been used to identify pain-related brain activity in various animal models, such as migraine [35], neuropathic pain [27,29,51], inflammatory bowel disease [52], brachial plexus avulsion injury [42,53], and fibromyalgia [54]. In line with this, we identified hierarchical regions of the brain activated in response to mechanical allodynia in neuropathic pain model rats that are closely similar to the pain matrix defined in the human neuroimaging studies in the present study. These observations suggest that FDG PET imaging in rodents could provide a comparable objective biomarker for the consistent evaluation of pain in small animals and humans that may accelerate translational research from the preclinical to the clinical stage and increase the success rate of the development of new therapeutic drugs. Moreover, since similar regions of the brain can be identified in animal studies, molecular/cellular mechanisms of the complex signature of pain can be elucidated in animals using modern neurophysiological approaches, such as genetic manipulation.

A major limitation of neuroimaging studies in preclinical animal models is the requirement of immobilization of the animals while scanning. In general, neuroimaging studies in laboratory animals requires the restricting of the head of the animal with anesthesia or a specific head-fix system that induces a reduction of neuronal activity [55,56]. Pain is a subjective experience where consciousness is essential for its processing. A previous neuroimaging study on neuropathic pain model rats has demonstrated that the pain-evoked activation in the somatosensory region was eliminated by anesthesia [51]. Recently, an alternative neuroimaging method based on the FDG PET scan has been widely used in small animals to avoid anesthesia and restraint stress [29–32]. In this FDG PET imaging procedure, FDG is injected under free-moving conditions and the animal can be housed in the home cage or engage in behavior tests during a certain uptake period. Subsequently, an

FDG PET scan is performed under anesthesia. Since FDG is taken up by the active regions of the brain and remains within the regions for at least an hour [33], the accumulated FDG could reflect brain activity during the uptake period under conscious conditions before the PET scan. Using this alternative FDG PET imaging method, we successfully identified mechanical allodynia-related brain activity in several representative pain-related regions of the brain in neuropathic pain rats and found that brain activity in these brain regions may encode multidimensional pain aspects. Hence, the FDG PET imaging method used in the present study enabled the evaluation of pain-related brain activity without anesthesia, which might be crucial for evaluating pain processing in preclinical investigations where consciousness is necessary.

A limitation of the present study should be considered. As a representative pain assessment method, the reflex-based von Frey test was used to evaluate the pain in the SNL rats in the present study. However, such a reflex-based pain assessment is known to indicate functional alteration of the brainstem or spinal cord but not high-order neuropsychological processing [22]. This may also be a reason why the brain activity in the identified pain-related regions showed a weak positive correlation with allodynia-related behavioral changes in the present study (Figure 4). More specific behavioral assessment for high-order pain processing is needed in the future, such as a reward and escape-based operant test or a conditioned place preference test.

5. Conclusions

The development of a consistent biomarker for the objective assessment of pain in preclinical and clinical studies is urgently needed. In the present study, we successfully identified several regions of the brain activated by mechanical allodynia in neuropathic pain rats using an alternative neuroimaging method based on an FDG-PET scan. Moreover, activated brain activity in the sensory-discrimination (S1HL), cognitive evaluation (mPFC), and emotional affection (CL) regions correlated with mechanical allodynia-related behavioral changes. These results indicate that the brain activity in these areas may encode different dimensions of pain components, and current alternative FDG PET imaging procedures in rodents could be a powerful tool for providing a consistent biomarker for the objective assessment of pain throughout preclinical to clinical studies. Thus, our study will lead to the elucidation of the complex signature of pain and help in the management of patients with chronic pain.

Author Contributions: Conceptualization, Y.C.; methodology, D.H., T.H., Y.W. (Yasuhiro Wada) and Y.C.; investigation, D.H., T.H., E.H. and Y.W. (Yasuhiro Wada); formal analysis, T.H., E.H., Y.W. (Yasuhiro Wada) and H.N.; writing—original draft preparation, Y.C.; writing—review and editing, H.N., Y.C. and Y.W. (Yasuyoshi Watanabe); supervision, Y.C.; funding acquisition, Y.C. and Y.W. (Yasuyoshi Watanabe). All authors have read and agreed to the published version of the manuscript.

Funding: This work was supported in part by JSPS KAKENHI Grant Numbers 15K14328, 17H02172 and 20K21777 to Y.C.

Institutional Review Board Statement: The animal study was conducted in accordance and approved by the Institutional Animal Care and Use Committee (IACUC) of RIKEN, Kobe Branch, protocol No. MA2009-16-25.

Informed Consent Statement: Not applicable.

Data Availability Statement: The data that support the findings of this study are available from the corresponding author upon reasonable request.

Conflicts of Interest: The authors declare that they have no conflict of interest.

References

1. Melzack, R.; Casey, K.L. Sensory, Motivational, and Central Control Determinants of Pain: A New Conceptual Model. In *The Skin Senses*; Kenshalo, D.R., Ed.; Charles, C. Thomas: Springfield, IL, USA, 1968; pp. 423–443.
2. Tracey, I. Neuroimaging enters the pain biomarker arena. *Sci. Transl. Med.* **2021**, *13*, eabj7358. [CrossRef] [PubMed]
3. Davis, K.D.; Aghaeepour, N.; Ahn, A.H.; Angst, M.S.; Borsook, D.; Brenton, A.; Burczynski, M.E.; Crean, C.; Edwards, R.; Gaudilliere, B.; et al. Discovery and validation of biomarkers to aid the development of safe and effective pain therapeutics: Challenges and opportunities. *Nat. Rev. Neurol.* **2020**, *16*, 381–400. [CrossRef] [PubMed]
4. Davis, K.D.; Flor, H.; Greely, H.T.; Iannetti, G.D.; Mackey, S.; Ploner, M.; Pustilnik, A.; Tracey, I.; Treede, R.D.; Wager, T.D. Brain imaging tests for chronic pain: Medical, legal and ethical issues and recommendations. *Nat. Rev. Neurol.* **2017**, *13*, 624–638. [CrossRef] [PubMed]
5. Martucci, K.T.; Mackey, S.C. Neuroimaging of Pain: Human Evidence and Clinical Relevance of Central Nervous System Processes and Modulation. *Anesthesiology* **2018**, *128*, 1241–1254. [CrossRef]
6. Mouraux, A.; Iannetti, G.D. The search for pain biomarkers in the human brain. *Brain J. Neurol.* **2018**, *141*, 3290–3307. [CrossRef]
7. Moisset, X.; Bouhassira, D. Brain imaging of neuropathic pain. *NeuroImage* **2007**, *37* (Suppl. 1), S80–S88. [CrossRef]
8. Apkarian, A.V.; Bushnell, M.C.; Treede, R.D.; Zubieta, J.K. Human brain mechanisms of pain perception and regulation in health and disease. *Eur. J. Pain* **2005**, *9*, 463–484. [CrossRef]
9. Baliki, M.N.; Petre, B.; Torbey, S.; Herrmann, K.M.; Huang, L.; Schnitzer, T.J.; Fields, H.L.; Apkarian, A.V. Corticostriatal functional connectivity predicts transition to chronic back pain. *Nat. Neurosci.* **2012**, *15*, 1117–1119. [CrossRef]
10. Tracey, I.; Woolf, C.J.; Andrews, N.A. Composite Pain Biomarker Signatures for Objective Assessment and Effective Treatment. *Neuron* **2019**, *101*, 783–800. [CrossRef]
11. Apkarian, A.V.; Sosa, Y.; Sonty, S.; Levy, R.M.; Harden, R.N.; Parrish, T.B.; Gitelman, D.R. Chronic back pain is associated with decreased prefrontal and thalamic gray matter density. *J. Neurosci. Off. J. Soc. Neurosci.* **2004**, *24*, 10410–10415. [CrossRef]
12. Peyron, R.; Garcia-Larrea, L.; Gregoire, M.C.; Convers, P.; Lavenne, F.; Veyre, L.; Froment, J.C.; Mauguiere, F.; Michel, D.; Laurent, B. Allodynia after lateral-medullary (Wallenberg) infarct. A PET study. *Brain J. Neurol.* **1998**, *121 Pt 2*, 345–356. [CrossRef] [PubMed]
13. Albe-Fessard, D.; Berkley, K.J.; Kruger, L.; Ralston, H.J., 3rd; Willis, W.D., Jr. Diencephalic mechanisms of pain sensation. *Brain Res.* **1985**, *356*, 217–296. [CrossRef] [PubMed]
14. Rainville, P.; Duncan, G.H.; Price, D.D.; Carrier, B.; Bushnell, M.C. Pain affect encoded in human anterior cingulate but not somatosensory cortex. *Science* **1997**, *277*, 968–971. [CrossRef] [PubMed]
15. Casey, K.L. Forebrain mechanisms of nociception and pain: Analysis through imaging. *Proc. Natl. Acad. Sci. USA* **1999**, *96*, 7668–7674. [CrossRef]
16. Peyron, R.; Garcia-Larrea, L.; Gregoire, M.C.; Costes, N.; Convers, P.; Lavenne, F.; Mauguiere, F.; Michel, D.; Laurent, B. Haemodynamic brain responses to acute pain in humans: Sensory and attentional networks. *Brain J. Neurol.* **1999**, *122 Pt 9*, 1765–1780. [CrossRef]
17. Bennett, G.J.; Xie, Y.K. A peripheral mononeuropathy in rat that produces disorders of pain sensation like those seen in man. *Pain* **1988**, *33*, 87–107. [CrossRef]
18. Decosterd, I.; Woolf, C.J. Spared nerve injury: An animal model of persistent peripheral neuropathic pain. *Pain* **2000**, *87*, 149–158. [CrossRef]
19. Kim, S.H.; Chung, J.M. An Experimental-Model for Peripheral Neuropathy Produced by Segmental Spinal Nerve Ligation in the Rat. *Pain* **1992**, *50*, 355–363. [CrossRef]
20. Seltzer, Z.; Dubner, R.; Shir, Y. A novel behavioral model of neuropathic pain disorders produced in rats by partial sciatic nerve injury. *Pain* **1990**, *43*, 205–218. [CrossRef]
21. Stephenson, D.T.; Arneric, S.P. Neuroimaging of pain: Advances and future prospects. *J. Pain* **2008**, *9*, 567–579. [CrossRef]
22. Vierck, C.J.; Hansson, P.T.; Yezierski, R.P. Clinical and pre-clinical pain assessment: Are we measuring the same thing? *Pain* **2008**, *135*, 7–10. [CrossRef] [PubMed]
23. Birnie, K.A.; Hundert, A.S.; Lalloo, C.; Nguyen, C.; Stinson, J.N. Recommendations for selection of self-report pain intensity measures in children and adolescents: A systematic review and quality assessment of measurement properties. *Pain* **2019**, *160*, 5–18. [CrossRef] [PubMed]
24. Main, C.J. Pain assessment in context: A state of the science review of the McGill pain questionnaire 40 years on. *Pain* **2016**, *157*, 1387–1399. [CrossRef] [PubMed]
25. Thompson, S.J.; Bushnell, M.C. Rodent functional and anatomical imaging of pain. *Neurosci. Lett.* **2012**, *520*, 131–139. [CrossRef] [PubMed]
26. Borsook, D.; Becerra, L. CNS animal fMRI in pain and analgesia. *Neurosci. Biobehav. Rev.* **2011**, *35*, 1125–1143. [CrossRef] [PubMed]
27. Chang, P.C.; Centeno, M.V.; Procissi, D.; Baria, A.; Apkarian, A.V. Brain activity for tactile allodynia: A longitudinal awake rat functional magnetic resonance imaging study tracking emergence of neuropathic pain. *Pain* **2017**, *158*, 488–497. [CrossRef]
28. Mizuma, H.; Shukuri, M.; Hayashi, T.; Watanabe, Y.; Onoe, H. Establishment of in vivo brain imaging method in conscious mice. *J. Nucl. Med. Off. Publ. Soc. Nucl. Med.* **2010**, *51*, 1068–1075. [CrossRef]
29. Kim, C.E.; Kim, Y.K.; Chung, G.; Im, H.J.; Lee, D.S.; Kim, J.; Kim, S.J. Identifying neuropathic pain using (18)F-FDG micro-PET: A multivariate pattern analysis. *NeuroImage* **2014**, *86*, 311–316. [CrossRef]

30. Kobayashi, M.; Cui, Y.; Sako, T.; Sasabe, T.; Mizoguchi, N.; Yamamoto, K.; Wada, Y.; Kataoka, Y.; Koshikawa, N. Functional neuroimaging of aversive taste-related areas in the alert rat revealed by positron emission tomography. *J. Neurosci. Res.* **2013**, *91*, 1363–1370. [CrossRef]
31. Sung, K.K.; Jang, D.P.; Lee, S.; Kim, M.; Lee, S.Y.; Kim, Y.B.; Park, C.W.; Cho, Z.H. Neural responses in rat brain during acute immobilization stress: A [F-18]FDG micro PET imaging study. *NeuroImage* **2009**, *44*, 1074–1080. [CrossRef]
32. Zeng, Y.; Hu, D.; Yang, W.; Hayashinaka, E.; Wada, Y.; Watanabe, Y.; Zeng, Q.; Cui, Y. A voxel-based analysis of neurobiological mechanisms in placebo analgesia in rats. *NeuroImage* **2018**, *178*, 602–612. [CrossRef] [PubMed]
33. Schiffer, W.K.; Mirrione, M.M.; Dewey, S.L. Optimizing experimental protocols for quantitative behavioral imaging with 18F-FDG in rodents. *J. Nucl. Med. Off. Publ. Soc. Nucl. Med.* **2007**, *48*, 277–287.
34. Chaplan, S.R.; Bach, F.W.; Pogrel, J.W.; Chung, J.M.; Yaksh, T.L. Quantitative assessment of tactile allodynia in the rat paw. *J. Neurosci. Methods* **1994**, *53*, 55–63. [CrossRef] [PubMed]
35. Cui, Y.; Toyoda, H.; Sako, T.; Onoe, K.; Hayashinaka, E.; Wada, Y.; Yokoyama, C.; Onoe, H.; Kataoka, Y.; Watanabe, Y. A voxel-based analysis of brain activity in high-order trigeminal pathway in the rat induced by cortical spreading depression. *NeuroImage* **2015**, *108*, 17–22. [CrossRef] [PubMed]
36. Coghill, R.C.; Sang, C.N.; Maisog, J.M.; Iadarola, M.J. Pain intensity processing within the human brain: A bilateral, distributed mechanism. *J. Neurophysiol.* **1999**, *82*, 1934–1943. [CrossRef]
37. Saade, N.E.; Al Amin, H.; Abdel Baki, S.; Chalouhi, S.; Jabbur, S.J.; Atweh, S.F. Reversible attenuation of neuropathic-like manifestations in rats by lesions or local blocks of the intralaminar or the medial thalamic nuclei. *Exp. Neurol.* **2007**, *204*, 205–219. [CrossRef]
38. Becerra, L.; Morris, S.; Bazes, S.; Gostic, R.; Sherman, S.; Gostic, J.; Pendse, G.; Moulton, E.; Scrivani, S.; Keith, D.; et al. Trigeminal neuropathic pain alters responses in CNS circuits to mechanical (brush) and thermal (cold and heat) stimuli. *J. Neurosci. Off. J. Soc. Neurosci.* **2006**, *26*, 10646–10657. [CrossRef]
39. Huang, J.; Gadotti, V.M.; Chen, L.; Souza, I.A.; Huang, S.; Wang, D.; Ramakrishnan, C.; Deisseroth, K.; Zhang, Z.; Zamponi, G.W. A neuronal circuit for activating descending modulation of neuropathic pain. *Nat. Neurosci.* **2019**, *22*, 1659–1668. [CrossRef]
40. Lorenz, J.; Cross, D.J.; Minoshima, S.; Morrow, T.J.; Paulson, P.E.; Casey, K.L. A unique representation of heat allodynia in the human brain. *Neuron* **2002**, *35*, 383–393. [CrossRef]
41. Zhang, Z.; Gadotti, V.M.; Chen, L.; Souza, I.A.; Stemkowski, P.L.; Zamponi, G.W. Role of Prelimbic GABAergic Circuits in Sensory and Emotional Aspects of Neuropathic Pain. *Cell Rep.* **2015**, *12*, 752–759. [CrossRef]
42. Huo, B.B.; Zheng, M.X.; Hua, X.Y.; Shen, J.; Wu, J.J.; Xu, J.G. Metabolic Brain Network Analysis with (18)F-FDG PET in a Rat Model of Neuropathic Pain. *Front. Neurol.* **2021**, *12*, 566119. [CrossRef] [PubMed]
43. Burns, E.; Chipchase, L.S.; Schabrun, S.M. Primary sensory and motor cortex function in response to acute muscle pain: A systematic review and meta-analysis. *Eur. J. Pain* **2016**, *20*, 1203–1213. [CrossRef] [PubMed]
44. Schabrun, S.M.; Christensen, S.W.; Mrachacz-Kersting, N.; Graven-Nielsen, T. Motor Cortex Reorganization and Impaired Function in the Transition to Sustained Muscle Pain. *Cereb Cortex* **2016**, *26*, 1878–1890. [CrossRef] [PubMed]
45. Chang, W.J.; O'Connell, N.E.; Beckenkamp, P.R.; Alhassani, G.; Liston, M.B.; Schabrun, S.M. Altered Primary Motor Cortex Structure, Organization, and Function in Chronic Pain: A Systematic Review and Meta-Analysis. *J. Pain* **2018**, *19*, 341–359. [CrossRef]
46. Liu, J.; Hao, Y.; Du, M.; Wang, X.; Zhang, J.; Manor, B.; Jiang, X.; Fang, W.; Wang, D. Quantitative cerebral blood flow mapping and functional connectivity of postherpetic neuralgia pain: A perfusion fMRI study. *Pain* **2013**, *154*, 110–118. [CrossRef]
47. Desouza, D.D.; Moayedi, M.; Chen, D.Q.; Davis, K.D.; Hodaie, M. Sensorimotor and Pain Modulation Brain Abnormalities in Trigeminal Neuralgia: A Paroxysmal, Sensory-Triggered Neuropathic Pain. *PLoS ONE* **2013**, *8*, e66340. [CrossRef]
48. Kobayashi, Y.; Kurata, J.; Sekiguchi, M.; Kokubun, M.; Akaishizawa, T.; Chiba, Y.; Konno, S.; Kikuchi, S. Augmented cerebral activation by lumbar mechanical stimulus in chronic low back pain patients: An FMRI study. *Spine* **2009**, *34*, 2431–2436. [CrossRef]
49. Pijnenburg, M.; Brumagne, S.; Caeyenberghs, K.; Janssens, L.; Goossens, N.; Marinazzo, D.; Swinnen, S.P.; Claeys, K.; Siugzdaite, R. Resting-State Functional Connectivity of the Sensorimotor Network in Individuals with Nonspecific Low Back Pain and the Association with the Sit-to-Stand-to-Sit Task. *Brain Connect.* **2015**, *5*, 303–311. [CrossRef]
50. Dolgin, E. Fluctuating baseline pain implicated in failure of clinical trials. *Nat. Med.* **2010**, *16*, 1053. [CrossRef]
51. Thompson, S.J.; Millecamps, M.; Aliaga, A.; Seminowicz, D.A.; Low, L.A.; Bedell, B.J.; Stone, L.S.; Schweinhardt, P.; Bushnell, M.C. Metabolic brain activity suggestive of persistent pain in a rat model of neuropathic pain. *NeuroImage* **2014**, *91*, 344–352. [CrossRef]
52. Huang, T.; Okauchi, T.; Hu, D.; Shigeta, M.; Wu, Y.; Wada, Y.; Hayashinaka, E.; Wang, S.; Kogure, Y.; Noguchi, K.; et al. Pain matrix shift in the rat brain following persistent colonic inflammation revealed by voxel-based statistical analysis. *Mol. Pain* **2019**, *15*, 1744806919891327. [CrossRef] [PubMed]
53. Shen, J.; Huo, B.B.; Hua, X.Y.; Zheng, M.X.; Lu, Y.C.; Wu, J.J.; Shan, C.L.; Xu, J.G. Cerebral (18)F-FDG metabolism alteration in a neuropathic pain model following brachial plexus avulsion: A PET/CT study in rats. *Brain Res.* **2019**, *1712*, 132–138. [CrossRef] [PubMed]
54. Neyama, H.; Nishiyori, M.; Cui, Y.; Watanabe, Y.; Ueda, H. Lysophosphatidic acid receptor type-1 mediates brain activation in micro-positron emission tomography analysis in a fibromyalgia-like mouse model. *Eur. J. Neurosci.* **2022**, *56*, 4224–4233. [CrossRef] [PubMed]

55. Franks, N.P. General anaesthesia: From molecular targets to neuronal pathways of sleep and arousal. *Nat. Rev. Neurosci.* **2008**, *9*, 370–386. [CrossRef]
56. Onoe, H.; Inoue, O.; Suzuki, K.; Tsukada, H.; Itoh, T.; Mataga, N.; Watanabe, Y. Ketamine increases the striatal N-[11C]methylspiperone binding in vivo: Positron emission tomography study using conscious rhesus monkey. *Brain Res.* **1994**, *663*, 191–198. [CrossRef]

Disclaimer/Publisher's Note: The statements, opinions and data contained in all publications are solely those of the individual author(s) and contributor(s) and not of MDPI and/or the editor(s). MDPI and/or the editor(s) disclaim responsibility for any injury to people or property resulting from any ideas, methods, instructions or products referred to in the content.

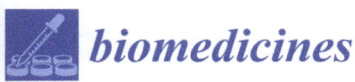

Article

Association of Pain Phenotypes with Risk of Falls and Incident Fractures

Maxim Devine [1,†], Canchen Ma [1,†], Jing Tian [1], Benny Antony [1], Flavia Cicuttini [2], Graeme Jones [1] and Feng Pan [1,*]

[1] Menzies Institute for Medical Research, University of Tasmania, Hobart 7000, Australia
[2] Department of Epidemiology and Preventive Medicine, Monash University Medical School, Commercial Road, Melbourne 3181, Australia
* Correspondence: feng.pan@utas.edu.au; Tel.: +61-3-6226-7700; Fax: +61-3-6226-7704
† These authors contributed equally to this work.

Abstract: Objective: To compare whether falls risk score and incident fracture over 10.7 years were different among three previously identified pain phenotypes. **Methods:** Data on 915 participants (mean age 63 years) from a population-based cohort study were studied at baseline and follow-ups at 2.6, 5.1 and 10.7 years. Three pain phenotypes were previously identified using the latent class analysis: Class 1: high prevalence of emotional problems and low prevalence of structural damage; Class 2: high prevalence of structural damage and low prevalence of emotional problems; Class 3: low prevalence of emotional problems and low prevalence of structural damage. Fractures were self-reported and falls risk score was measured using the Physiological Profile Assessment. Generalized estimating equations model and linear mixed-effects model were used to compare differences in incident fractures and falls risk score over 10.7 years between pain phenotypes, respectively. **Results:** There were 3 new hip, 19 vertebral, and 121 non-vertebral fractures, and 138 any site fractures during 10.7-year follow-up. Compared with Class 3, Class 1 had a higher risk of vertebral (relative risk (RR) = 2.44, 95% CI: 1.22–4.91), non-vertebral fractures (RR = 1.20, 95% CI: 1.01–1.42), and any site fractures (RR = 1.24, 95% CI: 1.04–1.46) after controlling for covariates, bone mineral density and falls risk score. Class 2 had a higher risk of non-vertebral and any site fracture relative to those in Class 3 (non-vertebral: RR = 1.41, 95% CI: 1.17–1.71; any site: RR = 1.44, 95% CI: 1.20–1.73), but not vertebral fracture. Compared with Class 3, Class 1 had a higher falls risk score at baseline (β = 0.16, 95% CI: 0.09–0.23) and over 10.7-year (β = 0.03, 95% CI: 0.01–0.04). **Conclusions:** Class 1 and/or Class 2 had a higher risk of incident fractures and falls risk score than Class 3, highlighting that targeted preventive strategies for fractures and falls are needed in pain population.

Keywords: falls risk; incident fractures; pain phenotypes

1. Introduction

Musculoskeletal pain is common in older adults with a prevalence ranging from 61% to 74% [1,2] and causes a significant burden on both individual and societal healthcare. The 2016 Global Burden of Disease Study has reported low back and neck pain ranking as 1st and 6th causes of years lived with disability among 30 leading diseases and injuries [3]. The burden of musculoskeletal pain and related health outcomes has been projected to rise continually by reducing physical function and quality of life, increasing rates of disability, and developing mortality in older adults [4,5].

As the major symptom of osteoarthritis (OA), musculoskeletal pain is highly heterogenous and affected by multiple factors, including peripheral, psychological, and neurological factors [6]. Studies have shown that 20% of musculoskeletal pain is ascribed to OA [7]. The heterogeneity of pain imposes difficulty in the effective intervention of pain conditions. Indeed, the "one-size-fits-all" approach may overlook the heterogeneity of pain and interactions between pain-related factors. Thus, identification of pain subgroups has been suggested as a novel approach to tailored pain management and decision-making for preventing related clinical outcomes [8]. Observational studies have demonstrated different health-related quality of life, disease activity, and mortality risk across musculoskeletal pain subgroups/phenotypes [8–10].

Fracture is a critical healthcare issue worldwide, resulting in recurrent fractures and subsequent mortality [11–13]. Ageing, osteoporosis, and falls are the major risk factors for fractures [14,15]. Musculoskeletal pain has been linked to an increased risk of falls, due to local joint pathology, muscle weakness, reduced neuromuscular response and slowed cognition, greater difficulty mobilising [16–19]. Pain has been suggested as an independent risk factor for fractures, although the results were contradictory. It has been proposed that inflammation related to pain is likely to play a role in the process of bone remodelling and thereby increasing the risk of fractures [20,21]. A previous large cohort study reported an association between severity of knee pain and non-vertebral and hip fractures, and our recent study demonstrated a dose-manner relationship between the number of painful sites and increased risk of fractures at both vertebral and non-vertebral sites [22,23]. In contrast, no associations between pain and incident hip or non-vertebral fractures were observed in men aged over 65 years with a 9.7-year follow-up time from a large multicentre prospective study [24].

Our recent study has identified three distinctive knee pain phenotypes by considering a broad range of pain-related factors, including structural abnormalities on magnetic resonance imaging (MRI), emotional issues, body mass index (BMI): Class 1: high prevalence of emotional problems and low prevalence of structural damage (38%); Class 2: high prevalence of structural damage and low prevalence of emotional problems (17%); Class 3: low prevalence of emotional problems and low prevalence of structural damage (45%) [25,26]. Further, pain severity and number of painful sites were found to be different between the classes/subgroups [26]. Given the link between pain and an increased risk of falls and fracture and the heterogeneity of pain, we hypothesised that the risk of falls and/or incident fractures was phenotype-specific in pain population. Therefore, this study was to compare whether falls and incident fractures risk over 10.7 years were different among the three knee pain phenotypes we previously identified.

2. Method

2.1. Participants

This study was conducted as part of the Tasmanian Older Adult Cohort Study (TASOAC). Participants aged 50–80 years [median (interquartile range), 62 (57–69) years] were randomly selected from the electoral roll in Southern Tasmania (43° S, southern part of island state in Australia, population 229,000), using sex-stratified random sampling. Participants were studied at baseline (n = 1099), 2.6 (n = 875), 5.1 (n = 768) and 10.7 (n = 563) years. The current study consisted of 915 participants who had been identified pain phenotypes and had complete data on interview and general questionnaires, bone mineral density (BMD), falls, and fractures. The study was approved by the Southern Tasmanian Health and Medical Human Research Ethics Committee (Ref. No: H0006488), and written informed consent was obtained from all participants.

2.2. Measurements for Factors to Identify Pain Phenotypes

Measurements of knee structural abnormalities on MRI, emotional problems, number of painful sites, BMI, sex, education level, and comorbidities, which were measured by trained observer(s) or self-report questionnaires at baseline, were used to identify pain phenotypes. The details of each measurement have been described elsewhere [25,26]. In brief, each participant had an MRI scan on their right knee in the sagittal plane on a 1.5-T whole body MR unit (Picker, OH) using a commercial transmit–receive extremity coil. The sequences used have been previously described [27]. Cartilage defects, bone marrow lesions (BMLs), and effusion-synovitis were assessed on MR images at the medial tibial, medial femoral, lateral tibial, and lateral femoral sites. Emotional problems were assessed by using one single mental health item from the short form-8 [28]. Participants reported whether they had pain (yes/no) occurring at their neck, back, hands, shoulders, hips, knees, or feet. A total number of painful sites was created by summing each site (ranging 0–7). Weight and height were measured, then BMI was calculated (kg/m^2). Sex was collected during interview. Highest education level was self-reported and grouped into three categories (low, medium, high). Common conditions including diabetes, myocardial infarction, hypertension, thrombosis, asthma, bronchitis/emphysema, osteoporosis, hyperthyroidism, hypothyroidism, and rheumatoid arthritis were recorded using a self-reported comorbidity questionnaire. Heart attack, hypertension, diabetes and rheumatoid arthritis have been reported to be linked to musculoskeletal pain [29]. Therefore, the presence of comorbidity was defined as participants having any of these four comorbidities.

2.3. Measurements for Outcomes

2.3.1. Incident Fractures

Fractures were self-reported at baseline, approximately 2.6-, 5- and 10.7-year follow-up. Participants responded to the following question: "List any fracture you may have had since your previous interview for this study. Please list these by the location of the fractures (e.g., left thumb, right wrist)" [30]. Incident fractures were classified as non-vertebral, vertebral, and any site fractures.

2.3.2. Falls Risk Score

Falls risk score was estimated from the physical profile assessment (PPA) at each time-point [31]. Performance in five physiological domains, including knee extension strength, balance, proprioception, reaction time, and edge contrast sensitivity, was assessed to calculate standardized Z-score for falls risk [31].

2.4. Measurements for Other Related Factors

At baseline, PA was measured by steps per day over seven consecutive days using a pedometer (Omron HJ-003 & HJ-102; Omron Healthcare, Kyoto, Japan). Our criteria for the inclusion of pedometer estimates have been described previously [32]. Hip BMD was measured by the dual-energy X-ray absorptiometry (Hologic, Waltham, MA, USA). The Hologic densitometer was calibrated automatically using the internal software system [33]. Age, smoking history, and pain medication use were recorded via a questionnaire at baseline.

2.5. Statistical Analysis

2.5.1. Identifying Pain Phenotypes

Methods for identifying pain phenotypes in this cohort have been described in detail [25,26]. Briefly, latent class analysis (LCA) was applied to identify groups of participants with similar profiles according to their baseline characteristics related to pain (i.e., sex, BMI, emotional problems, education level, comorbidities, number of painful sites, and MRI-detected knee structural damage). Three knee pain phenotypes were identified: Class 1: high prevalence of emotional problems and low prevalence of structural damage (38%); Class 2: high prevalence of structural damage and low prevalence of emotional problems (17%); Class 3: low prevalence of emotional problems and low prevalence of structural damage (45%). Pain severity in Class 1 and Class 2 was greater than that in Class 3.

2.5.2. Comparing Risks of Falls and Incident Fractures over 10.7 Years across Three Knee Pain Phenotypes

The characteristics of participants were compared across the pain phenotypes identified from the LCA using analysis of variance or multi-nominal logistic regression.

Falls risk score was normally distributed; therefore, linear mixed-effects model with a fixed effect for age, physical activity, smoking history, pain medication use at baseline, and random intercepts for follow-ups was used to compare the differences in falls risk score over 10.7-year between pain phenotypes. In the same mixed-effects model, the interaction term of pain phenotypes and follow-ups was used to compare the differences in change of falls risk score over 10.7-year between pain phenotypes.

Generalized estimating equations (GEE) log-binomial models with robust standard errors and adjustment for age, physical activity, smoking history, pain medication use, falls risk score, and hip BMD at baseline were used to compare the differences in incident fractures between pain phenotypes.

Stata V.15 was used for the analyses, and LCA analysis was performed using LCA Stata Plugin [34]. p values less than 0.05 (two-tailed) were regarded as statistically significant.

3. Results

The characteristics of the participants within each class are shown in Table 1. Classes 1, 2, 3 consisted of 38%, 17%, 45% of participants in this study. Compared with Classes 2 and 3, participants in Class 1 were more likely to be female, had lower hip BMD. Participants in Class 2 were older, more likely to be male, had higher BMI, and higher hip BMD than participants in Class1 and 3. Participants in Class 3 tended to have lower BMI than those in Class 1 and 2. There were 3 new hip, 19 vertebral, and 121 non-vertebral fractures, and 138 any site fractures during 10.7-year follow-up. Participants in Class 1 had higher incidences of non-vertebral and any site fractures than Class 3.

Table 1. Characteristics of the participants by three pain phenotypes.

	Class 1 ($n = 345$)	Class 2 ($n = 157$)	Class 3 ($n = 413$)	p-Value		
				C1 vs. C2	C1 vs. C3	C2 vs. C3
Age (years)	62.2 (7.5)	64.0 (7.0)	62.6 (7.3)	**0.01**	0.44	**0.047**
Female sex, n (%)	242 (70)	44 (28)	179 (43)	**<0.001**	**<0.001**	**0.001**
BMI (kg/m^2)	28.4 (5.1)	29.3 (4.5)	26.4 (3.9)	**0.04**	**<0.001**	**<0.001**
WOMAC pain score (0–45)	6.2 (7.3)	3.8 (6.3)	1.0 (2.1)	**0.001**	**<0.001**	**<0.001**
Number of painful sites (0–7)	5.0 (1.5)	2.7 (1.7)	1.8 (1.6)	**<0.001**	**<0.001**	**<0.001**
Hip BMD (g/cm^3)	0.95 (0.14)	1.02 (0.16)	0.96 (0.15)	**<0.001**	0.18	**<0.001**
Falls risk score (zscore)	0.26 (0.90)	0.05 (0.81)	0.10 (0.76)	**0.009**	**0.007**	0.56
Incident fractures from baseline to phase 4, n (%)						
Hip fracture	1 (0.3)	1 (0.6)	1 (0.2)	0.53	0.91	0.44
Vertebral fracture	10 (3)	5 (3)	4 (1)	0.84	0.10	0.06
Nonvertebral fracture	58 (17)	19 (12)	44 (11)	0.15	**0.01**	0.65
Any site fracture	66 (19)	24 (15)	48 (12)	0.26	**0.04**	0.27

Values are presented as mean (stand deviation) unless stated otherwise. BMI: body mass index; BMD: bone mineral density; C: Class; WOMAC: Western Ontario and McMaster Universities Arthritis Index. p-values are from post hoc testing for comparisons between classes determined by analysis of variance or logistic regression as appropriate. Bold denotes statistical significance.

Figure 1 shows changes in falls risk score over 10.7-year. Participants in Class 1 had a larger increase in falls risk score compared with Class 2 and 3 (Figure 1). When comparing the differences in falls risk score over 10.7 years between classes, participants in Class 1 had a higher falls risk score relative to those in Class 2 and 3 (Table 2). Participants in Class 2 had a lower falls risk score than those in Class 3. There was a greater change in falls risk score in Class 1 compared with Class 3. Changes in the falls risk score were not different between Class 1 and 2 and between Class 2 and 3.

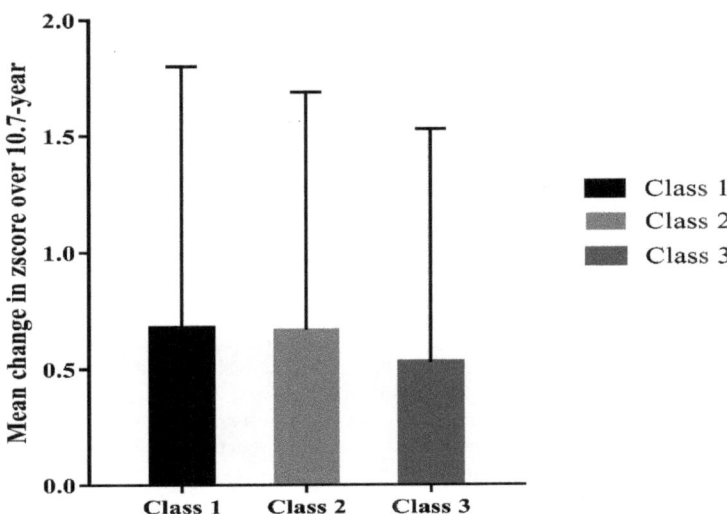

Figure 1. Mean change of falls risk score over 10.7-year in each class.

Table 2. The differences in falls risk scores over 10.7-year follow-up and changes in falls risk score among three pain phenotypes.

	Zscore over 10.7-Year Follow-Up β * (95% CI)	Change in Zscore from Baseline to 10.7-Year Follow-Up β † (95% CI)
Class 1 vs. Class 3	**0.16 (0.09, 0.23)**	**0.03 (0.01, 0.04)**
Class 2 vs. Class 3	**−0.09 (−0.18, −0.002)**	0.02 (−0.003, 0.04)
Class 1 vs. Class 2	**0.25 (0.15, 0.34)**	0.006 (−0.02, 0.03)

* Mixed-effects model including fixed effects for age, physical activity, smoking history, pain medication use at baseline, and random intercepts for follow-ups. † The interaction terms of pain phenotypes and follow-ups. Bold denotes statistical significance.

Table 3 shows the differences in incident fracture risks between classes after controlling for covariates, BMD, and falls risk score. Compared with Class 3, participants in Class 1 had a higher risk of vertebral, non-vertebral, and any site fractures. Participants in Class 2 had a higher risk of non-vertebral and any site fractures than those in Class 3, but not vertebral fracture. There were no differences in risks of vertebral, non-vertebral and any site fractures between Class 1 and Class 2.

Table 3. The differences in incident fracture risks over 10.7-year follow-up among three pain phenotypes.

	Incident Fractures over 10.7-Year Follow-Up		
	Vertebral RR * (95% CI)	Non-Vertebral RR * (95% CI)	Any Site RR * (95% CI)
Class 1 vs. Class 3	**2.44 (1.22, 4.91)**	**1.20 (1.01, 1.42)**	**1.24 (1.04, 1.46)**
Class 2 vs. Class 3	1.47 (0.64, 3.36)	**1.41 (1.17, 1.71)**	**1.44 (1.20, 1.73)**
Class 1 vs. Class 2	1.66 (0.73, 3.82)	0.85 (0.70, 1.04)	0.86 (0.71, 1.04)

* Generalized estimating equations log-binomial model included age, physical activity, smoking history, pain medication use, falls risk score, and hip BMD at baseline. Bold denotes statistical significance.

4. Discussion

This study found that falls risk score and risks of incident fracture differ across the three knee pain phenotypes. Class 1 (high prevalence emotional problems/low prevalence structural damage) was associated with a higher risk of falls compared to Class 2 (high prevalence structural damage/low prevalence emotional problems), and Class 3 (low prevalence emotional problems/low prevalence of structural damage). Participants in Classes 1 and 2 suffered from greater pain severity than those in Class 3, had a higher risk of incident fractures than those in Class 3, independent of falls risk score, BMD and covariates. These findings suggest that falls risk score and risks of incident fractures are manifested differently across pain phenotypes, and highlight that targeted preventive strategy for fractures and falls is needed in a specific pain phenotype.

Pain and the risk of falls have been suggested to have a link [16,17,35–39] due to joint pathology, muscle weakness, or slowed neuromuscular responses and cognitive/executive function [18,19]. The current study found a higher falls risk score in Class 1, compared with Classes 2 and 3. In addition, Class 1 had a greater change in falls risk score over 10.7 years, compared with Class 3. One of explanations for a greater falls risk score observed in Class 1 may be due to a greater pain severity in Class 1 at each time-point compared with Classes 2 and 3. This is supported by a 4-year follow-up cohort study including 765 participants aged over 70 years, which reported that presence of moderate-to-severe pain (yes/no) was associated with an increased risk of falls occurrence [40]. Similarly, a cross-sectional study from Framingham of older adults with a mean age of 69 years showed that severity of pain in foot was associated with a higher risk of falls occurrence [41]. However, we found that participants in Class 2 with distinctive structural damages had a lower falls risk score than Class 3, although Class 2 had a greater pain score than Class 3. This suggests that falls risk is not fully determined by pain itself but mediated by other factors. A recent study with compelling data reported that concerns about falls, knee strength, and standing balance were mediators of the relationship between knee pain and multiple falls [42]. The current study also found that the knee pain population with more emotional problems rather than structural damages was more likely to have a higher falls risk score. The plausible mechanisms between psychological problems and falls risk involve low self-efficacy, executive dysfunction, gait change, impairment of balance performance [43]. These findings suggest that psychological problems are more likely to drive the falls than pain resulting from structural damages. Intervention for psychological health in pain population may be effective in reducing falls risk.

Falls risk has been suggested as a major cause of fractures, but an increased risk of falls cannot fully explain relationships between pain and fractures. Indeed, our results found that different fractures risk were observed in different pain phenotypes independent of falls risk, suggesting that relationships between pain phenotypes and risk of fractures may not be mediated by pain-related falls risk. In line with a 3-year follow-up study on the relationship between severity of knee pain and risk of hip fracture in 6641 participants aged over 75 years [23], our study found an overall higher risk of incident fractures in Class 1 and Class 2 compared to Class 3. Similarly, Tatsuhiko et al found an association between the presence of back pain and vertebral fractures in 818 postmenopausal women with a mean 5.7-year follow-up [44]. In a community-based US cohort study with a mean 6.6-year follow-up, the presence of pain symptoms in knee OA had increased risk of non-vertebral fractures in 288 men aged over 70 years [45]. These findings reflect that experiencing pain may be a risk factor for fractures. In contrast, data from the MrOS cohort including 5993 community-dwelling men aged over 65 years reported no association between presence of knee pain and hip and non-spine fractures [24]. This discrepancy might be due to different study designs, pain assessment, and fracture sites assessed.

The current study further showed that associations between pain phenotypes and risk of incident fractures varied depending on fracture sites. The knee pain population classified with most pronounced emotional problems had a relatively higher risk of vertebral than non-vertebral fracture. Few studies have reported associations between psychological problems and vertebral and non-vertebral fracture. In a Danish cohort study of 4114 participants with a mean 7.8-year follow-up period, post-traumatic stress disorder was found to be associated with a higher incidence rate of spine and pelvis fractures than non-vertebral fractures, e.g., hand and wrist, and femur [46]. Similarly, a 13-year follow-up cohort study reported depressive disorders increased the risk of a subsequent new-onset vertebral fracture in adults aged ≥50 years [47]. One possible mechanism underlying the link of pain-related psychological factors and increased risk of fractures, particularly vertebral fracture, may be mediated through inflammatory response and stress hormones such as glucocorticoids, catecholamines, vitamin D [48]. Another possible mechanism is that pain-related psychological factors affect physical function, thereby leading to an increased risk of fractures [49]. In addition, participants classified with structural damages were more likely to have a higher risk of non-vertebral fractures, the reason for this is unclear. Taken together our findings suggest that a specific knee pain phenotype has a predisposition to fractures at a specific site. Targeted prevention for fractures at different sites may be beneficial for a specific pain phenotype.

The strengths of this study are a large sample and an extended follow-up period of 10.7 years. However, there are several limitations in this study. Firstly, self-reported fractures in this study without X-ray confirmation may have led to an overreporting of fractures [50]. Secondly, there were only three incident hip fracture during follow-ups. Thus, the risk of hip fracture across pain phenotypes cannot be estimated in this study.

In conclusion, Class 1 and/or Class 2 had a higher risk of incident fractures and falls risk score than Class 3, highlighting that targeted preventive strategies for fractures and falls are needed in pain population.

Author Contributions: Study design and conduct: F.P., F.C. and G.J.; Data collection: F.P., F.C. and G.J.; Data analysis: C.M., F.P. and J.T.; Data interpretation: M.D., C.M., F.P., J.T., F.C. and G.J.; Drafting and Revising manuscript: M.D., C.M., J.T., B.A., F.C., G.J. and F.P.; G.J. and F.P. take responsibility for the integrity of the data analysis. All authors have read and agreed to the published version of the manuscript.

Funding: This work was supported by the National Health and Medical Research Council of Australia (NHMRC) (302204) and Arthritis Australia (P0027184). JT is funded by the National Heart Foundation Fellowship; FC is funded by the NHMRC Leadership Fellowship; GJ is funded by the NHMRC Practitioner Fellowship; FP is funded by the NHMRC Early Career Fellowship.

Institutional Review Board Statement: The study was conducted in accordance with the Declaration of Helsinki, and approved by the Southern Tasmanian Health and Medical Human Research Ethics Committee (reference number H0006488 and date of approval 24 August 2001).

Informed Consent Statement: Written informed consent was obtained from all participants.

Data Availability Statement: The datasets generated during and/or analyzed during the current study are available from the corresponding author on reasonable request.

Acknowledgments: We would like to thank the participants who made this study possible, and we gratefully acknowledge the role of TASOAC staff and volunteers in collecting the data.

Conflicts of Interest: Maxim Devine, Canchen Ma, Jing Tian, Benny Antony, Flavia Cicuttini, Graeme Jones, and Feng Pan declare that they have no conflict of interest.

References

1. Lehti, T.E.; Rinkinen, M.O.; Aalto, U.; Roitto, H.M.; Knuutila, M.; Öhman, H.; Kautiainen, H.; Karppinen, H.; Tilvis, R.; Strandberg, T.; et al. Prevalence of Musculoskeletal Pain and Analgesic Treatment Among Community-Dwelling Older Adults: Changes from 1999 to 2019. *Drugs Aging* **2021**, *38*, 931–937. [CrossRef] [PubMed]
2. Karttunen, N.M.; Turunen, J.H.; Ahonen, R.S.; Hartikainen, S.A. Persistence of noncancer-related musculoskeletal chronic pain among community-dwelling older people: A population-based longitudinal study in Finland. *Clin. J. Pain* **2015**, *31*, 79–85. [CrossRef] [PubMed]
3. Disease, G.B.D.; Injury, I.; Prevalence, C. Global, regional, and national incidence, prevalence, and years lived with disability for 328 diseases and injuries for 195 countries, 1990–2016: A systematic analysis for the Global Burden of Disease Study 2016. *Lancet* **2017**, *390*, 1211–1259. [CrossRef]
4. Briggs, A.M.; Cross, M.J.; Hoy, D.G.; Sànchez-Riera, L.; Blyth, F.M.; Woolf, A.D.; March, L. Musculoskeletal Health Conditions Represent a Global Threat to Healthy Aging: A Report for the 2015 World Health Organization World Report on Ageing and Health. *Gerontologist* **2016**, *56* (Suppl 2), S243–S255. [CrossRef]

5. Blyth, F.M.; Briggs, A.M.; Schneider, C.H.; Hoy, D.G.; March, L.M. The Global Burden of Musculoskeletal Pain-Where to from Here? *Am. J. Public Health* **2019**, *109*, 35–40. [CrossRef]
6. Kittelson, A.J.; George, S.Z.; Maluf, K.S.; Stevens-Lapsley, J.E. Future directions in painful knee osteoarthritis: Harnessing complexity in a heterogeneous population. *Phys. Ther.* **2014**, *94*, 422–432. [CrossRef]
7. Butler, S. The impact of chronic pain—European patients' perspective over 12 months. *Scand. J. Pain* **2012**, *3*, 21–22. [CrossRef]
8. Meisingset, I.; Vasseljen, O.; Vøllestad, N.K.; Robinson, H.S.; Woodhouse, A.; Engebretsen, K.B.; Glette, M.; Øverås, C.K.; Nordstoga, A.L.; Evensen, K.A.I.; et al. Novel approach towards musculoskeletal phenotypes. *Eur. J. Pain* **2020**, *24*, 921–932. [CrossRef]
9. ten Klooster, P.M.; de Graaf, N.; Vonkeman, H.E. Association between pain phenotype and disease activity in rheumatoid arthritis patients: A non-interventional, longitudinal cohort study. *Arthritis Res. Ther.* **2019**, *21*, 257. [CrossRef]
10. Smith, D.; Wilkie, R.; Croft, P.; McBeth, J. Pain and Mortality in Older Adults: The Influence of Pain Phenotype. *Arthritis Care Res.* **2018**, *70*, 236–243. [CrossRef]
11. Center, J.R.; Bliuc, D.; Nguyen, T.V.; Eisman, J.A. Risk of subsequent fracture after low-trauma fracture in men and women. *JAMA* **2007**, *297*, 387–394. [CrossRef] [PubMed]
12. Center, J.R.; Nguyen, T.V.; Schneider, D.; Sambrook, P.N.; Eisman, J.A. Mortality after all major types of osteoporotic fracture in men and women: An observational study. *Lancet* **1999**, *353*, 878–882. [CrossRef]
13. Klotzbuecher, C.M.; Ross, P.D.; Landsman, P.B.; Abbott, T.A., 3rd; Berger, M. Patients with prior fractures have an increased risk of future fractures: A summary of the literature and statistical synthesis. *J. Bone Miner. Res.* **2000**, *15*, 721–739. [CrossRef] [PubMed]
14. Stone, K.L.; Seeley, D.G.; Lui, L.Y.; Cauley, J.A.; Ensrud, K.; Browner, W.S.; Nevitt, M.C.; Cummings, S.R.; Osteoporotic Fractures Research, G. BMD at multiple sites and risk of fracture of multiple types: Long-term results from the Study of Osteoporotic Fractures. *J. Bone Miner. Res.* **2003**, *18*, 1947–1954. [CrossRef] [PubMed]
15. Vranken, L.; Wyers, C.E.; van den Bergh, J.P.W.; Geusens, P. The Phenotype of Patients with a Recent Fracture: A Literature Survey of the Fracture Liaison Service. *Calcif. Tissue Int.* **2017**, *101*, 248–258. [CrossRef]
16. Dore, A.L.; Golightly, Y.M.; Mercer, V.S.; Shi, X.A.; Renner, J.B.; Jordan, J.M.; Nelson, A.E. Lower-extremity osteoarthritis and the risk of falls in a community-based longitudinal study of adults with and without osteoarthritis. *Arthritis Care Res. (Hoboken)* **2015**, *67*, 633–639. [CrossRef]
17. Gale, C.R.; Westbury, L.D.; Cooper, C.; Dennison, E.M. Risk factors for incident falls in older men and women: The English longitudinal study of ageing. *BMC Geriatr.* **2018**, *18*, 117. [CrossRef]
18. Leveille, S.G.; Jones, R.N.; Kiely, D.K.; Hausdorff, J.M.; Shmerling, R.H.; Guralnik, J.M.; Kiel, D.P.; Lipsitz, L.A.; Bean, J.F. Chronic musculoskeletal pain and the occurrence of falls in an older population. *JAMA* **2009**, *302*, 2214–2221. [CrossRef]
19. Welsh, V.K.; Clarson, L.E.; Mallen, C.D.; McBeth, J. Multisite pain and self-reported falls in older people: Systematic review and meta-analysis. *Arthritis Res. Ther.* **2019**, *21*, 67. [CrossRef]
20. Cauley, J.A.; Barbour, K.E.; Harrison, S.L.; Cloonan, Y.K.; Danielson, M.E.; Ensrud, K.E.; Fink, H.A.; Orwoll, E.S.; Boudreau, R. Inflammatory Markers and the Risk of Hip and Vertebral Fractures in Men: The Osteoporotic Fractures in Men (MrOS). *J. Bone Miner. Res.* **2016**, *31*, 2129–2138. [CrossRef]
21. Eriksson, A.L.; Movérare-Skrtic, S.; Ljunggren, Ö.; Karlsson, M.; Mellström, D.; Ohlsson, C. High-Sensitivity CRP Is an Independent Risk Factor for All Fractures and Vertebral Fractures in Elderly Men: The MrOS Sweden Study. *J. Bone Miner. Res.* **2014**, *29*, 418–423. [CrossRef] [PubMed]
22. Pan, F.; Tian, J.; Aitken, D.; Cicuttini, F.; Jones, G. Pain at multiple sites is associated with prevalent and incident fractures in older adults. *J. Bone Miner. Res.* **2019**, *34*, 2012–2018. [CrossRef] [PubMed]
23. Arden, N.K.; Crozier, S.; Smith, H.; Anderson, F.; Edwards, C.; Raphael, H.; Cooper, C. Knee pain, knee osteoarthritis, and the risk of fracture. *Arthritis Care Res.* **2006**, *55*, 610–615. [CrossRef]
24. Munch, T.; Harrison, S.L.; Barrett-Connor, E.; Lane, N.E.; Nevitt, M.C.; Schousboe, J.T.; Stefanick, M.; Cawthon, P.M. Pain and falls and fractures in community-dwelling older men. *Age Ageing* **2015**, *44*, 973–979. [CrossRef] [PubMed]
25. Pan, F.; Tian, J.; Munugoda, I.P.; Graves, S.; Lorimer, M.; Cicuttini, F.; Jones, G. Do Knee Pain Phenotypes Have Different Risks of Total Knee Replacement? *J. Clin. Med.* **2020**, *9*, 632. [CrossRef] [PubMed]
26. Pan, F.; Tian, J.; Cicuttini, F.; Jones, G.; Aitken, D. Differentiating knee pain phenotypes in older adults: A prospective cohort study. *Rheumatology* **2019**, *58*, 274–283. [CrossRef] [PubMed]
27. Doré, D.A.; Winzenberg, T.M.; Ding, C.; Otahal, P.; Pelletier, J.-P.; Martel-Pelletier, J.; Cicuttini, F.M.; Jones, G. The association between objectively measured physical activity and knee structural change using MRI. *Ann. Rheum. Dis.* **2013**, *72*, 1170–1175. [CrossRef]
28. Pan, F.; Laslett, L.; Blizzard, L.; Cicuttini, F.; Winzenberg, T.; Ding, C.; Jones, G. Associations Between Fat Mass and Multisite Pain: A Five-Year Longitudinal Study. *Arthritis Care Res.* **2017**, *69*, 509–516. [CrossRef]
29. Hoogeboom, T.J.; den Broeder, A.A.; Swierstra, B.A.; de Bie, R.A.; van den Ende, C.H. Joint-pain comorbidity, health status, and medication use in hip and knee osteoarthritis: A cross-sectional study. *Arthritis Care Res.* **2012**, *64*, 54–58. [CrossRef]
30. Knoop, J.; van der Leeden, M.; Thorstensson, C.A.; Roorda, L.D.; Lems, W.F.; Knol, D.L.; Steultjens, M.P.; Dekker, J. Identification of phenotypes with different clinical outcomes in knee osteoarthritis: Data from the Osteoarthritis Initiative. *Arthritis Care Res.* **2011**, *63*, 1535–1542. [CrossRef]

31. Lord, S.R.; Menz, H.B.; Tiedemann, A. A physiological profile approach to falls risk assessment and prevention. *Phys. Ther.* **2003**, *83*, 237–252. [CrossRef] [PubMed]
32. Scott, D.; Blizzard, L.; Fell, J.; Jones, G. Ambulatory activity, body composition, and lower-limb muscle strength in older adults. *Med. Sci. Sport. Exerc.* **2009**, *41*, 383–389. [CrossRef] [PubMed]
33. Scott, D.; Hayes, A.; Sanders, K.M.; Aitken, D.; Ebeling, P.R.; Jones, G. Operational definitions of sarcopenia and their associations with 5-year changes in falls risk in community-dwelling middle-aged and older adults. *Osteoporos. Int.* **2014**, *25*, 187–193. [CrossRef] [PubMed]
34. Lanza, S.T.; Dziak, J.J.; Huang, L.; Wagner, A.T.; Collins, L.M. *LCA Stata Plugin Users' Guide (Version 1.2)*; The Methodology Center: University Park, PA, USA, 2015.
35. Stubbs, B.; Schofield, P.; Binnekade, T.; Patchay, S.; Sepehry, A.; Eggermont, L. Pain is associated with recurrent falls in community-dwelling older adults: Evidence from a systematic review and meta-analysis. *Pain Med.* **2014**, *15*, 1115–1128. [CrossRef]
36. Stubbs, B.; Binnekade, T.; Eggermont, L.; Sepehry, A.A.; Patchay, S.; Schofield, P. Pain and the risk for falls in community-dwelling older adults: Systematic review and meta-analysis. *Arch. Phys. Med. Rehabil.* **2014**, *95*, 175–187.e179. [CrossRef]
37. Marshall, L.M.; Litwack-Harrison, S.; Makris, U.E.; Kado, D.M.; Cawthon, P.M.; Deyo, R.A.; Carlson, N.L.; Nevitt, M.C.; Osteoporotic Fractures in Men Study (MrOS) Research Group. A Prospective Study of Back Pain and Risk of Falls among Older Community-dwelling Men. *J. Gerontol. A Biol. Sci. Med. Sci.* **2017**, *72*, 1264–1269. [CrossRef]
38. Marshall, L.M.; Litwack-Harrison, S.; Cawthon, P.M.; Kado, D.M.; Deyo, R.A.; Makris, U.E.; Carlson, H.L.; Nevitt, M.C.; Study of Osteoporotic Fractures (SOF) Research Group. A Prospective Study of Back Pain and Risk of Falls among Community-dwelling Women. *J. Gerontol. A Biol. Sci. Med. Sci.* **2016**, *71*, 1177–1183. [CrossRef]
39. Kitayuguchi, J.; Kamada, M.; Inoue, S.; Kamioka, H.; Abe, T.; Okada, S.; Mutoh, Y. Association of low back and knee pain with falls in Japanese community-dwelling older adults: A 3-year prospective cohort study. *Geriatr. Gerontol. Int.* **2017**, *17*, 875–884. [CrossRef]
40. Cai, Y.; Leveille, S.G.; Shi, L.; Chen, P.; You, T. Chronic pain and circumstances of falls in community-living older adults: An exploratory study. *Age Ageing* **2022**, *51*, 1–6. [CrossRef]
41. Awale, A.; Hagedorn, T.J.; Dufour, A.B.; Menz, H.B.; Casey, V.A.; Hannan, M.T. Foot Function, Foot Pain, and Falls in Older Adults: The Framingham Foot Study. *Gerontology* **2017**, *63*, 318–324. [CrossRef]
42. Hicks, C.; Levinger, P.; Menant, J.C.; Lord, S.R.; Sachdev, P.S.; Brodaty, H.; Sturnieks, D.L. Reduced strength, poor balance and concern about falls mediate the relationship between knee pain and fall risk in older people. *BMC Geriatr.* **2020**, *20*, 94. [CrossRef] [PubMed]
43. Hadjistavropoulos, T.; Delbaere, K. The Psychology of Fall Risk: Fear, Anxiety, Depression, and Balance Confidence. In *Falls in Older People: Risk Factors, Strategies for Prevention and Implications for Practice*, 3rd ed.; Sherrington, C., Lord, S.R., Naganathan, V., Eds.; Cambridge University Press: Cambridge, UK, 2021; pp. 160–171. [CrossRef]
44. Kuroda, T.; Shiraki, M.; Tanaka, S.; Shiraki, Y.; Narusawa, K.; Nakamura, T. The relationship between back pain and future vertebral fracture in postmenopausal women. *Spine* **2009**, *34*, 1984–1989. [CrossRef] [PubMed]
45. Barbour, K.E.; Sagawa, N.; Boudreau, R.M.; Winger, M.E.; Cauley, J.A.; Nevitt, M.C.; Fujii, T.; Patel, K.V.; Strotmeyer, E.S. Knee Osteoarthritis and the Risk of Medically Treated Injurious Falls Among Older Adults: A Community-Based US Cohort Study. *Arthritis Care Res.* **2019**, *71*, 865–874. [CrossRef]
46. Yuan, S.; Chen, J.; Zeng, L.; Zhou, C.; Yu, S.; Fang, L. Association of bone mineral density and depression in different bone sites and ages: A meta-analysis. *Food Sci. Nutr.* **2021**, *9*, 4780–4792. [CrossRef] [PubMed]
47. Lee, S.C.; Hu, L.Y.; Huang, M.W.; Shen, C.C.; Huang, W.L.; Lu, T.; Hsu, C.L.; Pan, C.C. Risk of Vertebral Fracture in Patients Diagnosed with a Depressive Disorder: A Nationwide Population-Based Cohort Study. *Clinics* **2017**, *72*, 44–50. [CrossRef]
48. Kelly, R.R.; McDonald, L.T.; Jensen, N.R.; Sidles, S.J.; LaRue, A.C. Impacts of Psychological Stress on Osteoporosis: Clinical Implications and Treatment Interactions. *Front. Psychiatry* **2019**, *10*, 200. [CrossRef] [PubMed]
49. Talaei-Khoei, M.; Fischerauer, S.F.; Jha, R.; Ring, D.; Chen, N.; Vranceanu, A.-M. Bidirectional mediation of depression and pain intensity on their associations with upper extremity physical function. *J. Behav. Med.* **2018**, *41*, 309–317. [CrossRef]
50. Ivers, R.Q.; Cumming, R.G.; Mitchell, P.; Peduto, A.J. The accuracy of self-reported fractures in older people. *J. Clin. Epidemiol.* **2002**, *55*, 452–457. [CrossRef]

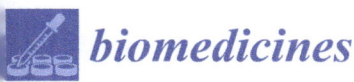

Article

Potential Effects of Non-Surgical Periodontal Therapy on Periodontal Parameters, Inflammatory Markers, and Kidney Function Indicators in Chronic Kidney Disease Patients with Chronic Periodontitis

Ahmed Chaudhry [1,2], Nur Karyatee Kassim [2,3,4,*], Siti Lailatul Akmar Zainuddin [1,2], Haslina Taib [1,2], Hanim Afzan Ibrahim [2,3,4], Basaruddin Ahmad [2,5], Muhammad Hafiz Hanafi [2,6] and Azreen Syazril Adnan [7]

1. Periodontic Unit, School of Dental Sciences, Universiti Sains Malaysia, Kubang Kerian 16150, Malaysia
2. Hospital Universiti Sains Malaysia, Kubang Kerian 16150, Malaysia
3. Basic Sciences and Medical Unit, School of Dental Sciences, Universiti Sains Malaysia, Kubang Kerian 16150, Malaysia
4. Chemical Pathology Department, School of Medical Sciences, Universiti Sains Malaysia, Kubang Kerian 16150, Malaysia
5. Biostatics Unit, School of Dental Sciences, Universiti Sains Malaysia, Kubang Kerian 16150, Malaysia
6. Department of Neurosciences, School of Medical Sciences, Universiti Sains Malaysia, Kubang Kerian 16150, Malaysia
7. Advanced Medical & Dental Institute, Universiti Sains Malaysia, Bertam, Jalan Tun Hamdan Sheikh Tahir, Pulau Pinang 13200, Malaysia
* Correspondence: karyatee@usm.my; Tel.: +60-199-822-305

Abstract: Chronic kidney disease (CKD) and chronic periodontitis (CP) contribute to the increased level of inflammatory biomarkers in the blood. This study hypothesized that successful periodontal treatment would reduce the level of inflammatory biomarkers in CKD patients. This prospective study recruited two groups of CP patients: 33 pre-dialysis CKD patients and 33 non-CKD patients. All patients underwent non-surgical periodontal therapy (NSPT). Their blood samples and periodontal parameters were taken before and after six weeks of NSPT. The serum level of high-sensitivity C-reactive protein (hs-CRP), interleukin 6 (IL-6), and periodontal parameters were compared between groups. On the other hand, kidney function indicators such as serum urea and estimated glomerular filtration rate (eGFR) were only measured in CKD patients. Clinical periodontal parameters and inflammatory markers levels at baseline were significantly higher ($p < 0.05$) in the CKD group than in the non-CKD group and showed significant reduction ($p < 0.05$) after six weeks of NSPT. CKD patients demonstrated a greater periodontitis severity and higher inflammatory burden than non-CKD patients. Additionally, CKD patients with CP showed a good response to NSPT. Therefore, CKD patients' periodontal health needs to be screened for early dental interventions and monitored accordingly.

Keywords: chronic kidney disease; inflammatory markers; periodontitis

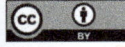

1. Introduction

Chronic periodontitis (CP) is a chronic inflammatory disease caused by bacteria and affects the periodontium's stability [1]. According to a report on the global economic impact of dental diseases, severe periodontitis is the sixth most prevalent disease globally, affecting 743 million people aged between 15 and 99 [2]. The development and maturation of plaque biofilm by bacterial colonization are considered the primary aetiological factor that contributes to periodontal disease's pathogenesis [3]. The appalling consequences of periodontal disease include edentulism (tooth loss) and systemic inflammation [4].

Chronic kidney disease (CKD) is defined as reduced kidney function as indicated by glomerular filtration rate (GFR) having a value less than 60 mL/min/1.73 m^2 and/or kidney damage for at least three months. Based on the degree of GFR reduction, CKD can be classified into five stages (stages I-V). The fifth stage (stage V) is considered an end-stage renal disease (ESRD), with a GFR value of less than 15 mL/min/1.73 m^2 and persistent bilateral damage of the nephrons, which are the basic functional units of the kidney [5]. According to the World Health Organization (WHO) global health estimates, CKD is the world's 14th leading cause of death [6]. In 2012, CKD caused 864,226 deaths (1.5% of deaths worldwide) [6]. CKD patients are susceptible to infection and atherosclerotic vascular disease, which are the major causes of morbidity and mortality in these patients. These two factors (i.e., infection and atherosclerotic vascular disease) were responsible for about 38% of annual deaths, with most of the deaths reported for ESRD patients [7]. A rise in inflammatory markers, such as interleukin 6 (IL-6) and C-reactive protein (CRP), are potent predictors of impaired kidney function and the development of cardiovascular disease in CKD patients [8,9].

Given the distinct pathogenesis of CKD and periodontitis, these two pathological conditions have been independent of each other. However, recent findings demonstrated a bidirectional relationship between CKD and periodontitis [10,11]. Moreover, clinical trials and cross-sectional studies suggested an association between CKD and the severity of periodontal problems [4,12,13]. CKD is responsible for a higher incidence of periodontal disease that is commonly manifested as plaque formation, calculus deposition, gingival hyperplasia, and increased gingival inflammation [14]. Furthermore, calculus and plaque build-ups have been associated with CKD patients' uremic syndrome [15]. In other studies, CKD and CP have been associated with several risk factors, including impaired immunity, diabetes mellitus, smoking, impaired oral hygiene, xerostomia, and malnutrition. This may account for a link between CP and its deleterious systemic effects in CKD patients [16,17].

Non-surgical periodontal therapy (NSPT) is the keystone of periodontal therapy and the first recommended approach to preventing periodontal infections. NSTP is defined as "plaque removal, plaque control, supragingival and subgingival scaling root planning (SRP), and adjunctive use of chemical agents" [18]. Apart from its evident benefits on oral health or clinical periodontal aspects [19,20], periodontal therapy also improved endothelial function, reduced systolic and diastolic blood pressure, increased heat shock protein 10 (HSP-10; an anti-inflammatory factor), decreased white blood cells count, and reduced arterial intima-media thickness [21,22]. In addition, earlier investigations have shown that starting NSPT with local SRP is potent to reduce inflammatory markers in CP and CKD patients [23–25].

Based on the above evidence, we hypothesized that CKD patients have a higher prevalence of periodontal infections than non-CKD patients. Periodontal infections worsen the systemic inflammatory status, leading to poor renal outcomes in CKD patients. Improving oral health care through NSPT may improve the systemic inflammatory status and improve renal function. However, there are limited studies regarding the effect of NSPT on CKD patients. Therefore, this study aimed to investigate the changes in periodontal parameters, serum inflammatory markers, and kidney function indicators in CKD patients with CP and non-CKD patients following NSPT. The evaluation of such inflammatory markers may serve as important biomarkers for the diagnosis and monitoring of CKD. Targeted therapy to enhance these inflammatory markers may serve as a useful adjunct for treating CKD in its early stages and slow its progression to ESRD, which has an irreversible threatening effect on CKD patients' morbidity and mortality.

2. Materials and Methods

2.1. Ethical Considerations

This study was submitted, reviewed, and approved by the Human Research Ethics Committee of Universiti Sains Malaysia (JEPeM USM code: USM/JEPeM/18020160). The study was conducted according to the guidelines described by the Helsinki Declaration of 1975, as revised in 2013. Informed consent was obtained from all patients prior to dental examination and the provision of periodontal therapy. All participants were aware of their right to withdraw from the study at any point during the study process.

A non-randomized clinical trial was conducted at Universiti Sains Malaysia (USM). A total of 66 subjects were divided equally into two groups. The non-CKD group comprised CP patients recruited from Dental Clinics Hospital USM, whereas the CKD group comprised CKD patients with CP recruited from the Nephrology Clinic and Chronic Kidney Disease Resource Centre, Hospital USM. The algorithm of patient recruitment in this study is presented in Figure 1.

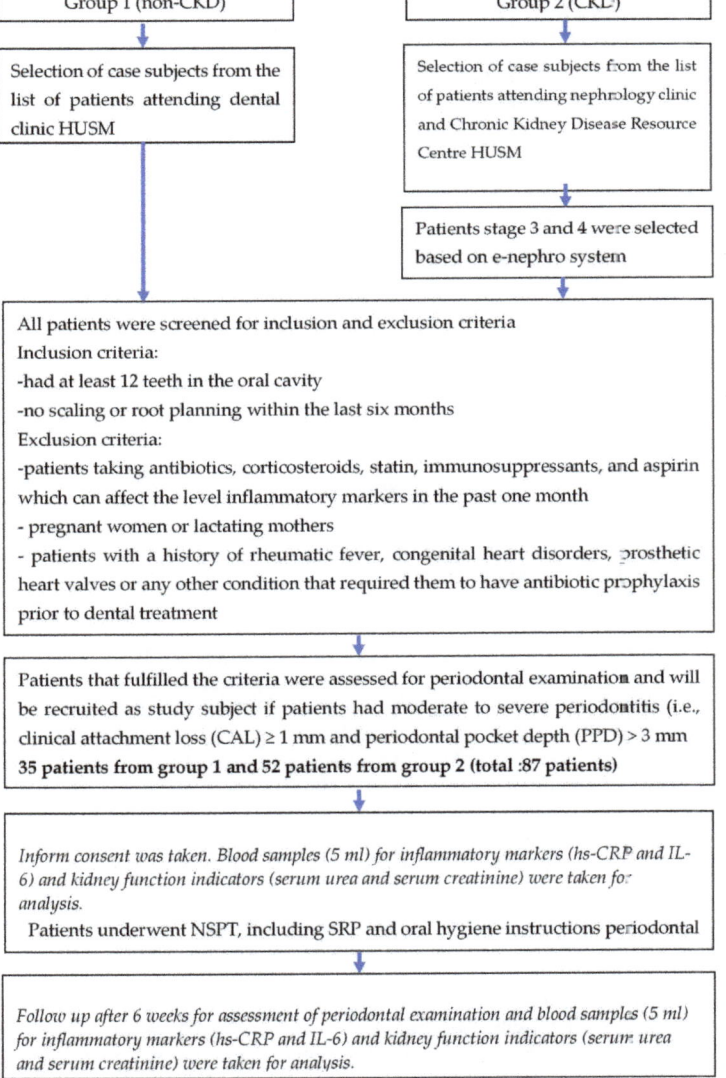

Figure 1. Algorithm of patient recruitment. HUSM, Hospital Universiti Sains Malaysia; CRP, C-reactive protein; IL-6, interleukin 6, NSPT, non-surgical periodontal therapy; SRP, scaling, and root planning.

2.2. Inclusion and Exclusion Criteria

The inclusion criteria for both groups were a) signing a written informed consent form, b) patients with moderate to severe periodontitis (i.e., clinical attachment loss (CAL) ≥ 1 mm and periodontal pocket depth (PPD) > 3 mm [26]), c) had at least 12 teeth in the oral cavity, and d) no scaling or root planning within the last six months. For the CKD group, only subjects in stage III and IV CKD determined based on the estimated glomerular filtration rate (eGFR) and had HbA1c levels < 7.5% were included [17].

The eGFR values were calculated to estimate the creatinine clearance using the Chronic Kidney Disease Epidemiology Collaboration (CKD-EPI) equation shown below:

$$eGFR = 141 \times \min(SCr/\kappa, 1)^\alpha \times \max(SCr/\kappa, 1)^{-1.209} \times 0.993^{age} \times 1.018 \text{ [if female]} \times 1.159 \text{ [if Black]} [27].$$

Exclusion criteria for both groups were (a) patients taking antibiotics, corticosteroids, statin, immunosuppressants, and aspirin which can affect the level of inflammatory markers in the past month, (b) pregnant women or lactating mothers, and (c) patients with a history of rheumatic fever, congenital heart disorders, prosthetic heart valves or any other condition that required them to have antibiotic prophylaxis prior to dental treatment.

2.3. Assessment of Clinical Periodontal Parameters

A proforma was used to collect patients' demographic details, such as age, gender, ethnicity, and other comorbidities. A coding system was used for patient identification to ensure that only the researchers had access to their information. Only one examiner was assigned for clinical periodontal examination. Clinical data acquired by the clinical examiner were calibrated by senior specialists. The intra- and inter-examiner observations indicated about 90% of the recording being reproduced within a ±1.0 mm range. Briefly, the clinical periodontal examination was performed by assessing the CAL and PPD. The assessments were done by measuring six points for every tooth (except the third molar) using the Michigan probe with Williams marking.

2.4. Collection of Blood Samples

Five mL of blood samples were drawn from the median cubital vein and collected in a plain tube for the analyses of inflammatory markers (hs-CRP and IL-6) and kidney function indicators (serum urea and serum creatinine).

2.5. Provision of NSPT

Patients subsequently underwent NSPT, including SRP and oral hygiene instructions. Full mouth SRP using an ultrasonic (EMS Piezon Master, Electro-Medical System, Nyon, Switzerland), and curettage at PPD sites with 5 mm or greater using hand scalers (Gracey, Dentsply, UK) were performed under local anesthesia (Mepivacaine 2.2 ml with adrenaline ratio 1:100,000). All treated sites were then irrigated with 0.2% chlorhexidine. Patients were also given oral hygiene instructions to brush their teeth at least twice a day using fluoridated toothpaste and a soft-bristled toothbrush and floss once daily. Patients from both groups were followed up six weeks after the NSPT. Clinical periodontal parameters and blood samples were analyzed.

2.6. Biochemical Assay

The collected blood samples were centrifuged at 3000 rpm, and the blood serum was stored at −80 °C until they were analyzed. The serum hs-CRP level was measured using the latex particle-enhanced immunoturbidimetric method in a COBAS INTEGRA 400 plus (Roche Diagnostics, Basle, Switzerland). On the other hand, the IL-6 was measured using the electrochemiluminescence immunoassay method in the COBAS 6000 analyzer (Roche Diagnostics, Rotkreuz, Switzerland). Serum creatinine and urea levels were measured using a spectrophotometric method in the Architect C8000 analyzer (Abbott, KC, USA).

2.7. Statistical Analysis

The summary statistics were obtained using mean (SD) and frequency (percentage) for all variables. The independent t-test and Chi-squared test were used for comparing the CKD and non-CKD groups. Repeated-measures analysis of variance was used for comparing the periodontal parameters from the baseline to six weeks and between the groups. Analyses were carried out using IBM SPSS 24.0 Armonk, NY, USA with the significance level set at 5%.

3. Results

3.1. Primary Characteristics of Study Participants

A total of 87 subjects were initially recruited for this study. However, only 66 (43 males and 23 females) participated in this study (33 patients in each group). The mean age of patients in the non-CKD and CKD groups was 49.18 ± 8.58 years and 55.96 ± 11.26 years, respectively. In total, 89.3% (n = 59) of the patients were Malay, and only 10.6% (n = 7) were Chinese. In the CKD group, 12 and 21 patients were in stages III and IV, respectively. Most of the patients were non-smokers, followed by ex-smokers and active smokers. The mean teeth count was significantly higher for the non-CKD group ($p < 0.05$) than for the (Table 1).

Table 1. Demographic profile and medical status of the study population.

Demographic Features	Study Groups		Significance
	Non-CKD Group n (%) (n = 33)	CKD Group n (%) (n = 33)	p-Value
Age (years) (mean ± SD)	49.18 ± 8.58	55.96 ± 11.26	0.1
Gender			
Male	16 (24.2)	27 (40.9)	
Female	17 (25.8)	6 (9.1)	0.004
Ethnicity			
Malay	28 (42.4)	31 (47)	
Chinese	5 (7.6)	2 (3)	0.4
Marital status			
Married	28 (42.4)	27 (40.9)	
Single	5 (7.6)	6 (9.1)	0.7
Mean number of teeth present	24.36 ± 3.89	19.51 ± 6.23	< 0.001
Smoking			
Non-smokers	22 (33.3)	25 (37.9)	
Ex-smokers	7 (10.6)	6 (9.1)	0.7
Active smokers	4 (6.1)	2 (3.0)	
CKD staging			
Stage-III	-	12 (36.4)	
Stage-IV	-	21 (63.6)	
Medical illness			
Diabetes mellitus	1	19	
Hypertension	9	23	
Ischemic heart disease	-	6	
Other medical illnesses	-	5	
No medical illness	23	-	

Data are presented as mean (SD). p-values were determined using the chi-squared test $p < 0.05$ was considered statistically significant. CKD, chronic kidney disease.

3.2. Clinical Periodontal Parameters

The PPD and CAL were significantly higher ($p < 0.05$) for the CKD group than the non-CKD group at the baseline level. Both groups showed significant improvement ($p < 0.05$) in the mean PPD and CAL after six weeks of NSPT. Nevertheless, there were no significant differences between groups when considering the mean of all periodontal variables during follow-up ($p > 0.05$). The mean baseline PPD for the non-CKD group was 4.76 ± 0.52 mm, while the mean PPD after NSPT was 2.97 ± 0.74 mm. On the other hand, the mean baseline PPD for the CKD group was 5.02 ± 0.50 mm, while the mean PPD after NSPT was 2.74 ± 0.50 mm. Apart from that, the mean CAL for the non-CKD group was 4.79 ± 0.52 mm and 3.20 ± 0.78 mm at baseline and post-treatment, respectively. In contrast, the mean CAL for the CKD group was 5.34 ± 1.06 mm and 3.26 ± 0.94 mm, respectively. Both groups demonstrated significant improvement in the plaque and gingival indicators after six weeks (Table 2).

Table 2. Clinical periodontal parameters of the study population.

Periodontal Parameters	Baseline	Six Weeks Follow-Up	p-Value
PPD (mm)			$p_{time}*_{group} = 0.002$
Non-CKD	4.76 ± 0.52	2.97 ± 0.74 *	$p_{time} < 0.001$
CKD	5.02 ± 0.50 †	2.74 ± 0.50 *	$p_{group} = 0.9$
p-value	0.046	0.15	
CAL (mm)			$p_{time}*_{group} = 0.02$
Non-CKD	4.79 ± 0.53	3.20 ± 0.152 *	$p_{time} < 0.001$
CKD	5.34 ± 1.06 †	3.27 ± 0.152 *	$p_{group} = 0.1$
p-value	0.01	0.77	
GBI (%)			$p_{time}*_{group} = 0.9$
Non-CKD	52.78 ± 22.33	19.68 ± 13.38 *	$p_{time} < 0.001$
CKD	56.12 ± 19.01	23.30 ± 5.81 *	$p_{group} = 0.3$
p-value	0.515	0.171	
PS (%)			$p_{time}*_{group} = 0.6$
Non-CKD	63.61 ± 18.41	23.49 ± 14.17 *	$p_{time} < 0.001$
CKD	61.53 ± 20.78	19.27 ± 8.16 *	$p_{group} = 0.3$
p-value	0.688	0.143	

Data are presented as mean (SD). p-values were determined using the independent t-test. $p < 0.05$ was considered statistically significant. * Statistically significant difference from baseline ($p < 0.05$). † Statistically significant difference from the non-CKD group at baseline ($p < 0.05$). PPD, periodontal pocket depth; CAL, clinical attachment loss; PS, plaque scores; GBI, gingival bleeding index; CKD, chronic kidney disease.

3.3. Inflammatory Markers

The results for hs-CRP and IL-6 are tabulated in Table 3. The mean baseline for hs-CRP and IL-6 in the CKD group were 3.07 ± 2.37 mg/L and 4.11 ± 2.84 pg/mL, respectively. On the other hand, the mean baseline for hs-CRP and IL-6 in the non-CKD group were 1.71 ± 1.64 mg/L and 2.54 ± 1.09 pg/mL, respectively. The independent samples t-test showed that the mean baseline for hs-CRP and IL-6 were significantly higher ($p < 0.05$) in the CKD group than in the non-CKD group. Analyses revealed a significant reduction ($p < 0.05$) in inflammatory marker levels when both groups are considered. For the CKD group, post-treatment measurements for hs-CRP and IL-6 were 1.50 ± 1.38 mg/L and 2.93 ± 1.47 pg/mL, respectively. For the non-CKD group, post-treatment measurements for hs-CRP and IL-6 were 0.82 ± 0.71 mg/L and 1.89 ± 0.63 pg/mL, respectively. Apart from that, kidney function indicators (eGFR and serum urea) showed improvement during the study's timeframe. However, these indicators did not show significant changes ($p > 0.05$) after NSPT.

Table 3. The value of inflammatory markers and kidney function indicator of the study population.

Variables	Baseline	Six Weeks Follow-Up	p-Value
hs-CRP (mg/L)			$p_{time}*_{group} = 0.2$
Non-CKD	1.71 ± 1.64	0.82 ± 0.71 *	$p_{time} < 0.001$
CKD	3.07 ± 2.37 †	1.50 ± 1.38 *	$p_{group} = 0.02$
p-value	0.03	0.041	

Table 3. *Cont.*

Variables	Baseline	Six Weeks Follow-Up	*p*-Value
IL-6 (pg/mL)			
Non-CKD	2.54 ± 1.09	1.89 ± 0.63 *	$p_{time\,*\,group} = 0.3$
CKD	4.11 ± 2.84 †	2.93 ± 1.47 *	$p_{time} = 0.001$
p-value	0.013	0.002	$p_{group} = 0.002$
Serum urea (mmol/L)			
Non-CKD	4.15 ± 1.23	4.04 ± 1.15	$p_{time\,*\,group} = 0.9$
CKD	12.57 ± 4.84 †	12.30 ± 5.35	$p_{time} = 0.8$
p-value	< 0.001	< 0.001	$p_{group} < 0.001$
eGFR (mL/min/1.73 m^2)			
Non-CKD	89.60 ± 21.33	92.21 ± 18.30	$p_{time\,*\,group} = 0.6$
CKD	25.96 ± 10.56 †	27.18 ± 12.17	$p_{time} = 0.1$
p-value	< 0.001	< 0.001	$p_{group} < 0.001$

Data are presented as mean (SD). *p*-values were determined using the independent *t*-test. $p < 0.05$ was considered statistically significant. * Statistically significant difference from baseline ($p < 0.05$). † Statistically significant difference from the non-CKD group at baseline ($p < 0.05$). hs-CRP, high sensitive-C reactive protein; IL-6, interleukin-6; eGFR, estimated glomerular filtration rate; CKD, chronic kidney disease.

4. Discussion

The NSPT was the first recommended approach to control periodontal infections. Notwithstanding its advancement over the years, NSPT remains the "gold standard" for which all treatment methods are compared. The main aim of NSPT is to restore gingival health by eliminating the factors responsible for gingival inflammation, such as endotoxins, plaque, and calculus in the oral cavity. This debridement procedure was carried out using hand instruments (i.e., curettes and scalers) and staged in different sessions [18]. Several researchers in the past have reported a decrease in gingival recession and probing depth after NSPT. They also indicated lesser bleeding during probing, lesser inflammation, and gingival redness [19,28,29]. Previous studies suggested that initial NSPT, comprising local SRP, is very potent in reducing inflammatory markers levels [30–32].

In this study, males were dominant in the CKD group since males are more susceptible to the disease than females [33]. This gender-specific finding of CKD progression and prevalence can be due to factors such as lifestyle, proteinuria, renal structure, body mass index, hypertension, sex hormones, and hyperglycemia [33–35]. Apart from that, we successfully ascertained the effects of NSPT in CKD subjects with CP and non-CKD subjects. Both groups showed major improvement in the clinical periodontal parameters and inflammatory markers after NSPT. Also, kidney function indicators have been shown to improve after NSPT. However, the observed difference was not significant. The results also showed an increased occurrence of tooth loss in patients suffering from CKD is associated with increased periodontal disease severity. Nevertheless, other factors, such as old age and concomitant medical problems such as diabetes, may exacerbate these problems [6,36].

Our study highlighted that CKD patients had a more severe form of periodontal disease than non-CKD patients. Overall, higher periodontal disease severity in CKD patients than in non-CKD patients can be associated with many risk factors, such as malnutrition, uremic syndrome, xerostomia, compromised immunity, and low oral health awareness [37,38]. In addition, the risk of diabetes mellitus was high in both groups. Previous research observed an independent link between diabetes and CP since diabetes is closely linked with reduced wound healing, increased monocyte response to dental plaque antigens, and impacted neutrophil chemotactic response. All these factors cause higher local tissue impairment [39]. Moreover, hyperglycemia may increase inflammation, oxidative stress, and apoptosis, contributing to increased periodontal destruction [40]. Additionally, diabetes has been known as one of the established primary aetiologies of CKD [6]. Hence, diabetes in the CKD subjects (Table 1) may also have caused additional damage to the periodontal tissues. Nguyen et al. (2017) suggested that the increased CAL status may be due to changes in salivary content (e.g., urea and calcium), thus contributing to the development of calculus in periodontal disease [4].

All periodontal aspects, such as PPD, CAL PS), and GBI, showed significant improvement in both groups after NSPT. The results were consistent with previous research that showed NSPT significantly improved CAL levels and reduced PPD in moderate or severe periodontitis [20,41]. NSPT is considered a gold standard for managing chronic periodontitis. Sanz et al. (2012) stated that numerous studies had reported its potency towards improving periodontal health through the mechanical debridement of subgingival plaque biofilms [20]. Clinical reports suggested that NSPT reduces the total number of gingival sites that bleed during probing, facilitating a transition of oral microbiota from gram-negative to gram-positive bacteria. Additionally, NSPT reduces the number of microorganisms, including black-pigmented species and spirochetes, with a concomitant increase in coccoid cells [42].

The findings from this study were similar to those reported by Artese et al. (2010), where periodontal therapy outcomes for CKD patients were analyzed [43]. The results of this study were also in agreement with other studies [44,45], which observed and recorded the differences in the clinical periodontal aspect before and after treatment for CKD patients with CP. Furthermore, advice on post-treatment oral healthcare given to patients in both groups may have played a role in improving oral health.

Inflammatory markers (IL-6 and CRP) were elevated in both CP and CKD conditions [36,37]. Our report highlighted a significant increase in baseline inflammatory marker levels for CKD patients than non-CKD patients. These observations may reflect the severity of systemic health problems. Pro-inflammatory cytokines (i.e., IL-6) accumulate within the body due to renal excretion failure caused by compromised renal function. These cytokines (IL-6) could also be attributed to the elevated production of CRP by hepatic cells [46]. Compromised immunity, atherosclerotic processes, cardiovascular disease, persistent infections, and gut microbiota dysbiosis have been reported as the factors responsible for the elevated inflammatory burden in CKD patients [47,48]. Such an inflammatory response is understood to be among the strongest predictors of diminished clinical outcomes for CKD patients [49].

As observed in this research, the significantly poor periodontal condition could also be related to the elevated production of IL-6 and hs-CRP in CP subjects. Several studies have documented CP as an infectious condition and a non-traditional risk factor for CKD due to high systemic inflammation loads. The high systemic inflammation loads arise from periodontal inflammation, locally generated inflammatory mediators, and acute phase reactants (IL-1, IL-6, tumor necrosis factor-alpha (TNF-α), and CRP) [10,37,50].

Accompanying the improvement in periodontal parameters after NSPT, both groups were observed to have significantly decreased serum inflammatory markers ($p < 0.05$). It was hypothesized that the control of local inflammation could result in a reduced systemic acute-phase response [51]. This may contribute to periodontal therapy's anti-inflammatory effects, which lead to a lesser overall pathogen load in the oral cavity, thus reducing systemic and local inflammatory markers.

Findings on inflammatory markers were also consistent with other studies [45,52]. By contrast, a study in Japan suggested a non-significant reduction in hs-CRP and IL-6 levels after NSPT in patients with periodontitis only. Nevertheless, the researchers asserted that Japanese people have lower serum hs-CRP and IL-6 levels relative to other populations. Furthermore, the small sample size used in their study may have contributed to the conflicting result. Although there was no significant difference in both inflammatory markers, an improvement trend was observed in hs-CRP levels after NSPT [53]. Ide et al. (2004) reported a clinically significant elevation in serum IL-6 and TNF-α levels after NSPT [54]. Specific studies have highlighted the beneficial aspects of NSPT as transitory and asserted that the clinical inflammatory indicators typically increased 12 months following the treatment [55,56]. Apart from that, NSPT has been observed to improve serum urea and eGFR levels in CKD patients. However, these findings were not statistically significant, possibly due to the premorbid medical condition and the small sample size.

These findings highlighted that periodontal therapy might have delayed CKD progression. Usually, CKD is progressive and associated with a sustained decline in renal function, as reflected by the reduction in eGFR. Its progression depends on CKD causes, albuminuria levels, acute kidney injury, uncontrolled blood sugar levels, and blood pressure dysregulation [6]. Hence, post-treatment improvement of mean eGFR for subjects in the CKD group suggested that NSPT may have reduced CKD progression. Existing literature concerning the effects of NSPT on the status of kidney indicators remains controversial. Previous research has observed significant benefits of periodontal therapy towards the improvement of eGFR in CKD patients [30,43]. Nevertheless, Chambrone et al. (2013) carried out a systemic review focusing on the effect of periodontal therapy on eGFR. The review concluded that there is a lack of evidence to support the hypothesis that periodontal treatment has positive effects on eGFR, considering the limited number of studies and varying methodologies.

This study provides a useful approach to the future management of CKD patients, focusing on the importance of monitoring oral hygiene which has often been neglected. Periodontal therapy should be part of the treatment in retarding the progression of CKD patients in the future. More studies should be performed to further enhance our knowledge in this research area to support the study findings.

5. Conclusions

Pre-dialysis CKD patients demonstrated good clinical periodontal and inflammatory responses after NSPT. Hence, an understanding of periodontal health and its benefits for pre-dialysis CKD patients should be emphasized. Multi-centered research with a large sample size is required to evaluate periodontal treatment effects on periodontal parameters, eGFR status, and inflammatory markers.

Author Contributions: Conceptualization, A.C., S.L.A.Z., M.H.H. and N.K.K.; methodology, A.C., N.K.K., A.S.A. and H.T.; validation, H.A.I. and B.A.; formal analysis, A.C. and B.A.; investigation, A.C. and S.L.A.Z.; resources, S.L.A.Z., M.H.H. and N.K.K.; data curation, A.C. and B.A.; writing—original draft preparation, A.C. and H.A.I.; writing—review and editing, A.C., S.L.A.Z., M.H.H. and N.K.K.; visualization, H.T. and H.A.I.; supervision, S.L.A.Z., N.K.K. and H.T.; project administration, A.C., S.L.A.Z., N.K.K. and H.T.; funding acquisition, S.L.A.Z. and N.K.K. All authors have read and agreed to the published version of the manuscript.

Funding: This research was funded by the Fundamental Research Grant Scheme (FRGS/1/2019 SKK08/USM/02/14) Ministry of Education, Malaysia. The reagent kits for the research partially supported by Roche Diagnostics Sdn Bhd, Malaysia.

Institutional Review Board Statement: The study was conducted in accordance with the Declaration of Helsinki and approved by the Ethics Committee of Universiti Sains Malaysia (JEPeM USM Code: USM/JEPeM/18020160).

Informed Consent Statement: Informed consent was obtained from all subjects involved in the study.

Data Availability Statement: Not applicable.

Acknowledgments: The authors would like to express appreciation to the staff from the School of Dental Sciences, USM) and Chronic Kidney Disease Resource Centre (Hospital USM) who provided help and assistance in the research.

Conflicts of Interest: The authors declare no conflict of interest.

References

1. Hajishengallis, G. Periodontitis: From microbial immune subversion to systemic inflammation. *Nat. Rev. Immunol.* **2015**, *15*, 30–44. [CrossRef] [PubMed]
2. Frencken, J.E.; Sharma, P.; Stenhouse, L.; Green, D.; Laverty, D.; Dietrich, T. Global epidemiology of dental caries and severe periodontitis—A comprehensive review. *J. Clin. Periodontol.* **2017**, *44*, S94–S105. [CrossRef] [PubMed]

3. Kinane, D.F.; Stathopoulou, P.G.; Papapanou, P.N. Periodontal diseases. *Nat. Rev. Dis. Prim.* **2017**, *3*, 17038. [CrossRef] [PubMed]
4. Nguyen, L.D.A.; Nguyen, T.T.T.; Pham, T.A.V. Periodontal Status in Chronic Kidney Disease Patients. *UI Proc. Health Med.* **2017**, *1*, 155–161. [CrossRef]
5. Clinical, K. K/DOQI clinical practice guidelines for chronic kidney disease: Evaluation, classification, and stratification. *Am. J. Kidney Dis.* **2002**, *39*, S1–S266.
6. Webster, A.C.; Nagler, E.V.; Morton, R.L.; Masson, P. Chronic Kidney Disease. *Lancet* **2017**, *389*, 1238–1252. [CrossRef]
7. Cengiz, M.I.; Bal, S.; Gökçay, S.; Cengiz, K. Does periodontal disease reflect atherosclerosis in continuous ambulatory peritoneal dialysis patients? *J. Periodontol.* **2007**, *78*, 1926–1934. [CrossRef]
8. Selim, G.; Stojceva-Taneva, O.; Zafirovska, K.; Sikole, A.; Gelev, S.; Dzekova, P.; Stefanovski, K.; Koloska, V.; Polenakovic, M. Inflammation predicts all-cause and cardiovascular mortality in haemodialysis patients. *Prilozi* **2006**, *27*, 133–144.
9. Stenvinkel, P.; Alvestrand, A. Inflammation in end-stage renal disease: Sources, consequences, and therapy. *Semin. Dial.* **2002**, *15*, 329–337. [CrossRef]
10. Fisher, M.A.; Taylor, G.W.; West, B.T.; McCarthy, E.T. Bidirectional relationship between chronic kidney and periodontal disease: A study using structural equation modeling. *Kidney Int.* **2011**, *79*, 347–355. [CrossRef]
11. Wahid, A.; Chaudhry, S.; Ehsan, A.; Butt, S.; Ali Khan, A. Bidirectional Relationship between Chronic Kidney Disease & Periodontal Disease. *Pak. J. Med. Sci.* **2013**, *29*, 211–215. [PubMed]
12. Oyetola, E.O.; Owotade, F.J.; Agbelusi, G.A.; Fatusi, O.A.; Sanusi, A.A. Oral findings in chronic kidney disease: Implications for management in developing countries. *BMC Oral Health* **2015**, *15*, 24. [CrossRef] [PubMed]
13. Choudhury, E.S. Periodontal Infections, Inflammatory Markers in Chronic Kidney Disease. Master's Thesis, University of Connecticut, Tolland, CT, USA, 2010.
14. Craig, R.G. Interactions between chronic renal disease and periodontal disease. *Oral Dis.* **2008**, *14*, 1–7. [CrossRef]
15. Dioguardi, M.; Caloro, G.A.; Troiano, G.; Giannatempo, G.; Laino, L.; Petruzzi, M.; Lo Muzio, L. Oral manifestations in chronic uremia patients. *Ren. Fail.* **2016**, *38*, 1–6. [CrossRef]
16. Chambrone, L.; Foz, A.M.; Guglielmetti, M.R.; Pannuti, C.M.; Artese, H.P.; Feres, M.; Romito, G.A. Periodontitis and chronic kidney disease: A systematic review of the association of diseases and the effect of periodontal treatment on estimated glomerular filtration rate. *J. Clin. Periodontol.* **2013**, *40*, 443–456. [CrossRef]
17. Kidney Disease: Improving Global Outcomes (KDIGO) CKD-MBD Work Group. KDIGO clinical practice guideline for the diagnosis, evaluation, prevention, and treatment of chronic kidney disease-Mineral and Bone Disorder (CKD-MBD). *Kidney Int. Suppl.* **2009**, *76*, S1–S130.
18. Tanwar, J.; Hungund, S.; Dodani, K. Nonsurgical periodontal therapy: A review. *J. Oral Res. Rev.* **2016**, *8*, 39–44. [CrossRef]
19. Son, A.; Pera, C.; Ueda, P.; Casarin, R.C.V.; Pimentel, S.P.; Cirano, F.R. Clinical effects of supragingival plaque control on uncontrolled type 2 diabetes mellitus subjects with chronic periodontitis. *Braz. J. Oral Sci.* **2016**, *47–51*, 1677–3225.
20. Sanz, I.; Alonso, B.; Carasol, M.; Herrera, D.; Sanz, M. Nonsurgical treatment of periodontitis. *J. Evid.-Based Dent. Pract.* **2012**, *12*, 76–86. [CrossRef]
21. Tonetti, M.S.; D'Aiuto, F.; Nibali, L.; Donald, A.; Storry, C.; Parkar, M.; Suvan, J.; Hingorani, A.D.; Vallance, P.; Deanfield, J. Treatment of periodontitis and endothelial function. *N. Engl. J. Med.* **2007**, *356*, 911–920. [CrossRef]
22. Ritam, S.; Jyoti, R. Effect of periodontal treatment on plasma fibrinogen, serum C-reactive protein and total white blood cell count in periodontitis patients: A prospective interventional trial. *Rom. J. Intern. Med.* **2013**, *51*, 45–51.
23. Mohammed, M.; Jesmin, F.; Kassim, N.K.; Zainuddin, S.L.; Hanafi, M.H.; Kamarudin, M.I.; Ahmad, F.; Sirajudeen, K. Levels of interleukins in patients with chronic kidney disease and periodontitis: A systematic review. *J. Int. Oral. Health* **2021**, *13*, 313–318.
24. Zhang, Q.; Chen, B.; Zhu, D.; Yan, F. Biomarker levels in gingival crevicular fluid of subjects with different periodontal conditions: A cross-sectional study. *Arch. Oral Biol.* **2016**, *72*, 92–98. [CrossRef]
25. Kumar, S.; Shah, S.; Budhiraja, S.; Desai, K.; Shah, C.; Mehta, D. The effect of periodontal treatment on C-reactive protein: A clinical study. *J. Nat. Sci. Biol. Med.* **2013**, *4*, 379–382. [CrossRef]
26. American Academy of Periodontology, O. American Academy of Periodontology Task Force report on the update to the 1999 classification of periodontal diseases and conditions. *J. Periodontol.* **2015**, *86*, 835–838.
27. Levey, A.S.; Stevens, L.A.; Schmid, C.H.; Zhang, Y.L.; Castro, A.F., 3rd; Feldman, H.I.; Kusek, J.W.; Eggers, P.; Van Lente, F.; Greene, T.; et al. A new equation to estimate glomerular filtration rate. *Ann. Intern. Med.* **2009**, *150*, 604–612. [CrossRef]
28. Ribeiro, É.D.P.; Bittencourt, S.; Nociti-Júnior, F.H.; Sallum, E.A.; Sallum, A.W.; Casati, M.Z. The effect of one session of supragingival plaque control on clinical and biochemical parameters of chronic periodontitis. *J. Appl. Oral Sci.* **2005**, *13*, 275–279. [CrossRef]
29. Haffajee, A.; Cugini, M.; Dibart, S.; Smith, C.; Kent Jr, R.; Socransky, S. The effect of SRP on the clinical and microbiological parameters of periodontal diseases. *J. Clin. Periodontol.* **1997**, *24*, 324–334. [CrossRef]
30. Graziani, F.; Cei, S.; La Ferla, F.; Vano, M.; Gabriele, M.; Tonetti, M. Effects of non-surgical periodontal therapy on the glomerular filtration rate of the kidney: An exploratory trial. *J. Clin. Periodontol.* **2010**, *37*, 638–643. [CrossRef]
31. Taylor, B.; Tofler, G.; Morel-Kopp, M.C.; Carey, H.; Carter, T.; Elliott, M.; Dailey, C.; Villata, L.; Ward, C.; Woodward, M. The effect of initial treatment of periodontitis on systemic markers of inflammation and cardiovascular risk: A randomized controlled trial. *Eur. J. Oral Sci.* **2010**, *118*, 350–356. [CrossRef]

32. Chakraborty, S.; Tewari, S.; Sharma, R.K.; Narula, S.C. Effect of non-surgical periodontal therapy on serum ferritin levels: An interventional study. *J. Periodontol.* **2014**, *85*, 688–696. [CrossRef]
33. Chang, P.Y.; Chien, L.N.; Lin, Y.F.; Wu, M.S.; Chiu, W.T.; Chiou, H.Y. Risk factors of gender for renal progression in patients with early chronic kidney disease. *Medicine* **2016**, *95*, e4203. [CrossRef] [PubMed]
34. Duru, O.K.; Li, S.; Jurkovitz, C.; Bakris, G.; Brown, W.; Chen, S.C.; Collins, A.; Klag, M.; McCullough, P.A.; McGill, J.; et al. Race and sex differences in hypertension control in CKD: Results from the Kidney Early Evaluation Program (KEEP). *Am. J. Kidney Dis.* **2008**, *51*, 192–198. [CrossRef] [PubMed]
35. Komura, H.; Nomura, I.; Kitamura, K.; Kuwasako, K.; Kato, J. Gender difference in relationship between body mass index and development of chronic kidney disease. *BMC Res. Notes* **2013**, *6*, 463. [CrossRef] [PubMed]
36. Chang, J.-F.; Yeh, J.-C.; Chiu, Y.-L.; Liou, J.-C.; Hsiung, J.-R.; Tung, T.-H. Periodontal pocket depth, hyperglycemia, and progression of chronic kidney disease: A population-based longitudinal study. *Am. J. Med.* **2017**, *130*, 61–69.e1. [CrossRef] [PubMed]
37. Fisher, M.A.; Taylor, G.W.; Papapanou, P.N.; Rahman, M.; Debanne, S.M. Clinical and serologic markers of periodontal infection and chronic kidney disease. *J. Periodontol.* **2008**, *79*, 1670–1678. [CrossRef] [PubMed]
38. Iwasaki, M.; Taylor, G.W.; Nesse, W.; Vissink, A.; Yoshihara, A.; Miyazaki, H. Periodontal disease and decreased kidney function in Japanese elderly. *Am. J. Kidney Dis.* **2012**, *59*, 202–209. [CrossRef]
39. Deshpande, K.; Jain, A.; Sharma, R.; Prashar, S.; Jain, R. Diabetes and periodontitis. *J. Indian Soc. Periodontol.* **2010**, *14*, 207–212. [CrossRef]
40. Genco, R.J.; Borgnakke, W.S. Risk factors for periodontal disease. *Periodontol. 2000* **2013**, *62*, 59–94. [CrossRef]
41. Badersten, A.; Nilveus, R.; Egelberg, J. Effect of nonsurgical periodontal therapy. *J. Clin. Periodontol.* **1984**, *11*, 63–76. [CrossRef]
42. Umeda, M.; Takeuchi, Y.; Noguchi, K.; Huang, Y.; Koshy, G.; Ishikawa, I. Effects of nonsurgical periodontal therapy on the microbiota. *Periodontol. 2000* **2004**, *36*, 98–120. [CrossRef] [PubMed]
43. Artese, H.P.C.; Sousa, C.O.; Luiz, R.R.; Sansone, C.; Torres, M.C.M. Effect of non-surgical periodontal treatment on chronic kidney disease patients. *Braz. Oral Res.* **2010**, *24*, 449–454. [CrossRef]
44. Fang, F.; Wu, B.; Qu, Q.; Gao, J.; Yan, W.; Huang, X.; Ma, D.; Yue, J.; Chen, T.; Liu, F. The clinical response and systemic effects of non-surgical periodontal therapy in end-stage renal disease patients: A 6-month randomized controlled clinical trial. *J. Clin. Periodontol.* **2015**, *42*, 537–546. [CrossRef] [PubMed]
45. Guo, N.; Lin, G. Effects of nonsurgical periodontal therapy on serum inflammatory factor levels in patients with chronic kidney disease and periodontitis. *Biomed. Res.-India* **2017**, *28*, 3899–3902.
46. Pecoits-Filho, R.; Heimburger, O.; Barany, P.; Suliman, M.; Fehrman-Ekholm, I.; Lindholm, B.; Stenvinkel, P. Associations between circulating inflammatory markers and residual renal function in CRF patients. *Am. J. Kidney Dis.* **2003**, *41*, 1212–1218. [CrossRef]
47. Mihai, S.; Codrici, E.; Popescu, I.D.; Enciu, A.-M.; Albulescu, L.; Necula, L.G.; Mambet, C.; Anton, G.; Tanase, C. Inflammation-Related Mechanisms in Chronic Kidney Disease Prediction, Progression, and Outcome. *J. Immunol. Res.* **2018**, *2018*, 16. [CrossRef] [PubMed]
48. Shrivastava, A.K.; Singh, H.V.; Raizada, A.; Singh, S.K. C-reactive protein, inflammation and coronary heart disease. *Egypt. Heart J.* **2015**, *67*, 89–97. [CrossRef]
49. Yeun, J.Y.; Levine, R.A.; Mantadilok, V.; Kaysen, G.A. C-Reactive protein predicts all-cause and cardiovascular mortality in hemodialysis patients. *Am. J. Kidney Dis.* **2000**, *35*, 469–476. [CrossRef]
50. Ismail, G.; Dumitriu, H.T.; Dumitriu, A.S.; Ismail, F.B. Periodontal disease: A covert source of inflammation in chronic kidney disease patients. *Int. J. Nephrol.* **2013**, *2013*, 515796. [CrossRef]
51. Hussain Bokhari, S.A.; Khan, A.A.; Tatakis, D.N.; Azhar, M.; Hanif, M.; Izhar, M. Non-Surgical Periodontal Therapy Lowers Serum Inflammatory Markers: A Pilot Study. *J. Periodontol.* **2009**, *80*, 1574–1580. [CrossRef]
52. Vilela, E.M.; Bastos, J.A.; Fernandes, N.; Ferreira, A.P.; Chaoubah, A.; Bastos, M.G. Treatment of chronic periodontitis decreases serum prohepcidin levels in patients with chronic kidney disease. *Clinics* **2011**, *66*, 657–662. [CrossRef] [PubMed]
53. Yamazaki, K.; Honda, T.; Oda, T.; Ueki-Maruyama, K.; Nakajima, T.; Yoshie, H.; Seymour, G.J. Effect of periodontal treatment on the C-reactive protein and proinflammatory cytokine levels in Japanese periodontitis patients. *J. Periodontal Res.* **2005**, *40*, 53–58. [CrossRef] [PubMed]
54. Ide, M.; Jagdev, D.; Coward, P.Y.; Crook, M.; Barclay, G.R.; Wilson, R.F. The short-term effects of treatment of chronic periodontitis on circulating levels of endotoxin, C-reactive protein, tumor necrosis factor-alpha, and interleukin-6. *J. Periodontol.* **2004**, *75*, 420–428. [CrossRef] [PubMed]
55. Piconi, S.; Trabattoni, D.; Luraghi, C.; Perilli, E.; Borelli, M.; Pacei, M.; Rizzardini, G.; Lattuada, A.; Eray, D.H.; Catalano, M. Treatment of periodontal disease results in improvements in endothelial dysfunction and reduction of the carotid intima-media thickness. *FASEB J.* **2009**, *23*, 1196–1204. [CrossRef] [PubMed]
56. Cobb, C.M. Microbes, inflammation, scaling and root planing, and the periodontal condition. *Am. Dent. Hyg. Assoc.* **2008**, *82*, 4–9.

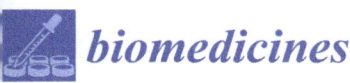

Article

Thrombin Activity in Rodent and Human Skin: Modified by Inflammation and Correlates with Innervation

Valery Golderman [1,2,†], Shani Berkowitz [1,2], Shani Guly Gofrit [1], Orna Gera [1,2], Shay Anat Aharoni [1], Daniela Noa Zohar [1], Daria Keren [1], Amir Dori [1,2,3], Joab Chapman [1,2,4,5] and Efrat Shavit-Stein [1,2,6,*]

1. Department of Neurology, The Chaim Sheba Medical Center, Ramat Gan 52626202, Israel; valery.rodionov@gmail.com (V.G.); shanihberkowitz@gmail.com (S.B.); shanygo@gmail.com (S.G.G.); geragra@post.tau.ac.il (O.G.); aharonianat@gmail.com (S.A.A.); zohardanielle@gmail.com (D.N.Z.); amir.dori@gmail.com (A.D.); dariaker9@gmail.com (D.K.); joabchapman@gmail.com (J.C.)
2. Department of Neurology and Neurosurgery, Sackler Faculty of Medicine, Tel Aviv University, Tel Aviv 6997801, Israel
3. Talpiot Medical Leadership Program, The Chaim Sheba Medical Center, Ramat Gan 52626202, Israel
4. Department of Physiology and Pharmacology, Sackler Faculty of Medicine, Tel Aviv University, Tel Aviv 6997801, Israel
5. Robert and Martha Harden Mental and Neurological Diseases, Sackler Faculty of Medicine, Tel Aviv University, Tel Aviv 6997801, Israel
6. The TELEM Rubin Excellence in Biomedical Research Program, The Chaim Sheba Medical Center, Ramat Gan 52621, Israel
* Correspondence: efrat.shavit.stein@gmail.com
† This work was performed in partial fulfillment of the requirement for the Ph.D. degree by Valery Golderman at the Sackler Faculty of Medicine, Tel-Aviv University, Israel.

Abstract: Thrombin is present in peripheral nerves and is involved in the pathogenesis of neuropathy. We evaluated thrombin activity in skin punch biopsies taken from the paws of male mice and rats and from the legs of patients with suspected small-fiber neuropathy (SFN). In mice, inflammation was induced focally by subcutaneous adjuvant injection to one paw and systemically by intraperitoneal lipopolysaccharides (LPS) administration. One day following injection, thrombin activity increased in the skin of the injected compared with the contralateral and non-injected control paws ($p = 0.0009$). One week following injection, thrombin increased in both injected and contralateral paws compared with the controls ($p = 0.026$), coupled with increased heat-sensitivity ($p = 0.009$). Thrombin activity in the footpad skin was significantly increased one week after systemic administration of LPS compared with the controls ($p = 0.023$). This was not accompanied by increased heat sensitivity. In human skin, a correlation was found between nerve fiber density and thrombin activity. In addition, a lower thrombin activity was measured in patients with evidence of systemic inflammation compared with the controls ($p = 0.0035$). These results support the modification of skin thrombin activity by regional and systemic inflammation as well as a correlation with nerve fiber density. Skin thrombin activity measurments may aid in the diagnosis and treatment of SFN.

Keywords: thrombin activity; skin; small-fiber neuropathy

1. Introduction

Neuroinflammation refers to the activation of an immune response in the nervous system and is commonly associated with neural destruction. The precise mechanisms that drive this process are not fully elucidated, and the coagulation system has been suggested to play a role. Inflammation upregulates the coagulation system in many systemic diseases and can be majorly activated, as seen in disseminated intravascular coagulation (DIC) during severe sepsis [1]. On the other hand, thrombin, a central coagulation factor, affects inflammation by several mechanisms through its cellular protease-activated receptors

(PARs), which are localized to various cell types such as endothelial, fibroblasts, smooth muscle, and sensory neurons [2,3].

Thrombin modulates long-term potentiation [4], synaptic transmission, and nerve conduction [5]. Excess thrombin activity is associated with numerous central nervous system (CNS) pathologies, including seizures, induced by lowering the epileptic threshold [4], glioblastoma multiforme edema formation [6,7], and primary inflammatory diseases of the brain such as multiple sclerosis [8]. In the peripheral nervous system (PNS), recent studies demonstrate the role of thrombin in the pathogenesis of diabetic neuropathy [9] and Guillain Barre syndrome (GBS) [10]. In the streptozotocin (STZ) diabetic neuropathy model in rats, and the animal model of GBS, increased thrombin activity in the sciatic nerve was found together with the destruction of the nodes of Ranvier structure, along with nerve conduction impairment [9–11]. These findings strongly implicate the cellular mediated thrombin pathway in the process and pathogenesis of neuropathy.

Thrombin has been found to play a significant role via several mechanisms in inflammatory processes of both the CNS and PNS. Thrombin can directly bind endothelial cells, leading to blood–brain barrier (BBB) breakdown; increasing antibodies permeability and lymphocyte infiltration to the CNS; and thus inducing edema, inflammation, and gliosis [12]. Injecting thrombin into peripheral tissues has been shown to induce neurogenic inflammation [13]. Cleavage of the thrombin receptor on sensory nerves stimulates the release of neuropeptides such as substance P, which interacts with neurokinin 1 (NK1R) on endothelial cells to induce extravasation of plasma proteins and edema [13]. Thrombin-activated PAR1 in small diameter nociceptive neurons causes sensitization of the capsaicin receptor transient receptor potential vanilloid subfamily 1 (TRPV1) and promotes the heat-dependent release of the pro-inflammatory neuropeptide calcitonin gene-related peptide (CGRP) [14], thereby suggesting that thrombin and PARs play a role in promoting inflammation and pain in the PNS.

Small-fiber neuropathy (SFN) occurs through various mechanisms including inflammatory processes found in diabetes, GBS, chronic inflammatory demyelinating polyneuropathy, and systemic autoimmune diseases [15]. SFN is a disorder characterized by damage to small, myelinated fibers (Aδ) or unmyelinated C fibers. These somatic fibers carry thermal and pain sensations from the skin to the CNS and their degeneration can lead to multiple symptoms including severe neuropathic pain and thermal allodynia [16]. Additionally, SFN patients are known to suffer from burning pain, shooting pain, allodynia, and hyperesthesia.

Previous studies indicate the presence and function of several coagulation factors in the skin, together with local PAR expression. Thus, it is interesting to study thrombin activity in the skin and whether it is modified locally in pathologies such as neuropathies. Measuring thrombin activity in the skin may serve as a highly accessible marker for the diagnosis and treatment of the coagulation-neuroinflammation process. The aim of our study was therefore to investigate whether thrombin activity can be detected and reliably measured in a skin biopsy and whether different pathological processes modify the activity.

2. Materials and Methods

2.1. Animals

Adult *Sprague Dawley (SD)* rats (10–12 weeks) and adult *ICR* and *C57BL/6J* mice (8–12 weeks) were housed in standard conditions and fed a standard diet with water available ad libitum. The ambient temperature was set to 22 °C to 23 °C with day/night light control. The protocols of this study were approved by the Sheba Medical Center Committee on the Use and Care of Animals (permit No: 1085-17,1000-15, 1191-19) according to the ARRIVE Guidelines.

For the skin biopsies, mice/rats were anesthetized using Pental (pentobarbital sodium 200 mg/mL); 3 mm punches were obtained from the right and left hind limbs.

2.2. Adjuvant-Induced Focal Inflammation

The right hind paw of the *ICR* mouse was injected subcutaneously (S.C.) with 50 µL Adjuvant Complete Freund (BD, 263810) or 50 µL saline. The mice were examined for pain responses using the hot-plate test 1 and 7 days following the injection. Mice were anesthetized using Pental, and skin biopsies for thrombin activity were obtained from the right and left hind paws.

2.3. LPS-Induced Systemic Inflammation

The systemic inflammation model in *C57BL/6J* mice was induced by intraperitoneal (I.P.) injection of lipopolysaccharides (LPS) (1 mg/kg, O111:B4, L4130, Sigma, Darmstadt, Germany). One week following injection, the pain response was examined using the hot-plate test. The mice were then anesthetized with Pental, and skin biopsies were obtained from the right hind paw for assessment of thrombin activity.

2.4. Hot-Plate Test

Hyper/hypoalgesia was evaluated using the hot-plate test, as previously described [17]. The mice were placed in an acrylic glass cylinder on a heated stage digitally maintained at 51 ± 0.1 °C. The time to heat-response indicated by paw licking, shaking, or jumping was measured. A maximum on-plate time was set to 30 s to prevent skin injury.

2.5. Thrombin Activity Measurement

Thrombin activity was assessed using a fluorogenic thrombin substrate (Bachem I-1560, excitation 360 nm; emission 465 nm), as previously described [18]. Human biopsies were thawed and washed 3 times for 5 min in Tris-buffer (contains in mM: 150 NaCl, 1 $CaCl_2$, 50 Tris-HCl: pH 8.0) on ice. Human and rodent biopsies were placed in a black 96-well microplate (Nunc, Roskilde, Denmark) containing Tris-buffer. The plate was incubated at 37 °C for 30 min before the addition of the substrate. To eliminate the effect of abundant endopeptidases in the assay, endopeptidase inhibitors (0.1 mg/mL, bestatin hydrochloride—B8385, Sigma; 200 µM prolyl endopeptidase inhibitor II, 537011, Merck Millipore) were added to the substrate. Known bovine thrombin concentrations (T-4648, Sigma) were used to create a calibration curve for each experiment. The specific thrombin inhibitor SIXAC (100 nM, American Peptide Company, Sunnyvale, CA, USA) [19] was added to chosen wells to assess the specificity of the assay. The cleavage of the substrate was measured using a microplate reader (Tecan; infinite 200; Männedorf, Switzerland). Each biopsy was weighed, and the measured thrombin activity was normalized to tissue weight. The results are presented as mU thrombin activity/mg of tissue or relative to the control.

2.6. Histology

Zamboni-fixed mouse and rat skin biopsies were sectioned into 16 µm sections and stained with Hematoxylin and Eosin (H&E). Briefly, tissue-containing slides were incubated for 10 s in Hematoxylin (Sigma, HHS-32); washed with water; dipped 3 times in Eosin Y (Sigma, HT110-2-32); washed with water; and dipped in 70% ethanol, 95% ethanol, and 100% ethanol. The slides were viewed using a microscope (Olympus, Tokyo, Japan). The images were analyzed using ImageJ software [20]. The thickness of the epidermis was measured in three independent sections. Epidermal thickness was defined as the distance between the distal border and the dermis–epidermis border.

For small-fiber staining, mouse and rat skin biopsies were fixed using Zamboni, sectioned into 16 µm sections, and adhered to charged slides. Slides were washed with PBS and incubated in a blocking solution (containing: 0.25 M Tris-buffered saline, 5% skim milk powder, 5% normal horse serum, and 0.3% Triton X-100) for 4 h at room temperature. The slides were then incubated with a primary antibody (rabbit anti-PGP9.5, SAB4503057, 1:200 in blocking solution diluted 1:1 in PBS) overnight at 4 °C. On the next day, the slides were washed and incubated with secondary antibody (DyLight488 conjugated donkey anti-rabbit IgG, Jackson ImmunoResearch,1:200 in blocking solution diluted 1:1 in PBS) for 1.5 h at room temperature. Following incubation, the slides were washed, dried, and mounted with an anti-fading mounting medium (DAKO Fluoromount). Sections from each animal were randomly analyzed using an Olympus microscope, and the IENFD, expressed as the average number of nerve fibers per millimeter epidermis, was quantified according to guidelines published by the European Federation of Neurological Societies [21].

2.7. Human Patients

Human skin biopsies were obtained following informed consent from 43 adults (age 25–78) who were referred due to pain complaints to determine evidence for skin denervation and assist with the diagnosis of SFN (<5th percentile of nerve fiber density normalized for age). SFN was identified in 14 out of 43 patients, and 19 out of 43 patients were suspected of having an inflammatory cause of neuropathy due to known autoimmune or inflammatory disease or by the presence of clearly elevated inflammatory markers (Table S1). Patients that were under anti-inflammatory and/or immunosuppression treatment were excluded from the "inflammatory group" and moved to the "non-inflammatory group".

The study was approved by the Chaim Sheba Medical Center Ethics Committee (6525-19-SMC). This work was reported according to the Strengthening the Reporting of Observational Studies in Epidemiology (STROBE) guidelines.

2.8. Skin Biopsy

Skin biopsies (two 3.0 mm punches) were obtained from the distal leg 10 cm above the lateral malleolus. One skin biopsy was fixed in Zamboni fixative and processed using standard procedures to determine the intra-epidermal nerve fiber density (IENFD) [21]. Skin IENFD quantitation was performed by A.D. employing immunofluorescence microscopy with the PGP9.5 pan-neuronal marker (Bio-rad, MCA4750GA). Normal IENFD values were based on published data [22] and adjusted according to controls at the Sheba Medical Center. IENFD below the 5th percentile for age was determined abnormal and consistent with skin denervation, indicating small-fiber sensory polyneuropathy. Another skin biopsy was kept unfixed at $-80\ °C$ for 3–8 weeks and then used for thrombin activity analysis.

2.9. Statistical Analysis

Unpaired t-tests and one-way ANOVA with Tukey post hoc analysis were conducted on normally distributed data. Linear regression was conducted for thrombin activity versus age and thrombin activity versus IENFD percentile. The results are expressed as the mean $\pm$ SEM, and p-values less than 0.05 were considered significant. All statistical analyses were conducted using Prism GraphPad (version 8.0.1 for Windows, GraphPad Software, La Jolla, CA, USA).

3. Results

3.1. Mouse versus Rat Skin

Thrombin activity was measured in the glabrous skin of rats and mice using an enzymatic specific fluorescent method. Skin biopsy was placed in a 96-well black plate, and the plate was incubated at 37 °C for 30 min to allow the thrombin to defuse out of the tissue. Following the incubation, a thrombin-specific substrate was added, and fluorescence intensity was measured for 50 min (Figure 1).

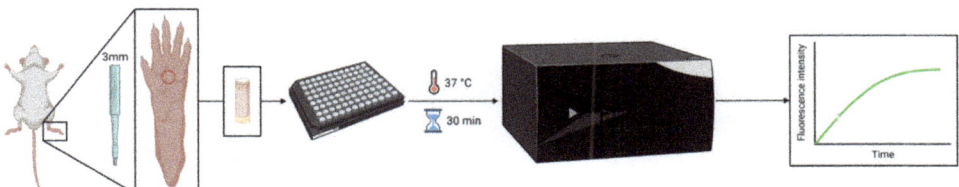

Figure 1. Thrombin activity in rodent skin-method flow diagram: for measuring thrombin activity in rodent skin, a 3 mm punch was obtained from the hind paw, placed in a 96-well black plate, and incubated at 37 °C for 30 min. Following the incubation, a specific thrombin substrate was added, and the fluorescence intensity over time was measured. Created with BioRender.com (accessed on 25 November 2021).

Both mice and rats showed detectable and specific thrombin activity in their hind paw skin, which was essentially abolished in the presence of SIXAC, a specific thrombin inhibitor (Figure 2A,B). In addition, we found that the rat skin biopsies weighed significantly more compared with the mouse skin (6.4 ± 0.25 and 4.7 ± 0.17 mg, respectively, $p < 0.0001$, Figure 2C). The measured thrombin activity was therefore normalized to the biopsy weight. Accordingly, significantly higher activity was measured in rats' skin compared with in the mice skin (2.5 ± 0.46 and 0.7 ± 0.13 mU/mg, respectively, $p = 0.0004$, Figure 2D).

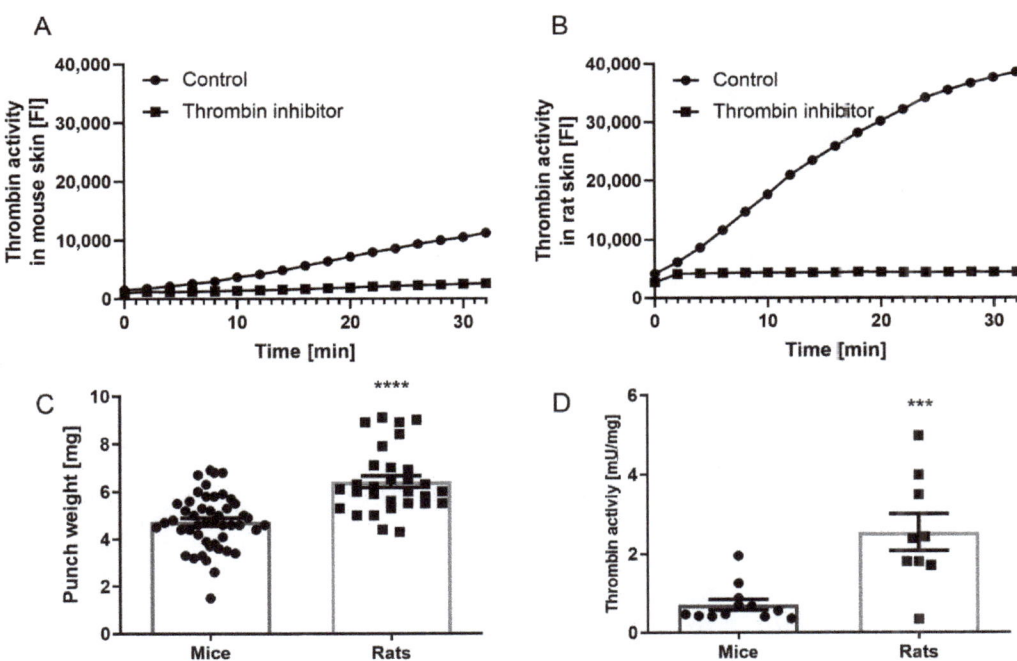

Figure 2. Thrombin activity in healthy mice and rats: representative graphs of measurable thrombin activity that was detected in mice (**A**) and rat (**B**) skin. This activity was fully inhibited by a specific thrombin inhibitor. (**C**) Biopsy weight was significantly lower in mice (n = 30) compared with in rats (n = 48). (**D**) Normalized thrombin activity was significantly higher in rats' skin (n = 9) compared with in the mice skin (n = 12). Results are presented as mean ± SEM, *** $p = 0.0004$, **** $p < 0.0001$. Scale bar—100 μm.

H&E skin staining revealed a significantly thicker epidermis layer in rats compared with in mice (97.23 ± 2.6 and 53.9 ± 2.3 μm, respectively, $p < 0.0001$, Figure 3A,B). In addition, staining of the small-fibers showed significantly higher fiber density in the rat skin compared with in the mouse skin (22.5 ± 1.2 and 12 ± 0.97, respectively, $p < 0.0001$, Figure 3C,D).

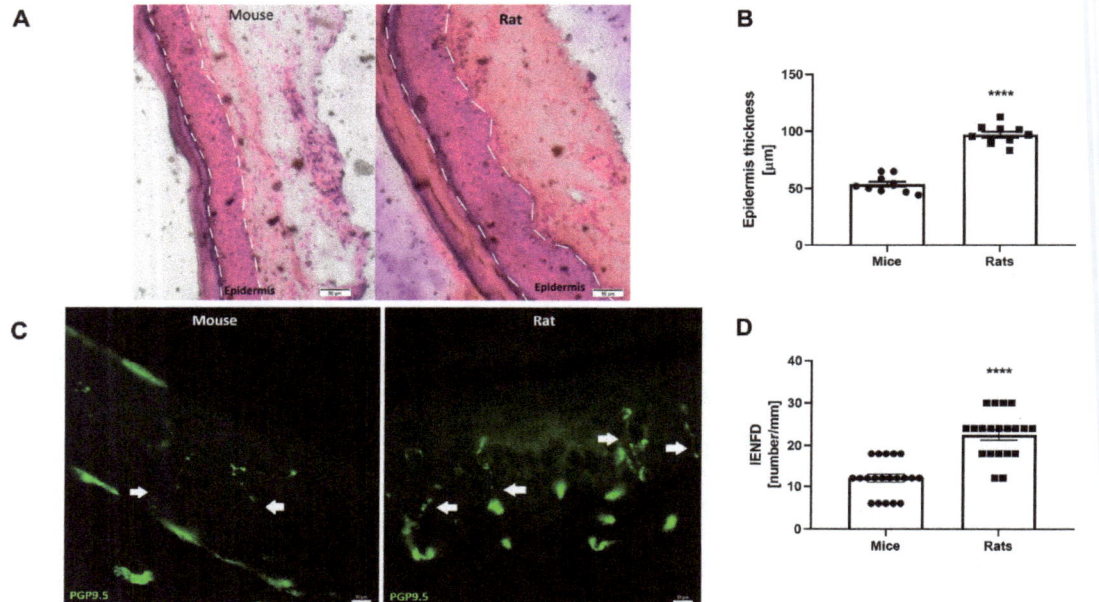

Figure 3. Structural differences between mouse and rat skin: (A) representative H&E staining of mouse and rat skin. Scale bar—50μm. White dashed lines represent the borders of the epidermis. Epidermis thickness was defined as the distance between the borders. (B) The epidermis layer was significantly thicker in rat skin compared with in mice skin, n = 10. (C) Representative PGP9.5 staining of mouse and rat skin. Scale bar—10μm. White arrowheads mark small-fibers. (D) The fiber density was significantly higher in rat skin compared with in mouse skin, n = 20. Results are presented as mean ± SEM, **** $p < 0.0001$.

3.2. Skin Thrombin Activity in Adjuvant-Induced Focal Inflammation

To examine the effect of focal inflammation on thrombin activity in the skin, we subcutaneously injected the adjuvant into the hind paw of ICR mice. After 24 h, adjuvant injected mice showed slightly higher heat sensitivity, which did not reach significance (Figure 4A). One week following the injection, the mice showed significantly higher heat sensitivity compared with the control (14.9 ± 2 and 25 ± 1.9 s, respectively, $p = 0.009$, Figure 4A).

We measured thrombin activity both in the skin of the adjuvant-injected and the contralateral paws as well as from the control mice. After 24 h, thrombin activity was higher in the skin of the adjuvant-injected paw, compared with that of the contralateral and control paws (3.7 ± 0.44, 0.82 ± 0.11 and 1 ± 0.22, respectively, $p = 0.0009$, Figure 4B). One week following adjuvant injection, thrombin activity in the skin of the injected paw declined, but both paws, i.e., injected and contralateral, showed significantly increased activity compared with the controls (2.7 ± 0.53, 2.3 ± 0.27, and 1 ± 0.24, respectively, $p = 0.026$, Figure 4B).

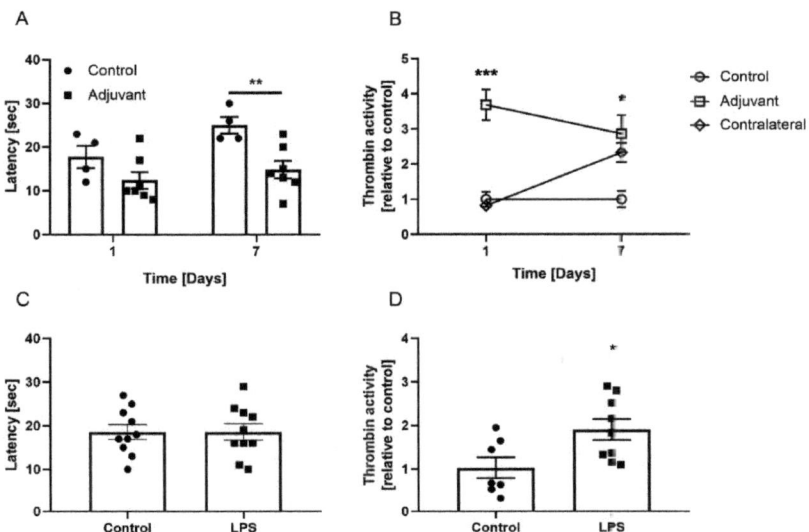

Figure 4. Heat sensitivity and thrombin activity in the skin of focal and systemic inflammation-induced mice. Adjuvant-induced focal inflammation in *ICR* mice: (**A**) Significantly higher heat sensitivity was found one week following adjuvant injection compared with the controls. n = 10 and 4, respectively. (**B**) Thrombin activity in the injected paw was significantly higher compared with the contralateral paw and the control group 24 h following adjuvant injection. Thrombin activity in the skin of the injected and the contralateral paws was significantly higher compared with the control group one week following adjuvant injection. n = 7 and 8. LPS-induced inflammation in *C57BL/6J* mice: (**C**) No difference in heat sensitivity between the groups was found one week following LPS injection. n = 10. (**D**) Significantly higher thrombin activity was found in the skin of LPS mice compared with that of the controls. n = 9 and 7, respectively. Thrombin activity results are presented relative to the controls. Results are presented as mean ± SEM, * $p < 0.025$, ** $p < 0.009$, *** $p < 0.0009$.

3.3. Skin Thrombin Activity in LPS-Induced Systemic Inflammation

To examine the effect of systemic inflammation on thrombin activity in the skin, we induced inflammation in the *C57BL/6J* mice using LPS injection. In contrast to focal inflammation, LPS mice did not show increased heat sensitivity one week following the induction compared with the controls (18.6 ± 1.89 and 18.6 ± 1.7 s, respectively, $p > 0.99$, Figure 4C). However, after one week, LPS-injected mice showed significantly higher thrombin activity in the skin compared with the controls (1.9 ± 0.24 and 1 ± 0.24, respectively, $p = 0.023$, Figure 4D). Nevertheless, this level of activity was not as high as the thrombin activity detected following focal inflammation.

3.4. Thrombin Activity in Human Skin

We extended our findings by measuring thrombin activity in human skin biopsies from patients with suspected SFN. The biopsy was taken from the leg, 10 cm above the lateral malleolus of the patient, classified as non-glabrous hairy skin. The skin was stored at −80 °C and analyzed after thawing. Some human skin biopsies contained blood; therefore, all biopsies were washed in a cold buffer before analysis (Figure 5).

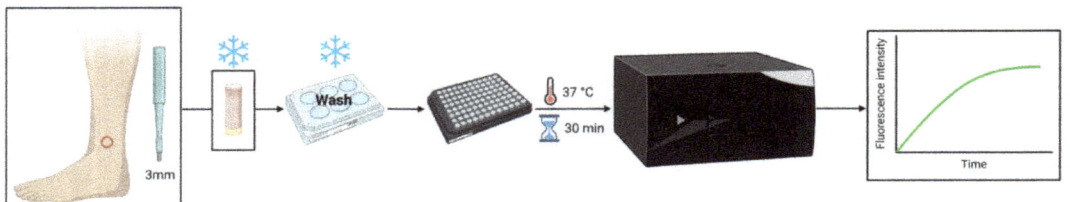

Figure 5. Thrombin activity in human skin—method flow diagram: For measuring thrombin activity in human skin, a 3 mm punch was obtained from the leg (10 cm above the lateral malleolus) and transferred to −80 °C until the thrombin activity assay. The biopsy was thawed and washed 3 times for 5 min on ice. Following this, it was placed in a 96-well black plate and incubated at 37 °C for 30 min. After incubation, a specific thrombin substrate was added and the fluorescence intensity over time was measured. Created with BioRender.com (accessed on 25 November 2021).

Patients were classified according to small-fiber density counts, determined as SFN patients when the small-fiber density was severely reduced, i.e., indicating skin denervation (<5% percentile normalized per age, Figure 6A). In addition, we classified patients as "inflammatory" according to known autoimmune inflammatory disease or the presence of inflammatory markers (Table S1). Those without evidence of inflammation were classified as idiopathic. We found no correlation between thrombin activity and age when we analyzed measurements from all patients ($p = 0.2034$, Figure 6B). We found a significant correlation between thrombin activity and the percentile of IENFD in all studied patients ($p = 0.0356$, Figure 6C). However, when skin showed severe denervation (SFN), no correlation between thrombin activity and percentile was seen ($p = 0.6491$, Figure 6D). Patients with inflammatory disorders/markers showed lower thrombin activity in the skin compared with idiopathic patients (0.595 ± 0.09 and 1.08 ± 0.12 mU/mg, respectively $p = 0.0035$, Figure 6E).

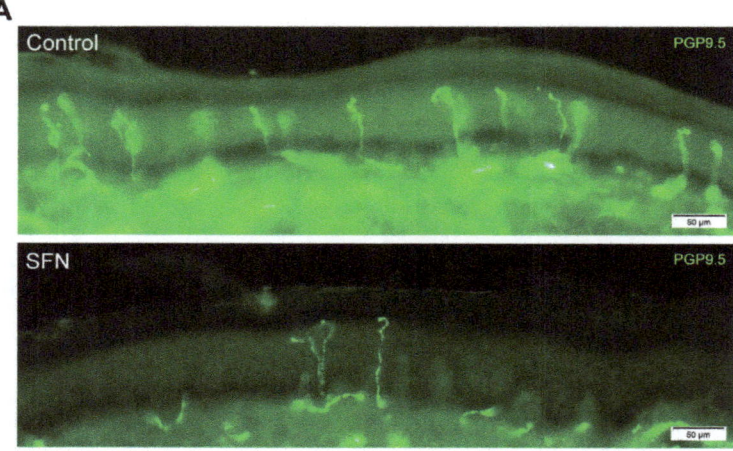

Figure 6. *Cont.*

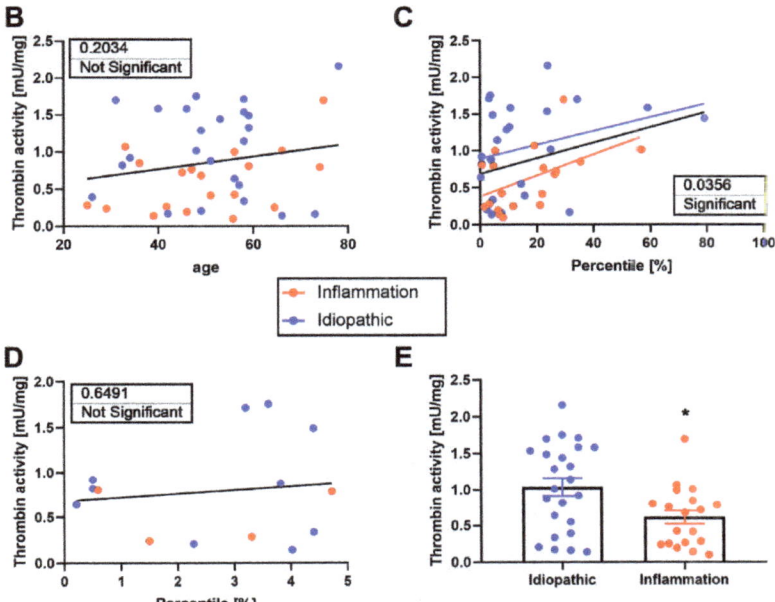

Figure 6. Thrombin activity in human skin: (**A**) Representative pictures of small-fiber staining of control (upper panel) and SFN (lower panel) patients. (**B**) No correlation was found between thrombin activity and age in all patients. $p = 0.2$, $R^2 = 0.04$, n = 43. (**C**) A significant correlation was found between thrombin activity and percentile in all patients. $p = 0.035$, $R^2 = 0.1$ for all patients; $p = 0.032$, $R^2 = 0.24$ for inflammation; and $p = 0.15$, $R^2 = 0.09$ for idiopathic. n = 43. (**D**) No correlation was found between thrombin activity and percentile in SFN patients. $p = 0.6$, $R^2 = 0.02$, n = 14. (**E**) Significantly increased thrombin activity was found in idiopathic patients (blue) compared with in inflammatory patients (red). n = 23 and 20, respectively. Results are presented as mean ± SEM, * $p = 0.0035$.

4. Discussion

In this study, we demonstrated intrinsic thrombin activity in the skin of rodents and humans for the first time. This activity was found to be correlated with the IENFD and modified by inflammation. We adapted our well-established method for thrombin activity measurement [18,23,24] by adding an incubation period to allow for the release of thrombin from the skin. We first demonstrated measurable thrombin activity in 3 mm biopsies from the glabrous skin of mice and rats. The specificity of the method was verified by adding SIXAC, a potent and specific thrombin inhibitor [19] that completely blocked the measurable thrombin activity. We found that rats have significantly higher thrombin activity in their skin in comparison with mice. H&E staining revealed that rats have a significantly thicker epidermis layer compared with mice, which is consistent with previous studies [25]. Thrombin activity in the skin may derive extrinsically from the blood or intrinsically from structures such as peripheral nerve and glial cells. Since in our hands, both mouse and rat biopsies contained undetectable levels of blood, we assume that the measured thrombin is mostly locally derived and released during the incubation period. In previously studied tissues, thrombin activity is locally produced by various neurons surrounding glia cells and its levels were modified in diseased states [24,26]. Analogously, in the skin, we assumed that thrombin activity is produced by neurons, glial cells, or local skin cells, which affects neural function. Both the dermis and epidermis contain nerve fibers that innervate the skin and its associated structures, such as sweat glands, hair follicles, and Meissner and Pacinian corpuscles [27]. In addition, we showed significantly higher IENFD in rat skin compared with in mouse skin, which is consistent with previous studies [28,29]. This may well explain the higher thrombin activity we found in the rat skin. The correlation between IENFD and thrombin activity was also currently demonstrated in normal human skin samples. It is thus suggested that in normal skin samples, the basal thrombin activity is correlated with small-fiber density and may serve as an alternative biomarker for relative denervation.

The link between inflammation and neuropathy is well established [30]; therefore, we tested thrombin activity using our novel method in two mice models of adjuvant-induced focal and LPS-induced systemic inflammation. We hypothesized that both focal and systemic inflammation cause peripheral neuronal damage, including to the small-fibers in the skin and, therefore, affect thrombin activity levels in the skin. We evaluated the functional neuronal damage using the hot-plate test [17]. In the adjuvant-induced model, we found significantly increased heat sensitivity one week, but not one day, following adjuvant injection. In contrast, significantly elevated thrombin activity was measured one-day post-adjuvant injection. followed by a significant but more modest increase one-week post-adjuvant injection. Moreover, one week following the adjuvant injection, the increase in thrombin activity was detected both in the injected foot skin and in the contralateral foot, which indicates that the focal inflammation spreads and becomes systemic over time, an interpretation supported by the increase in thrombin activity found in the systemic inflammatory LPS model. In contrast to the findings in the adjuvant focal inflammation model, we found no changes in heat sensitivity in the LPS model. Despite this, we were able to measure significantly increased thrombin activity in the skin. This important observation in both models points out the high sensitivity of this novel method to detect pathological processes before they can be assessed by behavioral tests. It is also important to note that the increased thrombin activity in the skin of the adjuvant-injected mice model (focal inflammation) was more significant than the increase in the LPS mice model (systemic inflammation). This suggests a correlation between the increase in thrombin activity and the level of the damage. To eliminate the possibility that the variance between the models is due to the strains of mice we used, we examined basal thrombin activity in these strains and found no significant difference (Figure S1). Further experiments are needed to determine the source of the excess thrombin activity. This increased activity can be due to physical damage to neurons and glia, glial activation, or increased neural activity as a compensatory feedback mechanism for fiber loss in the skin [31]. The role of high thrombin levels in neuropathy is supported by studies demonstrating that the inhibition of thrombin in inflammatory diseases protects from neural deficits [10]. We have found that nerve crush leads to increased intrinsic thrombin activity in the nerve [24]. The results of the present study extend the association between thrombin activity and small-fiber neuropathy in the skin.

Human skin biopsies are obtained routinely for the diagnosis of SFN. Therefore, we extended our study by testing thrombin activity in human skin biopsies from patients with suspected SFN. It is complex to directly compare the human and rodent skin thrombin levels since the human samples were first frozen and subsequently thawed. Based on our previous study with frozen tissue [32], we can assume that the measurable activity is lower compared with the activity in fresh tissue. We analyzed the data from patients and found a significant correlation between nerve-fiber density and thrombin activity. We hypothesize that in normal conditions (above the 5th percentile), thrombin is secreted from neurons or the surrounding glia and is a marker for the normal activity of the fibers. Decreased fiber density is probably associated with both fewer nerve fibers and glia accompanied by lower thrombin activity. It is reasonable to speculate that the main factor determining thrombin activity is the density of nerve fibers innervating the skin. The exact levels of skin thrombin activity may also be determined by local disease processes such as inflammation. Patients with inflammatory conditions have significantly lower thrombin activity in the skin compared with idiopathic patients. It is interesting to note the opposite effect of inflammation on thrombin activity in the skin of mice (increased activity) compared with humans (decreased activity). In well-defined inflammatory models conducted in mice, we examined the effects in a relatively short period following inflammation induction (up to one week). In contrast, in humans, the time period consists of different progression stages. Patients' skin biopsies are usually collected weeks, months, and even years after inflammation occurs. Therefore, we assume that an initial increase in thrombin activity occurs at the start of inflammation (as measured in mice skin), which is then followed by skin molecular and structural changes causing decreased thrombin activity (as measured in human skin). In addition, it is important to note that the skin we examined in rodents is glabrous and that the human skin of patients is hairy. It is well known that these two types of skin have different structures [33] and possibly different thrombin activity patterns. Furthermore, rodent punches are relatively clean and contain mostly skin layers and, in some cases, muscle fibers. In contrast, the punches obtained from humans sometimes had blood and a significant fat layer. This adds additional variation between patients and may add further complexity to the results. Furthermore, our data indicate a low but significant correlation between thrombin activity and IENFD percentile in the inflammatory group but not in the idiopathic group. We suggest that these groups differ in their clinical features, with the inflammatory group being better defined while the idiopathic group has patients with a variety of medical issues in different stages. In the inflammatory group at this stage of disease, low IENFD correlates with low thrombin activity. In the idiopathic group, there are a number of severely affected patients with high thrombin activity, possibly indicating an ongoing pathogenic process. The low correlation coefficient may be due to additional important factors affecting the neural integrity in the skin such as the specific pathogenesis, time course of the disease, regeneration, and treatments.

In conclusion, we have established a new specific method for measuring thrombin activity in rodent and human skin. We found that this method is sensitive enough to detect changes in thrombin activity in systemic and focal inflammation. Furthermore, changes in skin thrombin activity following inflammation precede changes in symptoms, such as heat sensitivity. In addition, we demonstrate a significant correlation between human skin thrombin activity and small-fiber density. Furthermore, we found decreased thrombin activity in the skin of patients with inflammatory conditions compared with that of idiopathic patients. Skin thrombin activity is therefore a useful novel marker linked to both inflammation and nerve fiber density. The elevated skin thrombin activity levels also suggest thrombin as a marker and therapeutic target in inflammatory neuropathies.

Supplementary Materials: The following supporting information can be downloaded at: https://www.mdpi.com/article/10.3390/biomedicines10061461/s1, Table S1: List of diseases and inflammatory markers of patients with an inflammatory cause of neuropathy. Figure S1: Thrombin activity in the skin of ICR VS C57BL/6J mice.

Author Contributions: V.G.: Conceptualization, Methodology, Visualization, Investigation, and Writing—Original draft preparation. S.B.: Methodology, Investigation, and Writing—Reviewing and Editing. S.G.G.: Conceptualization, Writing—Original draft preparation, and Writing—Reviewing and Editing. O.G.: Conceptualization, and Writing—Reviewing and Editing. S.A.A.: Investigation. D.N.Z.: Data Curation. D.K.: Methodology and Investigation. A.D.: Supervision, and Writing—Reviewing and Editing. J.C.: Conceptualization, Supervision, and Writing—Reviewing and Editing. E.S.-S.: Conceptualization, Supervision, and Writing—Reviewing and Editing. All authors have read and agreed to the published version of the manuscript.

Funding: This research received no external funding.

Institutional Review Board Statement: The study experiments involving animals were approved by the Sheba Medical Center Committee on the Use and Care of Animals (permit No: 1085-17, 1000-15, 1191-19).

Informed Consent Statement: The study experiments involving humans were approved by the Chaim Sheba Medical Center Ethics Committee (6525-19-SMC). Informed consent was obtained from all subjects involved in the study.

Data Availability Statement: All data are attached in the "Non-published Material".

Acknowledgments: We acknowledge Ramona Aronovich for her technical support and assistance in the rat and mouse skin biopsy processes and sectioning.

Conflicts of Interest: The authors declare no conflict of interest.

References

1. Iba, T.; Levi, M.; Levy, J.H. Sepsis-Induced Coagulopathy and Disseminated Intravascular Coagulation. *Semin. Thromb. Hemost.* **2020**, *46*, 89–95. [CrossRef] [PubMed]
2. Adams, M.N.; Ramachandran, R.; Yau, M.-K.; Suen, J.Y.; Fairlie, D.P.; Hollenberg, M.D.; Hooper, J.D. Structure, Function and Pathophysiology of Protease Activated Receptors. *Pharmacol. Ther.* **2011**, *130*, 248–282. [CrossRef] [PubMed]
3. Zhu, W.-J.; Yamanaka, H.; Obata, K.; Dai, Y.; Kobayashi, K.; Kozai, T.; Tokunaga, A.; Noguchi, K. Expression of mRNA for Four Subtypes of the Proteinase-Activated Receptor in Rat Dorsal Root Ganglia. *Brain Res.* **2005**, *1041*, 205–211. [CrossRef] [PubMed]
4. Maggio, N.; Shavit, E.; Chapman, J.; Segal, M. Thrombin Induces Long-Term Potentiation of Reactivity to Afferent Stimulation and Facilitates Epileptic Seizures in Rat Hippocampal Slices: Toward Understanding the Functional Consequences of Cerebrovascular Insults. *J. Neurosci.* **2008**, *28*, 732–736. [CrossRef] [PubMed]
5. Dutta, D.J.; Woo, D.H.; Lee, P.R.; Pajevic, S.; Bukalo, O.; Huffman, W.C.; Wake, H.; Basser, P.J.; SheikhBahaei, S.; Lazarevic, V.; et al. Regulation of myelin structure and conduction velocity by perinodal astrocytes. *Proc. Natl. Acad. Sci. USA* **2018**, *115*, 11832–11837. [CrossRef] [PubMed]
6. de Almeida, V.H.; Monteiro, R.Q. Protease-Activated Receptor 1 (PAR1): A Promising Target for the Treatment of Glioblastoma? *Transl. Cancer Res.* **2016**, *5*, S1274–S1280. [CrossRef]
7. Krenzlin, H.; Lorenz, V.; Alessandri, B. The Involvement of Thrombin in the Pathogenesis of Glioblastoma. *J. Neurosci. Res.* **2017**, *95*, 2080–2085. [CrossRef]
8. Han, M.H.; Hwang, S.I.; Roy, D.B.; Lundgren, D.H.; Price, J.V.; Ousman, S.S.; Fernald, G.H.; Gerlitz, B.; Robinson, W.H.; Baranzini, S.E.; et al. Proteomic Analysis of Active Multiple Sclerosis Lesions Reveals Therapeutic Targets. *Nature* **2008**, *451*, 1076–1081. [CrossRef]
9. Shavit-Stein, E.; Aronovich, R.; Sylantiev, C.; Gofrit, S.G.; Chapman, J.; Dori, A. The Role of Thrombin in the Pathogenesis of Diabetic Neuropathy. *PLoS ONE* **2019**, *14*, 0219453. [CrossRef]
10. Shavit-Stein, E.; Aronovich, R.; Sylantiev, C.; Gera, O.; Gofrit, S.G.; Chapman, J.; Dori, A. Blocking Thrombin Significantly Ameliorates Experimental Autoimmune Neuritis. *Front. Neurol.* **2018**, *9*, 1139. [CrossRef]
11. Shavit-Stein, E.; Beilin, O.; Korczyn, A.D.; Sylantiev, C.; Aronovich, R.; Drory, V.E.; Gurwitz, D.; Horresh, I.; Bar-Shavit, R.; Peles, E.; et al. Thrombin Receptor PAR-1 on Myelin at the Node of Ranvier: A New Anatomy and Physiology of Conduction Block. *Brain* **2008**, *131*, 1113–1122. [CrossRef] [PubMed]
12. Ebrahimi, S.; Jaberi, N.; Avan, A.; Ryzhikov, M.; Keramati, M.R.; Parizadeh, M.R.; Hassanian, S.M. Role of Thrombin in the Pathogenesis of Central Nervous System Inflammatory Diseases. *J. Cell Physiol.* **2017**, *232*, 482–485. [CrossRef] [PubMed]
13. De Garavilla, L.; Vergnolle, N.; Young, S.H.; Ennes, H.; Steinhoff, M.; Ossovskaya, V.S.; D'Andrea, M.R.; Mayer, E.A.; Wallace, J.L.; Hollenberg, M.D.; et al. Agonists of Proteinase-Activated Receptor 1 Induce Plasma Extravasation by a Neurogenic Mechanism. *Br. J. Pharmacol.* **2001**, *133*, 975–987. [CrossRef] [PubMed]
14. Vellani, V.; Kinsey, A.M.; Prandini, M.; Hechtfischer, S.C.; Reeh, P.; Magherini, P.C.; Giacomoni, C.; McNaughton, P.A. Protease Activated Receptors 1 and 4 Sensitize TRPV1 in Nociceptive Neurones. *Mol. Pain* **2010**, *6*, 61. [CrossRef] [PubMed]
15. Hovaguimian, A.; Gibbons, C.H. Diagnosis and Treatment of Pain in Small-Fiber Neuropathy. *Curr. Pain Headache Rep.* **2011**, *15*, 193–200. [CrossRef]
16. Lauria, G.; Lombardi, R. Skin Biopsy: A New Tool for Diagnosing Peripheral Neuropathy. *Br. Med. J.* **2007**, *334*, 1159–1162. [CrossRef]
17. Malmberg, A.B.; Bannon, A.W. Models of Nociception: Hot-Plate, Tail-Flick, and Formalin Tests in Rodents. In *Current Protocols in Neuroscience*; John Wiley & Sons, Ltd.: Hoboken, NJ, USA, 2001; Volume 6, pp. 8.9.1–8.9.15.
18. Bushi, D.; Chapman, J.; Katzav, A.; Shavit-Stein, E.; Molshatzki, N.; Maggio, N.; Tanne, D. Quantitative Detection of Thrombin Activity in an Ischemic Stroke Model. *J. Mol. Neurosci.* **2013**, *51*, 844–850. [CrossRef]
19. Shavit-Stein, E.; Sheinberg, E.; Golderman, V.; Sharabi, S.; Wohl, A.; Gofrit, S.G.; Zivli, Z.; Shelestovich, N.; Last, D.; Guez, D.; et al. A Novel Compound Targeting Protease Receptor 1 Activators for the Treatment of Glioblastoma. *Front. Neurol.* **2018**, *9*, 1087. [CrossRef]
20. Schneider, C.A.; Rasband, W.S.; Eliceiri, K.W. NIH Image to ImageJ: 25 Years of Image Analysis. *Nature Methods* **2012**, *9*, 671–675. [CrossRef]
21. Lauria, G.; Hsieh, S.T.; Johansson, O.; Kennedy, W.R.; Leger, J.M.; Mellgren, S.I.; Nolano, M.; Merkies, I.S.J.; Polydefkis, M.; Smith, A.G.; et al. European Federation of Neurological Societies/Peripheral Nerve Society Guideline on the Use of Skin Biopsy in the Diagnosis of Small Fiber Neuropathy. Report of a Joint Task Force of the European Federation of Neurological Societies and the Peripheral Ner. *J. Peripher. Nerv. Syst.* **2010**, *15*, 79–92. [CrossRef]

22. Lauria, G.; Bakkers, M.; Schmitz, C.; Lombardi, R.; Penza, P.; Devigili, G.; Smith, A.G.; Hsieh, S.T.; Mellgren, S.I.; Umapathi, T.; et al. Intraepidermal Nerve Fiber Density at the Distal Leg: A Worldwide Normative Reference Study. *J. Peripher. Nerv. Syst.* **2010**, *15*, 202–207. [CrossRef] [PubMed]
23. Gerasimov, A.; Golderman, V.; Gofrit, S.; Aharoni, S.; Zohar, D.; Itsekson-Hayosh, Z.; Fay-Karmon, T.; Hassin-Baer, S.; Chapman, J.; Maggio, N.; et al. Markers for Neural Degeneration and Regeneration: Novel Highly Sensitive Methods for the Measurement of Thrombin and Activated Protein C in Human Cerebrospinal Fluid. *Neural Regen. Res.* **2021**, *16*, 2086–2092. [CrossRef] [PubMed]
24. Gera, O.; Shavit-Stein, E.; Bushi, D.; Harnof, S.; Shimon, M.B.; Weiss, R.; Golderman, V.; Dori, A.; Maggio, N.; Finegold, K.; et al. Thrombin and Protein C Pathway in Peripheral Nerve Schwann Cells. *Neuroscience* **2016**, *339*, 587–598. [CrossRef] [PubMed]
25. Hanson, J. The Histogenesis of the Epidermis in the Rat and Mouse. *J. Anat.* **1947**, *81*, 174–17497. [PubMed]
26. Shavit Stein, E.; ben Shimon, M.; Artan Furman, A.; Golderman, V.; Chapman, J.; Maggio, N. Thrombin Inhibition Reduces the Expression of Brain Inflammation Markers upon Systemic LPS Treatment. *Neural Plast.* **2018**, *2018*, 7692182. [CrossRef] [PubMed]
27. Cobo, R.; García-Piqueras, J.; Cobo, J.; Vega, J.A. The Human Cutaneous Sensory Corpuscles: An Update. *J. Clin. Med.* **2021**, *10*, 227. [CrossRef]
28. Shavit-Stein, E.; Gofrit, S.G.; Gayster, A.; Teldan, Y.; Ron, A.; Bandora, E.A.; Golderman, V.; Gera, O.; Harnof, S.; Chapman, J.; et al. Treatment of Diabetic Neuropathy with A Novel PAR1-Targeting Molecule. *Biomolecules* **2020**, *10*, 1552. [CrossRef] [PubMed]
29. Hsieh, C.H.; Jeng, S.F.; Lu, T.H.; Yang, J.C.S.; Hsieh, M.W.; Chen, Y.C.; Rau, C.S. Correlation between Skin Biopsy with Quantification of Intraepidermal Nerve Fiber and the Severity of Sciatic Nerve Traction Injury in Rats. *J. Trauma* **2009**, *66*, 737–742. [CrossRef] [PubMed]
30. Marchand, F.; Perretti, M.; McMahon, S.B. Role of the Immune System in Chronic Pain. *Nat. Rev. Neurosci.* **2005**, *6*, 521–532. [CrossRef] [PubMed]
31. Gera, O.; Shavit-Stein, E.; Chapman, J. The Effect of Neuronal Activity on Glial Thrombin Generation. *J. Mol. Neurosci.* **2019**, *67*, 589–594. [CrossRef] [PubMed]
32. Reuveni, G.; Golderman, V.; Shavit-Stein, E.; Rosman, Y.; Shrot, S.; Chapman, J.; Harnof, S. Measuring Thrombin Activity in Frozen Brain Tissue. *NeuroReport* **2017**, *28*, 1176–1179. [CrossRef] [PubMed]
33. Mcglone, F.; Olausson, H.; Boyle, J.A.; Jones-Gotman, M.; Dancer, C.; Guest, S.; Essick, G. Touching and Feeling: Differences in Pleasant Touch Processing between Glabrous and Hairy Skin in Humans. *Eur. J. Neurosci.* **2012**, *35*, 1782–1788. [CrossRef] [PubMed]

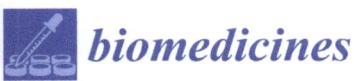

Article

Cerebrospinal Fluid in Classical Trigeminal Neuralgia: An Exploratory Study on Candidate Biomarkers

Teodor Svedung Wettervik [1,*], Dick Folkvaljon [1], Torsten Gordh [2], Eva Freyhult [3], Kim Kultima [4], Hans Ericson [1] and Sami Abu Hamdeh [1]

1. Department of Medical Sciences, Section of Neurosurgery, Uppsala University, SE-751 85 Uppsala, Sweden; d.folkvaljon@gmail.com (D.F.); hans.ericson@akademiska.se (H.E.); sami.abu.hamdeh@neuro.uu.se (S.A.H.)
2. Department of Surgical Sciences, Pain Research, Anesthesiology and Intensive Care, Uppsala University, SE-751 85 Uppsala, Sweden; torsten.gordh@surgsci.uu.se
3. Department of Cell and Molecular Biology, Uppsala University, 75124 Uppsala. Sweden; eva.freyhult@icm.uu.se
4. Department of Medical Sciences, Chemical Chemistry, Uppsala University, SE-751 85 Uppsala, Sweden; kim.kultima@medsci.uu.se
* Correspondence: teodor.svedung-wettervik@neuro.uu.se; Tel.: +46-18-558669

Abstract: Abstract: Background Trigeminal neuralgia (TN) is a severe type of facial pain. A neurovascular conflict between cranial nerve V and a nearby vessel is the main pathophysiological mechanism, but additional factors are likely necessary to elicit TN. In this study, the primary aim was to explore differences in protein expression in the cerebrospinal fluid (CSF) of TN patients in relation to controls. **Methods:** Sixteen TN patients treated with microvascular decompression and 16 control patients undergoing spinal anesthesia for urological conditions were included. Lumbar CSF was collected preoperatively for the TN patients and before spinal anesthesia for the controls. A multiplexed proximity extension analysis of 91 CSF proteins was conducted using Proseek Multiplex Development 96, including biomarkers of cell communication, cell death, neurogenesis, and inflammation **Results:** The TN patients and the controls were of similar age, sex, and burden of co-morbidities. The TN patients exhibited higher concentrations of Clec11a, LGMN, MFG-E8, and ANGPTL-4 in CSF than the controls (q < 0.05). **Conclusions:** TN patients exhibited increased CSF biomarkers indicative of peripheral demyelinating injury (Clec11a), immune tolerance and destruction of myelin (LGMN), neuronal cell death (MFG-E8), and disturbances in myelin clearance (ANGPTL-8). Our findings are hypothesis-generating for candidate biomarkers and pathophysiological processes in classical TN.

Keywords: cerebrospinal fluid; demyelination; neuroinflammation; trigeminal neuralgia

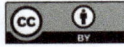

1. Introduction

Trigeminal neuralgia (TN) is characterized by brief and intense episodes of sharp facial pain, usually located in the V2/V3 dermatome of the trigeminal nerve (CN V) [1]. The estimated prevalence is between 0.1–0.3% [2,3] and the disease causes severe suffering for these patients with a significant reduction in the quality of life [4]. Classical TN has typically been attributed to a neurovascular conflict (NVC) between a cerebral vessel (most often the superior cerebellar artery) and CN V at the root entry zone (REZ) [5]. The NVC may induce dislocation, demyelination, and atrophy of CN V [6]. According to the ignition hypothesis, the injured, demyelinated CN V is susceptible to ephaptic transmission of innocuous somatosensory stimuli, which activate pain fibers and elicit severe facial pain in the corresponding nerve territory [6]. Still, it is evident that not all patients with NVC develop TN, since a simple neurovascular contact is also frequent in many asymptomatic cases [7,8]. It usually requires a pronounced NVC with additional morphological CN V changes such as distortion, dislocation, and atrophy, to develop classical TN [7,9]. However, it is likely that also other mechanisms than the mechanical, anatomical conflict are important in TN pathophysiology. For example, gene-related differences of the sodium channels of the axonal membrane influence their nerve transmission and affect the susceptibility to develop TN [10]. Furthermore, we recently found that TN patients exhibited elevated biomarkers of neuroinflammation and cell death in the cerebrospinal fluid (CSF) compared with controls, which normalized to the concentrations of controls after microvascular decompression (MVD) [11,12]. MVD is a surgical procedure that targets the NVC by dissecting CN V from the conflicting vessel and placing a material (e.g., Teflon) to reduce the risk of NVC recurrence, in medically refractory TN patients with radiological evidence of an NVC [13]. The role of neuroinflammation in classical TN is particularly interesting, since TN is also frequent in patients with the neuroinflammatory disease multiple sclerosis (MS) [1]. Although classical TN and MS-related TN are two distinct entities, they may share similar disease processes such as neuroinflammation, demyelination, and atrophy.

In the current study, the primary aim was to further explore potential pathophysiological mechanisms in classical TN by CSF analyses of protein biomarkers using the Proseek Multiplex Development 96 panel (Olink Bioscience, Uppsala, Sweden). The main findings were that TN patients exhibited elevated CSF biomarkers of neuroinflammation and neuronal injury.

2. Materials and Methods

2.1. Patients and Study Design

In this prospective observational study, patients referred to the Department of Neurosurgery at Uppsala University Hospital, who fulfilled the criteria for classical TN, according to the beta version of the International Classification of Headache disorders, third edition [14], and were candidates for surgical treatment with MVD between 2015 and 2017 were eligible for the study. The lumbar CSF of the TN patients was analyzed in relation to an aged-matched control group of 16 patients undergoing minor urological surgery under spinal anesthesia (University Hospital, Cluj, Romania).

2.2. CSF Collection

In the TN group, CSF was collected from the day before surgery by lumbar puncture without anesthesia. In the control group of urological patients, the lumbar CSF sample was collected by free flow into a sterile tube before the spinal anesthesia was administered. The CSF samples from both groups were handled according to the same protocol and were stored in a $-70\ °C$ freezer in both groups. The CSF samples from Cluj, Romania, were shipped to Uppsala, Sweden, by professional cargo, and kept frozen at $-70\ °C$ during delivery.

2.3. Proximity Extension Analysis

Multiplexed proximity extension analysis (PEA) was conducted using Proseek Multiplex Development 96 including 92 protein biomarkers. The Development panel analyzed a different subset of biomarkers as compared to the Inflammation panel that was used in a previous study by our group [12]. The current biomarker panel included a wide array of biological processes such as cell communication, cell death, neurogenesis, and inflammation (Supplementary Table S1). The protein biomarker neurofascin was excluded due to technical issues with the analysis. The PEA is a technique to analyze multiple biomarkers simultaneously, requires only a small sample volume (μL), and carries a high sensitivity and specificity. The proteins are reported in arbitrary units as normalized protein expression (NPX).

The procedure has been described in detail in a previous study by our group [12]. One μL CSF serum was mixed with a 3-μL incubation mix and incubated at $8\ °C$ overnight. A 96-mL extension mix based on PEA enzyme and PCR reagents were added, incubated for 5 min at room temperature, and the plate was then transferred to a thermal cycler for an extension reaction followed by 17 cycles of DNA amplification. A 96.96 Dynamic Array IFC (Fluidigm, South San Francisco, FL, CA) was prepared and primed. In a new plate, a

2.7 µL of sample mixture was mixed with a 7.2-µL detection mix, from which 5 µL was loaded into the right side of the primed 96.96 Dynamic Array IFC.

Five µL of the primer pairs were loaded into the left side of the 96.96 Dynamic Array IFC, and the protein expression program was run in a Fluidigm Biomark reader.

2.4. Statistical Analysis

The primary aim of this study was to explore potential CSF biomarkers in TN in relation to a control group. The categorical and ordinal/continuous variables were presented as numbers (proportions) and medians (interquartile range (IQR)), respectively. Differences in demographic variables between the TN patients and the controls were assessed with the Chi-square or Mann–Whitney U-test, depending on the type of data. A principal component analysis (PCA) was performed to investigate if there were global differences between TN and controls. Only biomarkers with less than 20% missing values were included.

Differences in CSF biomarker concentrations between TN and controls were assessed with linear regression analyses for each biomarker, adjusting for age and sex. To account for multiple comparisons, the false-discovery rate (FDR; Benjamini–Hochberg; q-values) procedure was used. Only biomarkers with a q-value < 0.05 were considered statistically significant. Furthermore, a multivariate partial least squares discriminant analysis (PLS-DA) classification model was trained to investigate if biomarker concentrations can be used to distinguish between TN and controls. Only biomarkers with less than 20% missing values were included in the model. The predictive ability of the PLS-DA models was evaluated by 10 5-fold cross-validations. The variable importance (VIP) was reported for the analyzed biomarkers.

2.5. Ethics

The study was conducted in accordance with the Helsinki declaration and its later amendments. The study was approved by the Regional Research Ethics Committee in Uppsala (Approval number 2014-178, date: 24 June 2014) for the TN patients and by the Institutional ethics committee of University of Medicine and Pharmacy, Cluj-Napoca, Romania (Approval number: Not applicable for this committee. Date: 20 May 2010) for the controls. Written informed consent was obtained by all study participants.

3. Results

Patients

Demographic details of the TN patients and the controls are described in Table 1. The TN patients and the controls were of a similar age (median 66 (IQR 55–69) vs. 67 (IQR 52–72) years) and female/male ratio (7/9 (44/56%) vs. 6/10 (38/63%)). Both groups also exhibited similar body mass index (BMI) and American Society of Anesthesiologist (ASA) grade.

Table 1. Demographic data in TN patients and controls.

Variables	TN	Controls	p-Value
Patients, n	16	16	
Age (years), median (IQR)	66 (55–69)	67 (52–72)	1.00
Sex (female/male), n (%)	7/9 (44/56%)	6/10 (38/63%)	0.72
BMI, median (IQR)	28 (24–31)	23 (24–31)	0.93
Tobacco use, n (%)	4 (25%)	8 (50%)	0.14
Hypertension, n (%)	8 (50%)	9 (56%)	0.72
Cardiovascular morbidity, n (%)	2 (13%)	5 (31%)	0.22
Ischemic heart disease, n (%)	1 (6%)	3 (19%)	
Stroke, n (%)	1 (6%)	1 (6%)	
Peripheral, n (%)	0 (0%)	1 (6%)	
Diabetes mellitus, n (%)	0 (0%)	3 (19%)	0.07
Pain other than TN, n (%)	4 (25%)	5 (31%)	0.69
Fibromyalgia, n (%)	1 (6%)	0 (0%)	

Table 1. *Cont.*

Variables	TN	Controls	*p*-Value
Osteoarthtritis, n (%)	2 (13%)	2 (13%)	
Lower back pain, n (%)	1 (6%)	2 (13%)	
Rheumatoid arthritis, n (%)	1 (6%)	1 (6%)	
ASA grade			0.83
1, n (%)	2 (13%)	2 (13%)	
2, n (%)	13 (81%)	12 (75%)	
3, n (%)	1 (6%)	2 (13%)	

Lumbar CSF—in TN patients and controls.

Of the 91 biomarkers measured using Proseek Multiplex Development 96, 20 were excluded from the analyses since more than 20% of the patients had missing values (under the limit of detection).

The PCA analysis of the CSF biomarker concentrations showed no clear differences between TN patients and controls (Figure 1).

The PCA analysis (Figure 1A) and the corresponding loadings (Figure 1B) of the CSF biomarker concentrations showed no clear differences between TN patients and controls.

To investigate if biomarker concentrations differed between TN patients and controls, a linear regression analysis was performed, adjusted for age and sex (Supplementary Table S2). Out of the 71 CSF biomarkers, four were significantly (q < 0.05) elevated in the TN patients (Table 2). These CSF biomarkers were Clec11a, LGMN, MFG-E8, and ANGPTL-4. None of the remaining 67 showed any tendency to differ between TN and controls.

Table 2. Differences in spinal CSF biomarker concentrations between TN patients and controls.

Biomarker	Coefficient	*p* (lm)	q (lm)
Clec11a	0.85	5.46×10^{-5}	0.0037
LGMN	0.59	0.00015	0.0037
MFG-E8	0.79	0.00016	0.0037
ANGPTL-4	0.60	0.00097	0.017

The table demonstrates the significant CSF biomarkers that differed between TN patients and controls. Each biomarker was analyzed using linear regression, adjusting for age and sex. The first column is the regression coefficient (positive value if higher biomarker concentration in the TN group), second column is the p- and third column contain q-values (FDR (Benjamini–Hochberg) adjusted *p*-values). Only proteins that were significant at the 5% FDR level are included in the table.

A PLS-DA model was trained to separate between TN and controls (Figure 2). The model showed good performance (mean error rate = 0.058) in separating between the two groups as evaluated in the cross-validation procedure.

The four most important proteins in the model all had a mean VIP score >1.5 (Figure 3), and were the same proteins (LGMN, Clec11a, MFG-E8, and ANGPTL-4) as found significantly elevated in the linear models.

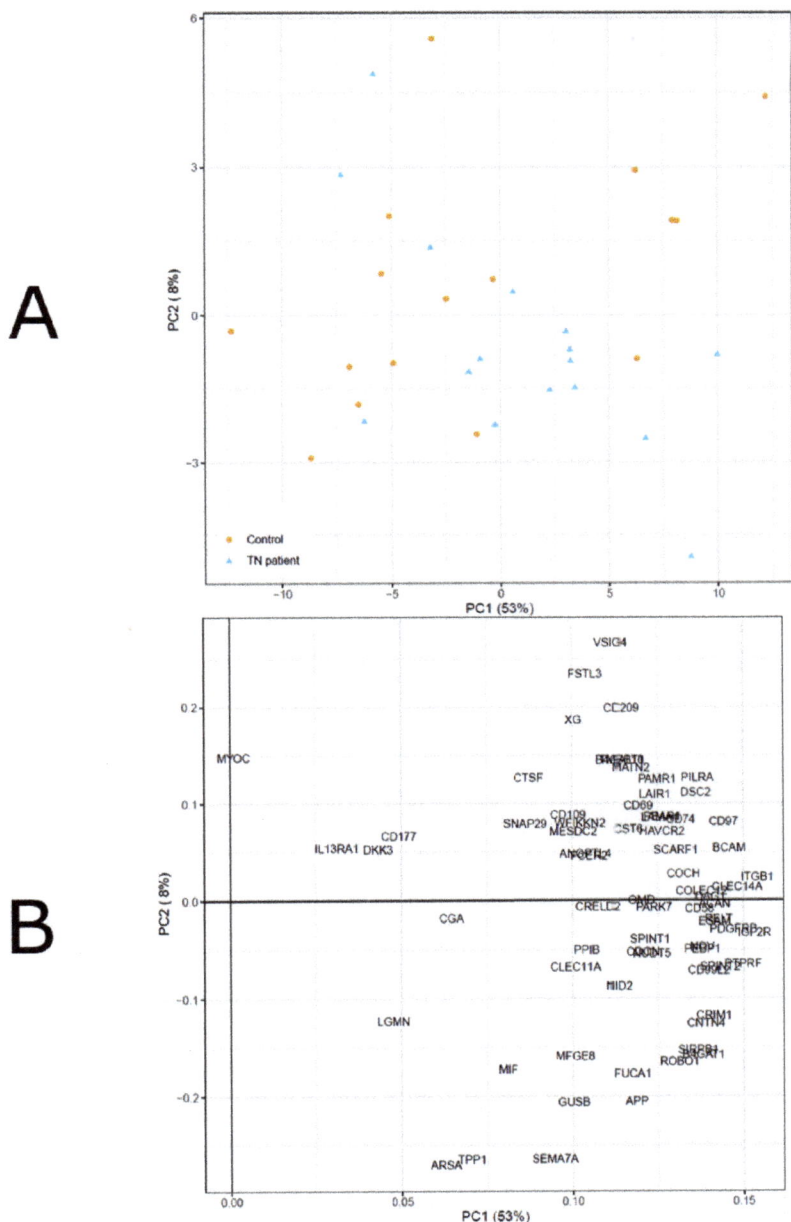

Figure 1. (**A**,**B**). CSF biomarkers in TN patients and controls—a PCA analysis.

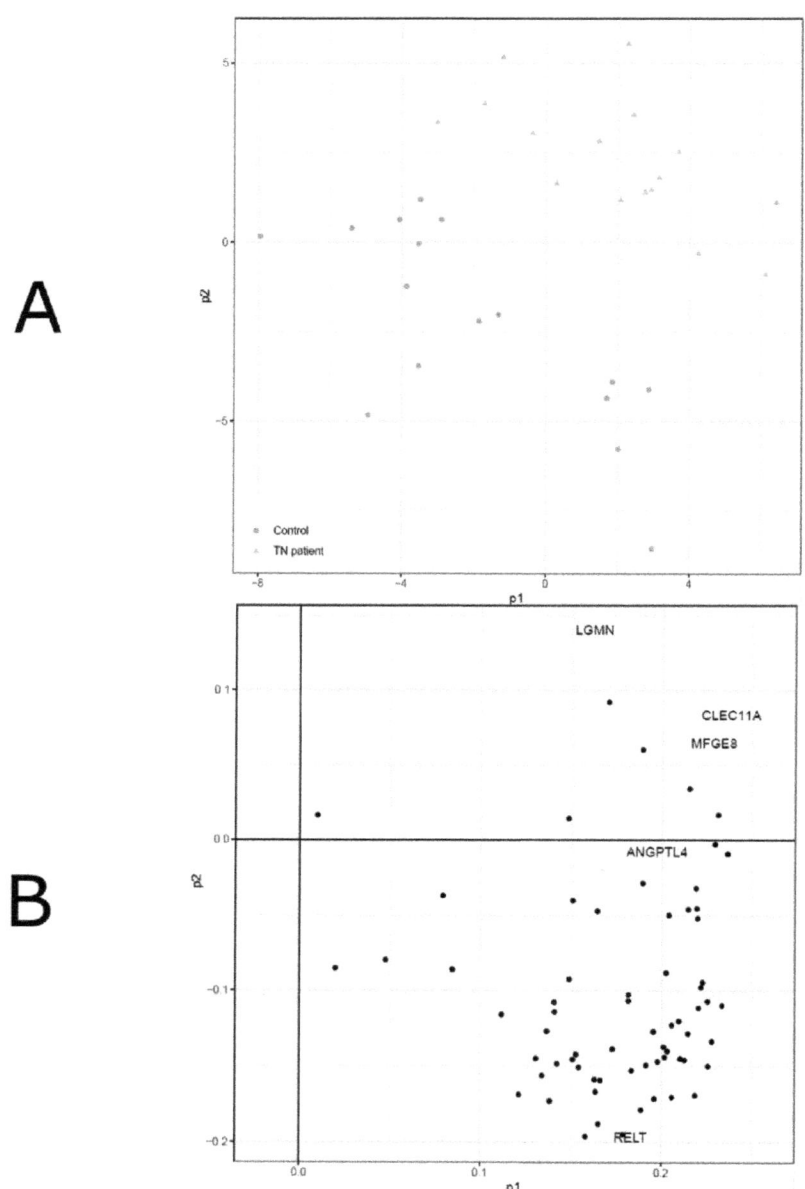

Figure 2. (**A**,**B**). CSF biomarkers in TN patients and controls—a PLS-DA analysis. A PLS-DA model (2A) and the corresponding loadings (2B) of CSF biomarkers in TN patients and controls are demonstrated. The model was trained to separate between TN and controls. The model showed good performance (mean error rate = 0.058) in separating between the two groups as evaluated in the cross-validation procedure. In the loadings plot, all proteins with VIP > 1.3 are named, and the remaining proteins are only shown as dots.

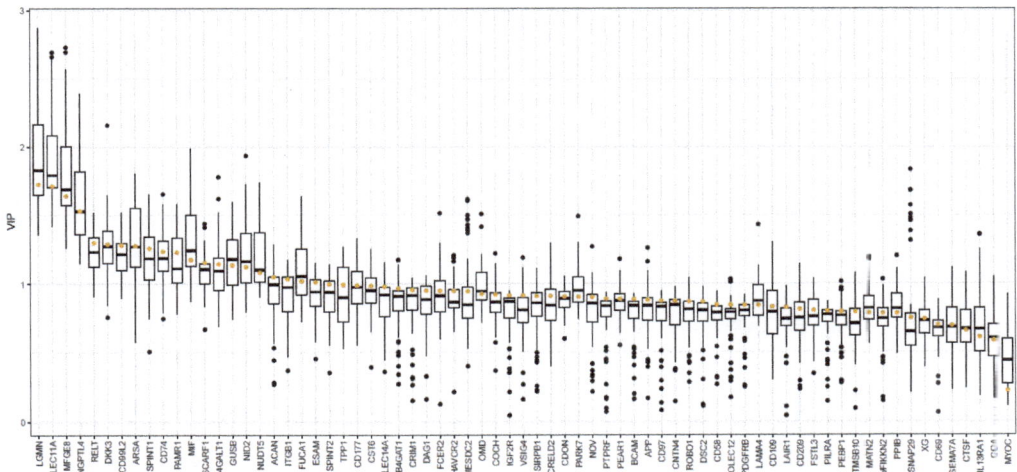

Figure 3. CSF biomarkers in TN patients and controls—a PLS-DA VIP analysis. The figure demonstrates the VIP values for clinical and biomarker variables in the PLS-DA model predicting patient or control CSF samples based on PEA data. The yellow dots represent the VIP for the full model (based on all data). The boxplots represent the VIP for the cross-validated models.

Figure 4 demonstrates differences in concentration of these four proteins between TN patients and controls.

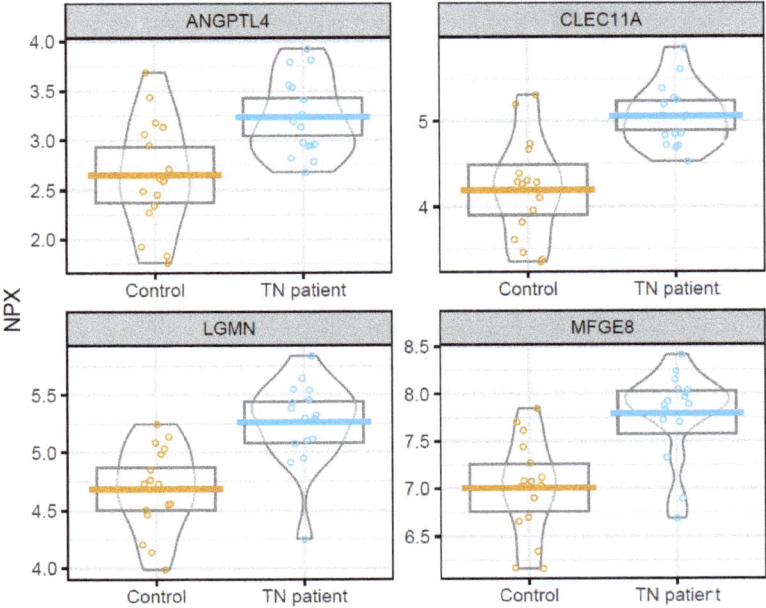

Figure 4. Elevated CSF biomarkers in TN patients. The figure demonstrates boxplots of ANGPTL-4, Clec11a, LGMN, and MFG-E8 in TN patients and controls.

4. Discussion

In this exploratory study of CSF biomarkers, we found that TN patients exhibited different protein concentration profiles as compared to controls. Particularly, Clec11a, LGMN, MFG-E8, and ANGPTL-4 were significantly higher in CSF in TN patients. These biomarkers are involved in neuroinflammation and myelin turnover and may reflect the demyelination and nerve atrophy that is commonly seen in TN.

Clec11a is generally known as a glycoprotein involved in hematopoiesis and osteoblast maturation [15]. There is a paucity of studies on Clec11a in CNS disorders. However, it seems that the CSF content of Clec11a is elevated in chronic inflammatory demyelinating disease (CIDP) compared to both MS and neurological conditions not primarily characterized by neuroinflammation [16]. The authors hypothesized that, considering the connection between Clec11a and hematopoiesis, Clec11a might particularly drive inflammation in peripheral nerves. This is interesting since the NVC in classical TN is located in the REZ and may affect both the central and peripheral component of the nerve. Elevated Clec11a in TN might hence reflect inflammatory injury to the peripheral part of CN V. Furthermore, in a study by Stein et al., blood levels of Clec11 gradually increased with time in patients with chronic spinal cord injury, possibly reflecting chronic nerve degeneration [17]. Altogether, Clec11a may reflect chronic CN V demyelination and nerve degeneration.

LGMN, also known as osteolectin, is a protease located in the endoplasmatic reticulum, golgi apparatus, and the lysosome. In pathological conditions, it may be translocated to the cytosol and extracellular compartment [18]. One major function is to regulate the lysosomal processing of proteins that are ultimately presented at the major histocompatibility complex II (MHC-II). Particularly, increased LGMN is associated with increased degradation of myelin based protein (MBP) in antigen-presenting immune cells. This can predispose for decreased MBP immune tolerance, leading to increased autoimmune T-cell activity and destruction of MBP [19]. Increased LGMN has also been found in active and chronic lesions of white matter in humans, suggesting ongoing neuroinflammation [20]. Hence, elevated LGMN may reflect an increased propensity to develop immune reactions towards the myelin and could indicate ongoing inflammation in the white matter.

MFG-E8 is a multifunctional glycoprotein that is mainly present in lactating mammary glands, but also in many other organs such as the heart, lungs, vessels, and the brain [21]. One function of MFG-E8 is to enhance phagocytosis of apoptotic cells, which also has an anti-inflammatory effect since it reduces the pro-inflammatory signaling cascade. Previous studies suggest that MFG-E8 mediates phagocytic neuronal cell death during neuroinflammation [22] and higher MFG-E8 in the TN patients may hence reflect trigeminal degeneration. Furthermore, we have previously found that the tumor necrosis factor (TNF)-β is elevated in CSF in TN patients [12]. TNF-β is known to contribute to the development of tertiary lymphoid organs. We speculated if this reflects the development of arachnoiditis that is often seen in association with CN V in TN. Interestingly, MFG-E8 is produced by these tertiary lymphoid organs [23] and elevated MFG-E8 might possibly be a reflection of such arachnoiditis. However, it should also be mentioned that MFG-E8 may be neuroprotective in some CNS diseases. In Alzheimer's disease, MFG-E8 increases beta-amyloid clearance and, in cerebral ischemia, it ameliorates neuroinflammation [21,24]. In addition, another role for MFG-E8 is in vascular ageing, as it promotes the development of atherosclerosis [21]. Classical TN typically occurs in older patients and may be associated with vascular ageing and degeneration, as indicated by a higher MFG-E8.

ANGPTL-4 is a glycoprotein [25,26] that is involved in angiogenesis, lipid metabolism, and inflammation [27]. Particularly in CNS diseases, increased ANGPTL-4 reduces macrophage and microglia clearance of damaged myelin [28,29]. In MS, ANGPTL-4 is reduced in active lesions, which is considered favorable since it increases clearance of damaged myelin and enhances remyelination and recovery [29]. Higher ANGPTL-4 in TN may therefore indicate disturbed myelin clearance with reduced chances of remyelination [30].

Altogether, our findings indicate increased neuroinflammation and disturbances in myelin turnover in TN. Particularly, many of these proteins have been studied in MS. This is interesting considering the relatively high burden of TN in MS patients.[1] Although TN is usually explained by demyelinating lesions of the trigeminal pathways in the pons in MS, an NVC at the REZ is occasionally present and has even been suggested to drive demyelination in some of these MS patients [31,32]. Hence, despite the fact that patients with classical and MS-related TN are considered two distinct disease entities, they may exhibit both similar and different underlying pathophysiological mechanisms. Since NVC does not always lead to development of TN, additional factors may be necessary. Based on our findings, patients with classical TN exhibited CSF biomarkers indicative of decreased immune tolerance towards MBP, and these patients may have an increased propensity towards neuroinflammatory reactions of CN V. Similar to MS, there may also be increased neuroinflammatory phagocytosis leading to atrophy of CN V in TN. However, in contrast to MS, we also found that CSF biomarkers related to demyelination of the peripheral nervous system were elevated in the patients with classical TN. The TN patients also exhibited increased ANGPTL-4, suggesting a reduced capacity to clear damaged myelin. These findings are hypothesis-generating for potential pathophysiological pathways in classical TN and highlight candidate biomarkers that may be relevant for future research efforts.

Lastly, our findings should also be viewed in light of important contributions regarding CSF analyses in TN patients. Others have found increases in substance P, calcitonin gene-related peptide (CGRP), and vasoactive intestinal peptide (VIP) as well as reductions in β-endorphin, serotonin, and dopamine in CSF [33,34], reflecting additional neurochemical pathophysiological mechanisms of relevance in this disease.

Methodological Considerations

It is evident that NVC is not sufficient to elicit classical TN, and there is a need to elucidate further pathophysiological mechanisms. There is so far a paucity of studies assessing CSF biomarkers that may be involved in these processes [12]. This observational, prospective study is therefore an important exploratory contribution to this field. However, there are some limitations. The relatively low number of patients in both the TN and the control group increases the risk of false positive findings. At the same time, many of the studied proteins were functionally related and statistical methods were applied to adjust for multiple comparisons. We therefore think reasonably safe conclusions can be made. Furthermore, it is a challenge to select and obtain CSF from an appropriate control group. In this study, we chose to include individuals of similar age, sex, and health (ASA) who also awaited surgery, but for urological conditions and from another country (Sweden vs. Romania). The controls were chosen to mimic the pre-surgery situation experienced by the TN patients. However, we cannot exclude that factors that were not accounted for between the groups affected the results to some extent. Furthermore, CSF samples were handled according to the same protocol for both the TN and control patients, although some minor differences could have occurred. Another limitation is that we only included TN patients at a stage with medically refractory pain, which predisposed for the indication to proceed with MVD surgery. It is possible that a different biomarker pattern would occur at another stage of the disease.

5. Conclusions

TN patients exhibited increased CSF biomarkers indicative of peripheral demyelinating injury (Clec11a), immune tolerance and destruction of myelin (LGMN), neuronal cell death (MFG-E8), and disturbances in myelin clearance (ANGPTL-8). Our findings are hypothesis-generating for candidate biomarkers and pathophysiological processes in classical TN.

Supplementary Materials: The following supporting information can be downloaded at: https://www.mdpi.com/article/10.3390/biomedicines10050998/s1, Table S1: Analyzed CSF biomarkers with the Proseek Multiplex Development 96; Table S2: Differences in spinal CSF biomarker concentrations between TN patients and controls–the entire analysis.

Author Contributions: Conceptualization, H.E., S.A.H. and T.G.; methodology, H.E., S.A.H., K.K., E.F. and T.S.W.; software, K.K. and E.F.; formal analysis, K.K., E.F. and T.S.W.; resources, H.E.; data curation, H.E., K.K., E.F. and T.S.W.; writing—original draft preparation, T.S.W.; writing—review and editing, H.E., S.A.H., K.K., E.F., T.G. and D.F.; visualization, K.K. and E.F.; supervision, H.E. and S.A.H. All authors have read and agreed to the published version of the manuscript.

Funding: This research was funded by the Uppsala University Hospital.

Institutional Review Board Statement: The study was conducted in accordance with the Declaration of Helsinki, and approved the Regional Research Ethics Committee in Uppsala (Approval number 2014-178, date: 24 June 2014) for the TN patients and by the Institutional ethics committee of University of Medicine and Pharmacy, Cluj-Napoca, Romania (Approval number: Not applicable for this committee. Date: 20 May 2010) for the controls.

Informed Consent Statement: Informed consent was obtained from all subjects involved in the study.

Data Availability Statement: The data are available from the authors upon reasonable request.

Acknowledgments: We thank Marie Essermark for acquisition of clinical data and handling of CSF samples. We also thank Constantin Bodolea, Cluj Napoca, Romania, for valuable collaboration and collection of the control CSF samples.

Conflicts of Interest: The authors declare no conflict of interest. The funders had no role in the design of the study; in the collection, analyses, or interpretation of data; in the writing of the manuscript, or in the decision to publish the results.

References

1. Bendtsen, L.; Zakrzewska, J.M.; Heinskou, T.B.; Hodaie, M.; Leal, P.R.L.; Nurmikko, T.; Obermann, M.; Cruccu, G.; Maarbjerg, S. Advances in diagnosis, classification, pathophysiology, and management of trigeminal neuralgia. *Lancet Neurol.* **2020**, *19*, 784–796. [CrossRef]
2. Sjaastad, O.; Bakketeig, L.S. The rare, unilateral headaches. Vågå study of headache epidemiology. *J. Headache Pain* **2007**, *8*, 19–27. [CrossRef] [PubMed]
3. Mueller, D.; Obermann, M.; Yoon, M.S.; Poitz, F.; Hansen, N.; Slomke, M.A.; Dommes, P.; Gizewski, E.; Diener, H.C.; Katsarava, Z. Prevalence of trigeminal neuralgia and persistent idiopathic facial pain: A population-based study. *Cephalalgia Int. J. Headache* **2011**, *31*, 1542–1548. [CrossRef] [PubMed]
4. Tölle, T.; Dukes, E.; Sadosky, A. Patient burden of trigeminal neuralgia: Results from a cross-sectional survey of health state impairment and treatment patterns in six European countries. *Pain Pract. Off. J. World Inst. Pain* **2006**, *6*, 153–160. [CrossRef]
5. Thomas, K.L.; Vilensky, J.A. The anatomy of vascular compression in trigeminal neuralgia. *Clin. Anat.* **2014**, *27*, 89–93. [CrossRef]
6. Gambeta, E.; Chichorro, J.G.; Zamponi, G.W. Trigeminal neuralgia: An overview from pathophysiology to pharmacological treatments. *Mol. Pain* **2020**, *16*, 1744806920901890. [CrossRef]
7. Antonini, G.; Di Pasquale, A.; Cruccu, G.; Morino, S.; Romano, A.; Trasimeni, G.; Vanacore, N.; Bozzao, A. Magnetic resonance imaging contribution for diagnosing symptomatic neurovascular contact in classical trigeminal neuralgia: A blinded case-control study and meta-analysis. *Pain* **2014**, *155*, 1464–1471. [CrossRef]
8. Maarbjerg, S.; Di Stefano, G.; Bendtsen, L.; Cruccu, G. Trigeminal neuralgia - diagnosis and treatment. *Cephalalgia* **2017**, *37*, 648–657. [CrossRef]
9. Leal, P.R.; Barbier, C.; Hermier, M.; Souza, M.A.; Sindou, M. Atrophic changes in the trigeminal nerves of patients with trigeminal neuralgia due to neurovascular compression and their association with the severity of compression and clinical outcomes. *J. Neurosurg.* **2014**, *120*, 1484–1495. [CrossRef]
10. Smith, C.A.; Paskhover, B.; Mammis, A. Molecular mechanisms of trigeminal neuralgia: A systematic review. *Clin. Neurol. Neurosurg.* **2021**, *200*, 106397. [CrossRef]
11. Abu Hamdeh, S.; Khoonsari, P.E.; Shevchenko, G.; Gordh, T.; Ericson, H.; Kultima, K. Increased CSF Levels of Apolipoproteins and Complement Factors in Trigeminal Neuralgia Patients-In Depth Proteomic Analysis Using Mass Spectrometry. *J. Pain* **2020**, *21*, 1075–1084. [CrossRef] [PubMed]
12. Ericson, H.; Abu Hamdeh, S.; Freyhult, E.; Stiger, F.; Bäckryd, E.; Svenningsson, A.; Gordh, T.; Kultima, K. Cerebrospinal fluid biomarkers of inflammation in trigeminal neuralgia patients operated with microvascular decompression. *Pain* **2019**, *160*, 2603–2611. [CrossRef] [PubMed]
13. Jannetta, P.J.; McLaughlin, M.R.; Casey, K.F. Technique of microvascular decompression. Technical note. *Neurosurg. Focus* **2005**, *18*, E5. [CrossRef] [PubMed]
14. Headache Classification Committee of the International Headache Society (IHS). The International Classification of Headache Disorders, 3rd edition (beta version). *Cephalalgia Int. J. Headache* **2013**, *33*, 629–808. [CrossRef]

15. Wang, M.; Guo, J.; Zhang, L.; Kuek, V.; Xu, J.; Zou, J. Molecular structure, expression, and functional role of Clec11a in skeletal biology and cancers. *J. Cell. Physiol.* **2020**, *235*, 6357–6365. [CrossRef]
16. Bonin, S.; Zanotta, N.; Sartori, A.; Bratina, A.; Manganotti, P.; Trevisan, G.; Comar, M. Cerebrospinal Fluid Cytokine Expression Profile in Multiple Sclerosis and Chronic Inflammatory Demyelinating Polyneuropathy. *Immunol. Investig.* **2018**, *47*, 135–145. [CrossRef] [PubMed]
17. Stein, A.; Panjwani, A.; Sison, C.; Rosen, L.; Chugh, R.; Metz, C.; Bank, M.; Bloom, O. Pilot study: Elevated circulating levels of the proinflammatory cytokine macrophage migration inhibitory factor in patients with chronic spinal cord injury. *Arch. Phys. Med. Rehabil.* **2013**, *94*, 1498–1507. [CrossRef]
18. Dall, E.; Brandstetter, H. Structure and function of legumain in health and disease. *Biochimie* **2016**, *122*, 126–150. [CrossRef]
19. Manoury, B.; Mazzeo, D.; Fugger, L.; Viner, N.; Ponsford, M.; Streeter, H.; Mazza, G.; Wraith, D.C.; Watts, C. Destructive processing by asparagine endopeptidase limits presentation of a dominant T cell epitope in MBP. *Nat. Immunol.* **2002**, *3*, 169–174. [CrossRef]
20. Oveland, E.; Ahmad, I.; Lereim, R.R.; Kroksveen, A.C.; Barsnes, H.; Guldbrandsen, A.; Myhr, K.M.; Bø, L.; Berven, F.S.; Wergeland, S. Cuprizone and EAE mouse frontal cortex proteomics revealed proteins altered in multiple sclerosis. *Sci. Rep.* **2021**, *11*, 7174. [CrossRef]
21. Li, B.Z.; Zhang, H.Y.; Pan, H.F.; Ye, D.Q. Identification of MFG-E8 as a novel therapeutic target for diseases. *Expert Opin. Ther. Targets* **2013**, *17*, 1275–1285. [CrossRef] [PubMed]
22. Fricker, M.; Neher, J.J.; Zhao, J.W.; Théry, C.; Tolkovsky, A.M.; Brown, G.C. MFG-E8 mediates primary phagocytosis of viable neurons during neuroinflammation. *J. Neurosci. Off. J. Soc. Neurosci.* **2012**, *32*, 2657–2666. [CrossRef] [PubMed]
23. Krautler, N.J.; Kana, V.; Kranich, J.; Tian, Y.; Perera, D.; Lemm, D.; Schwarz, P.; Armulik, A.; Browning, J.L.; Tallquist, M.; et al. Follicular dendritic cells emerge from ubiquitous perivascular precursors. *Cell* **2012**, *150*, 194–206. [CrossRef] [PubMed]
24. Cheyuo, C.; Aziz, M.; Wang, P. Neurogenesis in Neurodegenerative Diseases: Role of MFG-E8. *Front. Neurosci.* **2019**, *13*, 569. [CrossRef] [PubMed]
25. Chakraborty, A.; Kamermans, A.; van Het Hof, B.; Castricum, K.; Aanhane, E.; van Horssen, J.; Thijssen, V.L.; Scheltens, P.; Teunissen, C.E.; Fontijn, R.D.; et al. Angiopoietin like-4 as a novel vascular mediator in capillary cerebral amyloid angiopathy. *Brain J. Neurol.* **2018**, *141*, 3377–3388. [CrossRef]
26. Guo, L.; Li, S.Y.; Ji, F.Y.; Zhao, Y.F.; Zhong, Y.; Lv, X.J.; Wu, X.L.; Qian, G.S. Role of Angptl4 in vascular permeability and inflammation. *Inflamm. Res. Off. J. Eur. Histamine Res. Soc.* **2014**, *63*, 13–22. [CrossRef]
27. Yang, J.; Song, Q.Y.; Niu, S.X.; Chen, H.J.; Petersen, R.B.; Zhang, Y.; Huang, K. Emerging roles of angiopoietin-like proteins in inflammation: Mechanisms and potential as pharmacological targets. *J. Cell. Physiol.* **2021**, *237*, 98–117. [CrossRef]
28. Martin, N.A.; Nawrocki, A.; Molnar, V.; Elkjaer, M.L.; Thygesen, E.K.; Palkovits, M.; Acs, P.; Sejbaek, T.; Nielsen, H.H.; Hegedus, Z.; et al. Orthologous proteins of experimental de- and remyelination are differentially regulated in the CSF proteome of multiple sclerosis subtypes. *PLoS ONE* **2018**, *13*, e0202530. [CrossRef]
29. Kamermans, A.; Rijnsburger, M.; Chakraborty, A.; van der Pol, S.; de Vries, H.E.; van Horssen, J. Reduced Angiopoietin-Like 4 Expression in Multiple Sclerosis Lesions Facilitates Lipid Uptake by Phagocytes via Modulation of Lipoprotein-Lipase Activity. *Front. Immunol.* **2019**, *10*, 950. [CrossRef]
30. Bruce, K.D.; Gorkhali, S.; Given, K.; Coates, A.M.; Boyle, K.E.; Macklin, W.B.; Eckel, R.H. Lipoprotein Lipase Is a Feature of Alternatively-Activated Microglia and May Facilitate Lipid Uptake in the CNS During Demyelination. *Front. Mol. Neurosci.* **2018**, *11*, 57. [CrossRef]
31. Montano, N.; Rapisarda, A.; Ioannoni, E.; Olivi, A. Microvascular decompression in patients with trigeminal neuralgia and multiple sclerosis: Results and analysis of possible prognostic factors. *Acta Neurol. Belg.* **2020**, *120*, 329–334. [CrossRef] [PubMed]
32. Cruccu, G.; Biasiotta, A.; Di Rezze, S.; Fiorelli, M.; Galeotti, F.; Innocenti, P.; Mameli, S.; Millefiorini, E.; Truini, A. Trigeminal neuralgia and pain related to multiple sclerosis. *Pain* **2009**, *143*, 186–191. [CrossRef] [PubMed]
33. Strittmatter, M.; Grauer, M.; Isenberg, E.; Hamann, G.; Fischer, C.; Hoffmann, K.H.; Blaes, F.; Schimrigk, K. Cerebrospinal fluid neuropeptides and monoaminergic transmitters in patients with trigeminal neuralgia. *Headache* **1997**, *37*, 211–216. [CrossRef] [PubMed]
34. Qin, Z.L.; Yang, L.Q.; Li, N.; Yue, J.N.; Wu, B.S.; Tang, Y.Z.; Guo, Y.N.; Lai, G.H.; Ni, J.X. Clinical study of cerebrospinal fluid neuropeptides in patients with primary trigeminal neuralgia. *Clin. Neurol. Neurosurg.* **2016**, *143*, 111–115. [CrossRef] [PubMed]

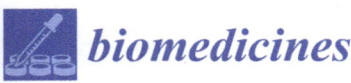

Review

The Role of miRNAs in Neuropathic Pain

Martina Morchio [1,2], Emanuele Sher [3], David A. Collier [3], Daniel W. Lambert [1,2] and Fiona M. Boissonade [1,2,*]

1. School of Clinical Dentistry, University of Sheffield, Sheffield S10 2TA, UK
2. The Neuroscience Institute, University of Sheffield, Sheffield S10 2TN, UK
3. UK Neuroscience Hub, Eli Lilly and Company, Bracknell RG12 1PU, UK
* Correspondence: f.boissonade@sheffield.ac.uk

Abstract: Neuropathic pain is a debilitating condition affecting around 8% of the adult population in the UK. The pathophysiology is complex and involves a wide range of processes, including alteration of neuronal excitability and synaptic transmission, dysregulated intracellular signalling and activation of pro-inflammatory immune and glial cells. In the past 15 years, multiple miRNAs–small non-coding RNA–have emerged as regulators of neuropathic pain development. They act by binding to target mRNAs and preventing the translation into proteins. Due to their short sequence (around 22 nucleotides in length), they can have hundreds of targets and regulate several pathways. Several studies on animal models have highlighted numerous miRNAs that play a role in neuropathic pain development at various stages of the nociceptive pathways, including neuronal excitability, synaptic transmission, intracellular signalling and communication with non-neuronal cells. Studies on animal models do not always translate in the clinic; fewer studies on miRNAs have been performed involving human subjects with neuropathic pain, with differing results depending on the specific aetiology underlying neuropathic pain. Further studies using human tissue and liquid samples (serum, plasma, saliva) will help highlight miRNAs that are relevant to neuropathic pain diagnosis or treatment, as biomarkers or potential drug targets.

Keywords: microRNA; chronic pain; neuropathic pain

1. Introduction

The perception of pain allows organisms to learn from noxious experiences and avoid harmful stimuli. It relies on the communication between neurons arising from the periphery of the body, which contain receptors specialised in sensing particular nociceptive inputs (chemical, mechanical, thermal), and neurons in the spinal cord, which relay the message to higher brain centres, where the signal can be processed and integrated with other sensory information. Impairment of this mechanism due to lesions to the somatosensory system results in a persistent perception of pain even in absence of painful stimuli. This condition is broadly termed neuropathic pain and includes chronic pain states caused by damage to nerves due to physical trauma and other conditions such as diabetes, cancer, herpes infection and multiple sclerosis. Currently, first-line treatments include tricyclic antidepressants, selective serotonin–noradrenaline reuptake inhibitors and calcium channel modulators (gabapentin and pregabalin); however, the efficacy is limited and varies considerably across patients, while side effects can be substantial [1,2].

Meanwhile, advances in the understanding of a class of regulatory short non-coding RNA molecules, known as microRNA (miRNA), have provided a new hope for treatment of various conditions including cancer, hepatitis C and cardiovascular diseases. Selected miRNA therapeutics are undergoing pre-clinical to phase II clinical trials [3], while the first small interfering RNA (siRNA) therapeutic received FDA approval in 2018 for the treatment of a rare polyneuropathy condition [4]. MicroRNAs are capable of inhibiting the translation of messenger RNA into proteins, inducing widespread changes in the proteome of a cell. In the past decade, increasing evidence of their role in neuropathic pain has

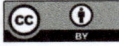

Citation: Morchio, M.; Sher, E.; Collier, D.A.; Lambert, D.W.; Boissonade, F.M. The Role of miRNAs in Neuropathic Pain. *Biomedicines* **2023**, *11*, 775. https://doi.org/10.3390/biomedicines11030775

Academic Editor: Mats Eriksson

Received: 13 January 2023
Revised: 27 February 2023
Accepted: 28 February 2023
Published: 3 March 2023

Copyright: © 2023 by the authors. Licensee MDPI, Basel, Switzerland. This article is an open access article distributed under the terms and conditions of the Creative Commons Attribution (CC BY) license (https://creativecommons.org/licenses/by/4.0/).

surfaced and has helped to identify molecular pathways and mechanisms important in the generation and persistence of chronic pain states [5,6].

The first evidence of a relationship between pain and microRNAs was found by Bai, et al. [7] in 2007, who identified seven dysregulated miRNAs following CFA injection in the masseter muscle of rats. The importance of miRNAs in inflammatory pain was shown in mice by Zhao, et al. [8] through the nociceptor-specific deletion of Dicer, an enzyme responsible for pre-miRNA cleavage into mature miRNA (Figure 1), which caused an attenuated response to CFA intraplanar injection compared to wild type. Several mRNA transcripts were found to be altered in the Dicer null mice, including pain-relevant molecules such as $Na_v1.7$, 1.8 and 1.9, and P2X3. Surprisingly, these transcripts were downregulated, suggesting that loss of miRNAs may lead to upregulation of transcriptional repressors which control the expression of these nociceptive genes [8].

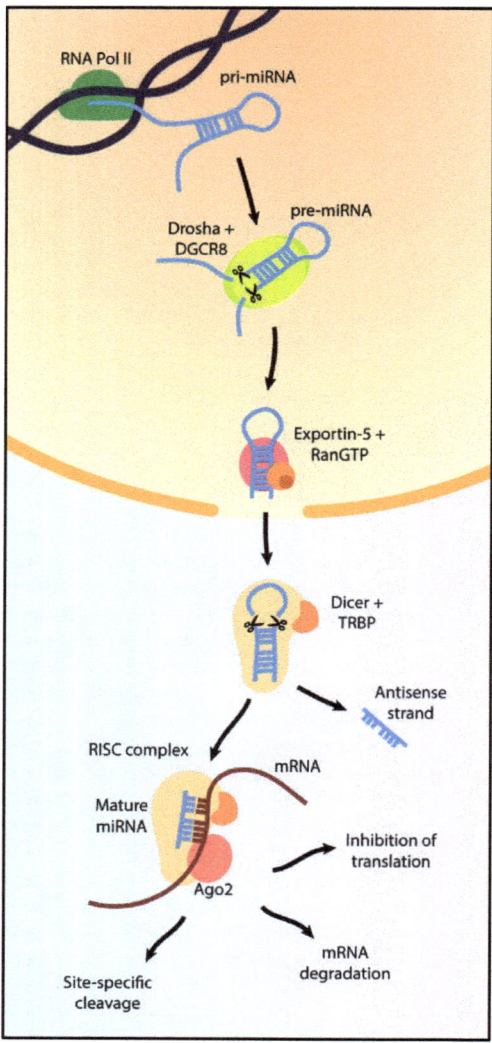

Figure 1. The canonical pathway of miRNA biogenesis.

Several miRNAs and their respective targets have been investigated in animal models of neuropathic pain during the past decade (Table 1). miRNA targets can be predicted using in silico models; however, experimental validation is necessary to prove the presence of interaction in biological systems and their physiological relevance. A target is deemed to be validated when (a) a reporter assay shows mRNA/miRNA interaction, (b) miRNA/mRNA co-expression is observed with RT-PCR (and possibly in situ hybridisation), (c) miRNA overexpression/knockdown has an effect on the target protein and its biological function [9].

Table 1. List of dysregulated miRNAs in various chronic pain animal models and the relevant validated targets. bCCI = bilateral CCI, BCP = bone cancer pain, CCI = chronic constriction injury, CIP = chemotherapy-induced pain, CIVP = chronic inflammatory visceral pain, DNP = diabetic neuropathic pain, DRG = dorsal root ganglion, iCCI = infraorbital CCI, pSNL = partial spinal nerve ligation, TG = trigeminal ganglion.

MicroRNA	Change	Injury Model	Localisation	Validated Target/s	Reference
miR-150 miR-20b	Down	CCI	DRG Spinal cord	AKT3	Cai, et al. [10] You, et al. [11]
miR-195	Up	SNL	Spinal microglia	ATG14	Shi, et al. [12]
miR-23	Up	SNI	DRG	A20	Zhang, et al. [13]
miR-142	Up	CCI	Sciatic nerve	AC9	Li, et al. [14]
miR-34c	Up	BCP	DRG	Cacna1e (Ca$_v$2.3)	Gandla, et al. [15]
miR-219 miR-103	Down Down	CFA SNL	Spinal cord Spinal cord	CAMKII Ca$_v$1.2	Pan, et al. [16] Favereaux, et al. [17]
miR-186-5p	Down	SNL	Spinal cord	CXCL13	Jiang, et al. [18]
miR-23a	Down	pSNL	Spinal cord	CXCR4	Pan, et al. [19]
miR-124	Down	SNL	Spinal cord and DRG	EGR1	Jiang, et al. [20]
miR-30a-5p	Down	CCI	Spinal cord	EP300	Tan, et al. [21]
miR-211	Down	CIVP	Spinal cord	ERK	Sun, et al. [22]
miR-124-3p	Down	CCI	Spinal cord	EZH2	Zhang, et al. [23]
miR-194	Down	CCI	Spinal cord	FOXA1	Zhang, et al. [24]
miR-500	Up	CIP	Spinal cord	GAD67	Huang, et al. [25]
miR-15a/16	Up	CCI	Spinal cord	GRK2	Li, et al. [26]
miR-129 miR-141 miR-142-3p miR-193 miR-381	Down	CCI CCI SNL DNP CCI	Spinal cord DRG DRG Spinal cord DRG	HMGB1	Ma, et al. [27] Zhang, et al. [28] Zhang, et al. [29] Wu, et al. [30] Xia, et al. [31]
miR-381	Down	CCI	Spinal cord	HMGB1, CXCR4	Zhan, et al. [32]
miR-124-3p	Down	CFA	Spinal cord	IL6R	Liu, et al. [33]
miR-146	Up	CCI	DRG, spinal cord	IRAK1, TRAF6	Wang, et al. [34]
miR-9 miR-29a	Up	DNP	Sciatic nerve	ISL1	Sun, et al. [35]
miR-124 miR-141	Down	CCI	Spinal cord	JAG1	Li, et al. [36]

Table 1. Cont.

MicroRNA	Change	Injury Model	Localisation	Validated Target/s	Reference
miR-17-92 cluster	Up	SNL	DRG	KCNA1, KCNA4, KCNC4, KCND3, KCNQ5, DPP10, SCN1B	Sakai, et al. [37]
miR-137a	Up	CCI	DRG, spinal cord	KCNA2	Zhang, et al. [38]
miR-216	Down	CCI	DRG, spinal cord	KDM3A	Wang and Li [39]
miR-152	Down	PNI	Spinal cord	MafB	Tozaki-Saitoh, et al. [40]
miR-26a	Down	CCI	Spinal cord	MAPK6	Zhang, et al. [41]
miR-223	Down	iCCI	TG	MKNK2	Huang, et al. [42]
miR-101	Up	CCI	Spinal cord and microglia	MKP4	Qiu, et al. [43]
miR-183	Down	CCI	Spinal cord	mTOR	Xie, et al. [44]
miR-125a-3p	Down	CFA	TG	p38 MAPK	Dong, et al. [45]
miR-195	Up	iCCI	Caudal medulla and CSF	Patched1	Wang, et al. [46]
miR-122	Down	CCI	Spinal cord	PDK4	Wan, et al. [47]
miR-1224	Down	CFA	Spinal cord	pre-circ-Filip1I	Pan, et al. [48]
miR-16	Up	CCI	Spinal cord	RAB23	Chen, et al. [49]
miR-202 miR-590	Down	bCCI DNP	Spinal cord DRG	RAP1A	Fang, et al. [50] Wu, et al. [51]
miR-144	Down	CCI	DRG	RASA1	Zhang, et al. [52]
miR-140	Down	CCI	DRG	S1PR1	Li, et al. [53]
miR-96 miR-384	Down	CCI	DRG	SCN3A	Chen, et al. [54] Ye, et al. [55]
miR-182 miR-30b	Down	CCI SNI	DRG	SCN9A	Jia, et al. [56] Cai, et al. [57] Shao, et al. [58]
miR-34 miR-448	Up	CFA CCI	Spinal cord	SIRT1	Chen, et al. [59] Chu, et al. [60]
miR-190a	Down	DNP	Spinal cord	SLC17A6, (VGLUT2)	Yang, et al. [61]
miR-135a	Up	CCI	Spinal cord	SLC24A2	Zhou, et al. [62]
miR-155 miR-221	Up	CCI	Spinal cord Spinal cord and microglia	SOCS1	Tan, et al. [63] Xia, et al. [64]
miR-218	Up	CCI	Spinal cord and microglia	SOCS3	Li and Zhao [65]
miR-93 miR-98 miR-544	Down	CCI	Spinal cord	STAT3	Yan, et al. [66] Zhong, et al. [67] Jin, et al. [68]
miR-124a	Down	BCP	Spinal cord	Synpo	Elramah, et al. [69]
miR-28	Down	CCI	Spinal cord	TF Zeb1	Bao, et al. [70]
miR-30c	Up	SNI	Spinal cord	TGFβ	Tramullas, et al. [71]
miR-451	Down	CFA	Spinal cord and microglia	TLR4	Sun and Zhang [72]
miR-154	Down	CCI	Spinal cord	TLR5	Wei, et al. [73]
miR-21	Up	SNL	DRG	TLR8	Zhang, et al. [74]

Table 1. *Cont.*

MicroRNA	Change	Injury Model	Localisation	Validated Target/s	Reference
miR-183	Down	CCI	DRG	TREK1	Shi, et al. [75]
miR-183	Down	CCI	Spinal cord	TXNIP	Miao, et al. [76]
miR-134	Down	CCI	Spinal cord	Twist1	Ji, et al. [77]
miR-34a	Down	CCI	DRG	VAMP2	Brandenburger, et al. [78]
miR-128	Down	CCI	Spinal cord and microglia	ZEB1	Zhang, et al. [79]
miR-150	Down	CCI	Spinal cord and microglia	Zeb1	Yan, et al. [80]
miR-206	Down	CCI	Spinal microglia	ZEB2	Chen, et al. [81]

The identified microRNAs and their putative targets belong to a wide variety of pain-relevant pathways that can be broadly classified into those related to neuronal excitability, intracellular signalling and interaction with non-neuronal cells. In this review, examples from each category will be presented. Another important question is how miRNAs are regulated themselves. The study of miRNAs involved in pain has contributed to our understanding of mechanisms underpinning modulation of miRNA levels, such as by sequestration in stress granules (assemblies of untranslated mRNA and RNA binding proteins formed in conditions of stress) and sponging by long non-coding RNA. Additionally, an alternative mode of action of miRNA, targeting proteins directly and causing their activation, will be presented in the context of pain. Finally, opportunities and difficulties relating to the application of miRNA therapeutics to the clinic will be discussed. Examples of miRNAs linked with chronic pain that have been identified in clinical human samples are shown in Table 2.

Table 2. List of studies on miRNA linked with chronic pain with a neuropathic component conducted on human samples. CRPS = complex regional pain syndrome, CiPN = chemotherapy-induced painful peripheral neuropathy, DN = diabetic neuropathy, PPN = painful peripheral neuropathy, sDSP = symptomatic distal sensory polyneuropathy, WBC = white blood cells.

Clinical Condition	Control	Sample Types	Significance	Reference
CiPN in patients with multiple myeloma	Myeloma patients without CiPN	Plasma	miR-22, -23a and -24a are clinically relevant biomarkers for CiPN.	Łuczkowska, et al. [82]
CRPS	Healthy	Whole blood	Exosomal miRNA signature is altered in CPRS patients.	McDonald, et al. [83] Orlova, et al. [84]
Diabetic neuropathy	Diabetic patients without neuropathy	WBCs	miR-128 is upregulated in diabetic neuropathy; miR-155 and -499 are downregulated.	Ciccacci, et al. [85]
Diabetic neuropathy	Healthy	Plasma and skin biopsy	miR-199-3p is increased in patients with DN and targets SERPINE2.	Li, et al. [86]
HIV-associated sDSP	Non-DSP and HIV	Plasma	Increased miR-455 expression is associated with reduced neurite growth.	Asahchop, et al. [87]

Table 2. *Cont.*

Clinical Condition	Control	Sample Types	Significance	Reference
Lingual nerve injury	Lingual nerve injury without pain	Neuroma	miR-29a and miR-500a are inversely correlated with clinical VAS scores.	Tavares-Ferreira, et al. [88]
Musculoskeletal pain	Healthy	Plasma	miR-320 and miR-98 successfully distinguish the origin of chronic pain in 70% of the patients.	Dayer, et al. [89]
Neuropathic pain of various origins	Healthy	Primary human CD4$^+$ T cells	Increased miR-124a and miR-155 levels promote Tregs differentiation.	Heyn, et al. [90]
Painful peripheral neuropathy	Painless peripheral neuropathy and healthy	WBCs and sural nerve biopsy	miR-132-3p is overexpressed in WBC and sural nerve of patients affected by peripheral neuropathies.	Leinders, et al. [91]
Painful peripheral neuropathy	Painless peripheral neuropathy and healthy	Plasma and sural nerve biopsy	miR-101 and -132 are altered in plasma and sural nerve of DN patients. miR-101 targets KPNB1.	Liu, et al. [92]
Painful peripheral neuropathy	Painless peripheral neuropathy and healthy	WBCs, sural nerve and skin biopsy	miR-21, -146 and -155 are differentially expressed in WBC, skin and sural nerve of patients affected by peripheral neuropathies.	Leinders, et al. [93]
Trigeminal neuralgia	Healthy	Serum	miR-132, -146, -155 and -384 are upregulated in patients with trigeminal neuralgia.	Li, et al. [94]
Neuropathic low back pain	Patients without neuropathic pain	Sinuvertebral nerve biopsy	TRPV1 upregulation is inversely correlated with miR-375 and -455 expression.	Li, et al. [95]

2. MicroRNA Biogenesis

MicroRNAs are transcribed by RNA Polymerase II—and occasionally by RNA Polymerase III—into a hairpin-like structure denominated primary miRNA (pri-miRNA) [96]. Drosha cleavage of the pri-miRNA leads to the formation of pre-miRNA, which is exported out of the nucleus via Ran-GTP and Exportin-5.

In the cytoplasm, Dicer, coupled with the RNA binding protein (TRBP), performs an additional cleavage at the loop terminal, resulting in the separation of a sense and antisense strand, which is commonly degraded. The resulting single strand of miRNA binds to AGO proteins, creating the RISC complex which is also stabilised by several other proteins including FMRP, R2D2 and the germin family.

Finally, the RISC complex binds to the 3′ UTR sequence of the target mRNA, preventing its translation [97]. The consensus sequence, named the "seed" region, is usually positioned between nucleotides 2 to 7 of the 5' end of the miRNA. Translational inhibition can occur in three ways: mRNA degradation, translational repression and site-specific cleavage [6].

Non canonical pathways have also been identified, including miRtrons, snoRNA and tRNA-derived miRNA, which are generated without Drosha cleavage, and miR-451, which is generated in a Dicer-independent way [98].

3. MicroRNA Involvement in Pain Pathways

Understanding the role of miRNAs in nociceptive pathways would contribute to a greater understanding of neuropathic pain development, enabling the identification of new druggable targets. Many studies have been performed in animal models to investigate the role of miRNAs and identify their targets in vivo. In this section, studies mostly from animal models will be discussed in the context of neuronal excitability, synaptic transmission, intracellular signalling and communication with non-neuronal cells. The potential of translating these studies to human disease will be discussed in Section 5, alongside additional findings regarding miRNAs relevant to pain from human tissues.

3.1. Neuronal Excitability

The transmission of information from the periphery of the body to the brain relies on the propagation of action potentials throughout the axon of sensory nerves. This is enabled by the presence of different classes of ion channels in the membrane that set the potential of a cell and allow the propagation of electrical impulses. MicroRNAs can alter the expression of ion channels, resulting in altered neuronal excitability and increased pain perception following nerve injury (Figure 2A).

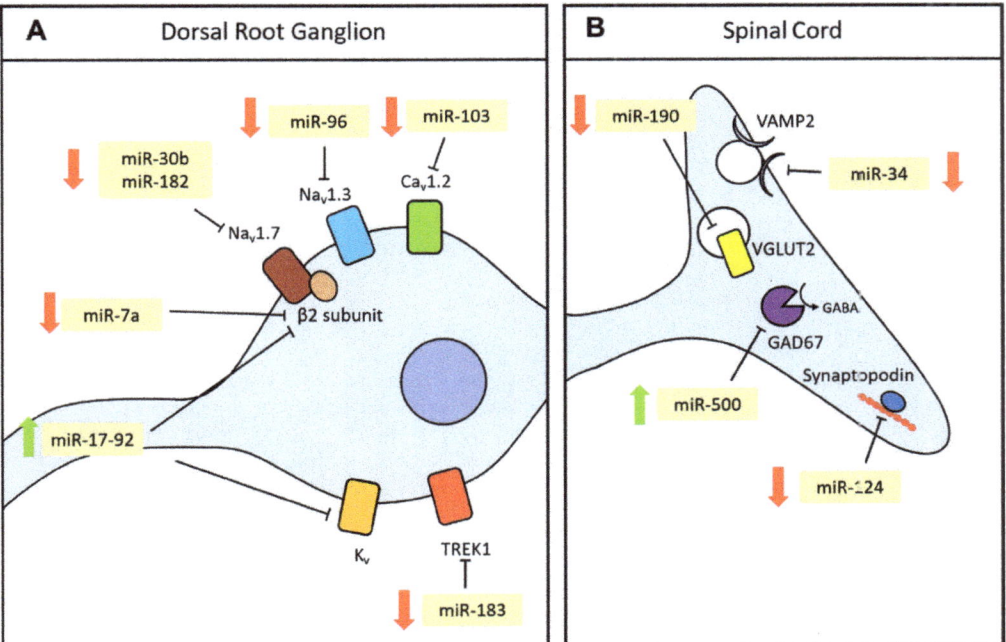

Figure 2. Diagram showing miRNAs dysregulated in neuropathic pain whose targets are directly involved in (**A**) cellular excitability and (**B**) synaptic transmission, verified in animal models. Red downward arrows indicate that the miRNA is downregulated during neuropathic pain, whilst upward green arrows indicate miRNA upregulation in neuropathic pain conditions.

Voltage-gated sodium channels (VGSC) allow the rapid inward entry of sodium ions that enable the generation and transmission of action potentials. They are located at the nodes of Ranvier on the axonal membrane and in DRGs. $Na_v1.7$, one of ten members of the VGSC family, was shown to be targeted by miR-30b and miR-182. These miRNAs are downregulated in the DRG following nerve injury, and, if administered intrathecally or injected in the DRG, respectively, they alleviate mechanical hypersensitivity [57,58]. Resveratrol, a natural polyphenol with anti-oxidant and anti-inflammatory properties, was shown to alleviate pain following CCI through miR-182 upregulation, which by inhibiting Nav1.7 may reduce neuronal excitability [56].

Another member of the VGSC family, $Na_v1.3$, is targeted by miR-96 and miR-384 in DRGs: when the miRNA mimics are administered intrathecally, the behavioural response indicative of hypersensitivity following nerve injury is alleviated [54,55]. Finally, miR-7a targets the β2 subunit of VGSCs, which is involved in transport and gating of sodium channels and is downregulated in neuronal cell bodies following nerve injury, causing hyper-excitability in C-fibres [99].

Another class of ion channels important in pain transmission are calcium channels, classified in various subtypes, which have different roles in excitable cells. $Ca_v1.2$ L-Type calcium channels regulate long-term changes in gene expression, inducing neuronal sensitisation in neuropathic pain. miR-103 modulates three $Ca_v1.2$ subunits ($Ca_v1.2$-α1, α2δ1 and β1) in spinal cord neurons, promoting mRNA decay. miR-103 is downregulated following nerve injury, concomitant with the upregulation of $Ca_v1.2$. Additionally, delivery of miR-103 mimic after SNL reduces pain sensitisation via $Ca_v1.2$ downregulation [17].

In addition to sodium and calcium channels, potassium channels also play an important role in neuronal excitability. Voltage-gated potassium channels play a role in setting the resting membrane potential, enabling the neuron to return to its resting state following depolarisation [100]. The miR-17-92 cluster was found to be upregulated following nerve injury and target several voltage-gated potassium channels (Kv1.1, Kv1.4, Kv3.4, Kv4.3, Kv7.5). miR-17-19 AAV injection causes the suppression of A-type potassium currents and induces mechanical allodynia. Administration of potassium channel activators reverses mechanical allodynia following miR-17-92 AAV injection, indicating that the cluster acts through the modulation of potassium channels [37]. More recently, Kv1.2 has been shown to be downregulated by miR-137a in neuropathic pain, contributing to pain hypersensitivity [38]. The authors have shown that cultured nociceptors from rats with CCI to the sciatic nerve display reduced potassium currents and increased neuronal excitability, which was rescued in nociceptors from rats treated with miR-137 antagomir. miR-137 inhibition following CCI resulted in increased Kv1.2 protein expression and pain relief [38].

Another potassium channel, TREK1, is regulated by miR-183. TREK1 is a mechano- and temperature-sensitive channel and contributes to the initiation of action potentials in C-fibres [101]. miR-183 is downregulated following nerve injury, whilst TREK1 is upregulated. miR-183 administration alleviates neuropathic pain through the inhibition of TREK1 [75].

Overall, the evidence suggests that several classes of ion channels are regulated by miRNAs. Due to the multitude of potential targets, miRNA-based therapeutics might also struggle to achieve specificity. However, studying miRNA dysregulation in chronic pain states will help to identify novel pathways that can be targeted pharmacologically with fewer side effects. Modulation of ion channels with specific inhibitors has proved to be a successful strategy in the development of analgesics. For example, pregabalin and gabapentin, currently first-line treatments for neuropathic pain, are calcium channels modulators. However, due to the presence of off-target effects and limited efficacy, there is an unmet need for better inhibitors [102].

3.2. Synaptic Transmission

Following the initiation and propagation of action potentials, the signal reaches the central terminals of nociceptors and is relayed to second-order neurons in the spinal cord through synaptic transmission. Modulating the components of this process allows fine-tuning of the amount of information that is transmitted further in the pathway. Various miRNAs have been shown to target genes involved in synaptic transmission in animal models, as shown in Figure 2B. For example, miR-190a is downregulated in diabetic peripheral neuropathy and targets SLC17A6, also known as VGLUT2, a glutamate transporter important in fast synaptic transmission [61]. Similarly, miR-34a undergoes long-term downregulation following CCI and targets VAMP2, belonging to the family of SNARE proteins, important for neurotransmitter release [78]. A study on cancer pain highlighted the role of miR-124 as a regulator of synaptopodin, a structural component of dendrites involved in the formation of strong excitatory synapses [69]. miR-500 is involved in chemotherapy-induced neuropathy, targeting GAD67, an enzyme necessary for the synthesis of GABA in inhibitory interneurons in the dorsal horn of the spinal cord. After paclitaxel injection, miR-500 was upregulated, causing a downregulation of GAD67. This resulted in a loss of inhibitory inputs, leading to an increase in excitatory nociceptive signals [25]. Both miR-124 and miR-500 dysregulation have been linked to nerve injury-induced neuropathic pain [88,103].

Overall, the evidence suggests that following the establishment of neuropathic pain, synaptic transmission is facilitated by the downregulation of miRNA targeting synaptic components, resulting in enhanced pain perception. Another mechanism that has been investigated in neuropathic pain is the loss of inhibitory inputs due to apoptosis of GABAergic interneurons [104]. The involvement of miRNA in this context should be investigated, as the initiation of apoptotic mechanisms requires extensive alteration of gene expression which could potentially be under the control of miRNAs, due to their ability to target multiple transcripts. Indeed, several miRNAs have already been linked to neuronal cell death in neurological diseases such as Alzheimer's [105], neuroblastoma [106] and ischemic disease [107].

3.3. Intracellular Signalling

A fundamental aspect in the establishment of neuropathic pain is the change in gene expression and post-translational modifications in the nociceptors which lead to a persistent alteration in neuronal excitability, a process known as peripheral sensitisation. This occurs through the activation of intracellular signalling pathways, such as the mitogen-activated protein kinases (MAPK), that are triggered by the activation of receptors by inflammatory mediators and cause the activation of kinases and transcription factors, resulting in the upregulation of ion channels and pro-nociceptive receptors (e.g., $Na_v1.8$ and TRPV1) [108]. The MAPK family is divided in three pathways: extracellular signal-regulated kinases (ERK), p38 and c-Jun N-terminal kinase (JNK) [109]. Various miRNAs have been found to be involved in the regulation of each of them in the context of pain (summarised in Figure 3).

The ERK pathway is activated in response to inflammation and growth factors, such as NGF, BDNF and other neurotrophins. It involves the sequential activation of Ras, Raf, MEK and ERK and leads to neuronal sensitisation [108]. MicroRNA-144 is downregulated in neuropathic pain and targets RASA1, a member of the Ras family, involved in the ERK activating cascade. Overexpression of miR-144 reverses nerve injury-induced mechanical allodynia and thermal hyperalgesia and leads to a reduction in pro-inflammatory cytokines in the DRG. The interaction between miR-144 and RASA1 was confirmed in satellite glial cells isolated from murine DRG. Furthermore, when miR-144 agomir was administered along with RASA1 lentiviral overexpression, the behavioural response to pain was indicative of increased hypersensitivity and the expression of pro-inflammatory cytokines was restored [52]. Another study highlights RASA1 interaction with miR-206 in PC12 cells and finds that miR-206 is also downregulated following CCI [110]. This study lacks the characterisation of miR-206 effect on RASA1 expression in vivo. However, it emerges that regulation of RASA1 by miRNAs plays an important role in neuropathic pain. miR-206 downregulation is also involved in neuropathic pain through brain-derived neurotrophic factors (BDNF) interaction, leading again to the activation of the MEK/ERK signalling pathway. Overexpression of miR-206 reverses the behavioural response to pain, leading to decreased hypersensitivity, and reduces neuroinflammation, resulting in decreased BDNF and MEK/ERK phosphorylation. When BDNF is also overexpressed, the effects of miR-206 injection are abrogated, concomitant with an upregulation of phospho-MEK and phospho-ERK [111]. Overall, ERK activation in neuropathic pain is facilitated by the downregulation of specific miRNAs, including miR-206 and miR-144.

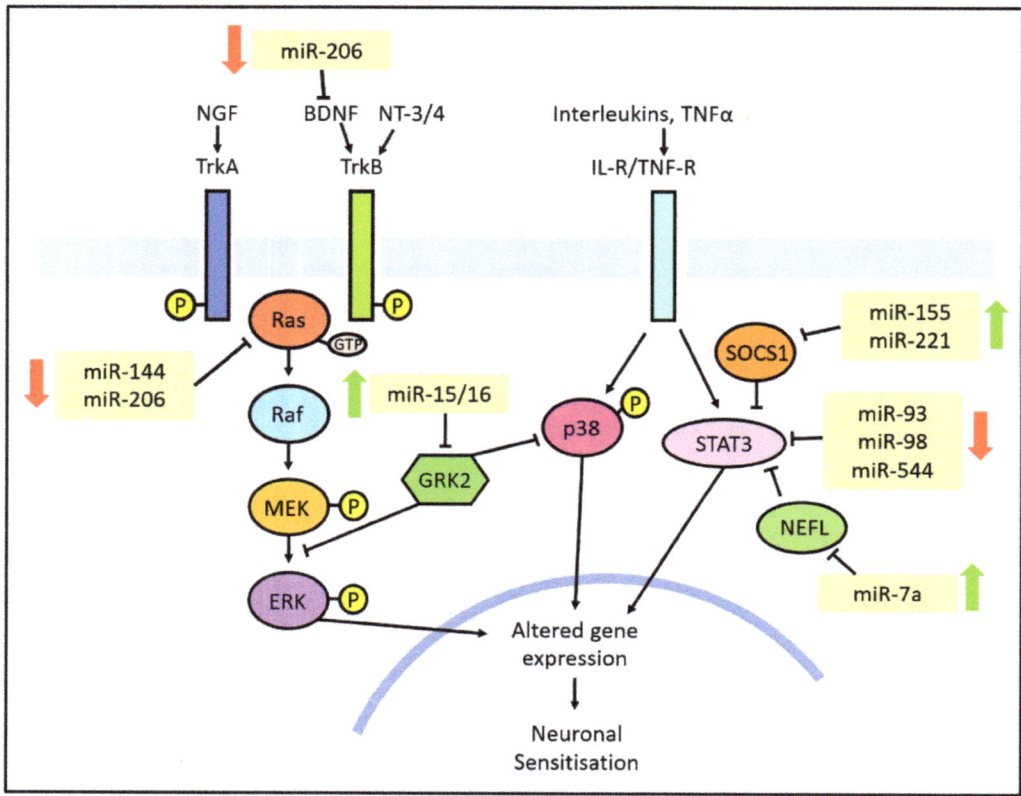

Figure 3. Diagram displaying miRNA dysregulated in neuropathic pain and their targets involved in intracellular signalling. Red downward arrows indicate that the miRNA is downregulated during neuropathic pain, whilst upward green arrows indicate miRNA upregulation in neuropathic pain.

Another important signalling pathway in the context of neuropathic pain is mediated by p38 activation in spinal microglia, following cellular stress and binding of inflammatory mediators to extracellular receptors [112]. Phosphorylated p38 is translocated into the nucleus where it activates transcription factors, such as NF-kB and STAT3, promoting the expression of inflammatory mediators such as TNFα and IL-1β [108].

Several regulators and downstream targets of p38 are targeted by miRNA. For example, miR-15/16 targets GRK2, a G-protein coupled receptor (GPCR) that inhibits p38. This miRNA cluster is upregulated following CCI in rats and its inhibition leads to reduced hyperalgesia, increased GRK2 expression and decreased phosphorylation of p38 and NF-kB p65. GRK2 knockdown leads to the abrogation of mir-15/16 inhibition, including restoration of p-p38 and p-NF-kB levels [26].

Similarly, miR-221 targets suppressor of cytokine 1 (SOCS1) and its upregulation following CCI causes increased NF-kB and p38 phosphorylation [64]. SOCS1 is also targeted by miR-155, upregulated following CCI [63]. miR-155 inhibition partially reverses changes seen in behavioural responses to thermal and mechanical stimuli, indicating a reduction in hyperalgesia. It also reduces phosphorylation of Ik-Bα and p38, whilst if SOCS1 was also knocked down, the effects of miR-155 inhibition are abrogated. These findings suggest that SOCS1 is involved in neuropathic pain through the regulation of the NF-kB and p38 pathways and is itself targeted by miR-155 and miR-221. miR-155 is also upregulated in neuropathic pain induced by the chemotherapeutic agent Bortezomib, causing increased JNK and p38 phosphorylation [113]. Inhibition of miR-155 causes a reduction in the behavioural response to mechanical stimuli and restoration of JNK and p38 phosphorylation levels [113].

Fewer studies have been performed on the role of JNK in chronic pain. Its activation in sensory neurons and spinal glia following nerve injury is known to be involved in the development of allodynia and hyperalgesia [114]. MicroRNA modulation of JNK, as well as other MAPKs, plays a role in trigeminal nerve injury induced by CCI to the infraorbital nerve. miR-223 is downregulated following CCI, along with an increase in ERK, p38 and JNK phosphorylation levels. miR-223 overexpression with a lentiviral vector improves the behavioural response to mechanical stimuli and restores MAPKs phosphorylation levels. The effect of miR-223 may occur through the direct interaction with the translational repressor MKNK2, involved in the MAPK pathways [42].

Finally, several miRNAs (miR-93, miR-98 and miR-544) have been found to target STAT3 and to be downregulated following nerve injury. STAT3 is an inflammatory transcription factor activated following phosphorylation by p38 [66–68]. miR-7a also indirectly regulates STAT3 by targeting neurofilament light polypeptide (NEFL), alleviating neuropathic pain [115].

ERK and p38 are only two of the pathways that are potentially targeted by miRNA to contribute to neuropathic pain. For example, bioinformatic evidence shows that miR-500 potentially targets proteins and transcription factors activated in response to cAMP alterations, another important secondary intracellular messenger [116]. Overall, there is now evidence that several miRNAs influence neuronal excitability through the regulation of intracellular signalling cascades. This could be an interesting route to investigate potential new analgesics. It also provides greater understanding of these mechanisms, which are relevant to a wide variety of human diseases.

3.4. Interaction with Non-Neuronal Cell Types

Non-neuronal cell types, including glial cells and immune cells, make up the environment surrounding neurons and contribute to the establishment of inflammation and alteration of excitability following nerve injury [117]. MicroRNAs can influence this environment through various means, inducing changes in several types of non-neuronal cells including macrophages, microglia, Schwann cells, astrocytes and lymphocytes.

3.4.1. Macrophages Communicate through miRNA-Containing Extracellular Vesicles

At the nerve injury site, macrophages are activated by pathogen-associated molecular patterns (PAMP) and damage-associated molecular patterns (DAMP) released in response to tissue injury. They contribute to the increased recruitment of immune cells via the secretion of MMPs and vasoactive mediators and establish tissue inflammation through the secretion of cytokines, interferons, interleukins, prostanoids, growth factors and nitrous oxide. Macrophages are also recruited in the dorsal root ganglia following nerve injury and cause additional secretion of pro-inflammatory cytokines that ultimately lead to a change in post-translational modifications and gene expression in neuronal cell bodies, resulting in increased excitability [118].

In addition to the secretion of cytokines and other well-known pro-inflammatory mediators, macrophages communicate with neuronal cell bodies through miRNA-containing exosomes. McDonald [83] showed that exosomes secreted by activated murine macrophages display a characteristic miRNA signature and induce NF-kB activation, a known pro-inflammatory intracellular mediator, in vitro. In vivo studies show that intraplanar injection of exosomes from LPS-treated macrophages induces increased thermal hyperalgesia shortly after CFA administration. However, over the course of 48 h, exosomes from both LPS+ and LPS- macrophages caused a decrease in the severity of thermal hyperalgesia. This indicates that macrophage activation might promote transient increase in inflammation and hyperalgesia, followed by resolution. Additionally, human patients suffering from CRPS show an increased level of miRNA in circulating exosomes, attesting the potential importance of these molecules.

Another piece of evidence supporting the concept of communication between neurons and macrophages through miRNA-containing exosomes following nerve injury has been described by Simeoli, et al. [119]. Cultured DRG neurons treated with capsaicin release exosomes which contain miR-21. When these exosomes are administered to macrophages, a switch to M1 pro-inflammatory phenotype is observed which is mediated by miR-21. In vivo miR-21 antagomir intrathecal injection causes decreased hyperalgesia and a lower number of M1 macrophages. This indicates that miR-21, secreted in exosomes by activated neuronal cell bodies, stimulates a pro-inflammatory phenotype in macrophages, which leads to increased inflammation and hyperalgesia. Zhang, et al. [13] identified a similar mechanism involving miR-23 and A20, a negative regulator of NF-kB which can induce M1 polarization. miR-23 was shown to be secreted in extracellular vesicles (EVs) from cultured DRG neurons explanted from SNI mice or following capsaicin administration. Macrophages cultured with miR-23-containing EVs displayed a downregulation of A20 protein level, increased NF-kB activation and increased expression of the M1 marker Nos2. Inhibition of miR-23 following SNI in mice resulted in reduced hyperalgesia and inflammation, as well as reduced macrophage infiltration in the DRG, which were more likely to display an M2 non-inflammatory phenotype.

3.4.2. Schwann Cell Proliferation Is Directed by miRNA

Schwann cells (SCs) are found in the peripheral nervous system wrapped around neuronal axons. Their role involves myelinating large-diameter axons and ensheathing small-diameter axons in structures known as Remak bundles, providing nourishment to the neurons and promoting peripheral nerve regeneration [120]. Following nerve injury, the interaction between Neuregulin on the axonal membrane and ERBB2/3 on SCs leads to demyelination, followed by SC proliferation. Additionally, SCs secrete NGF, BDNF, prostaglandins, MMPs and cytokines, which lead to peripheral sensitisation and altered neuronal gene expression [121].

The SC response following nerve injury consists of a de-differentiation and proliferation phase, followed by a remyelination phase. Several miRNAs have been implicated in the proliferation phase as described in a review by Sohn and Park [122]. Examples include let-7b, implicated in NGF inhibition and downregulated following nerve injury, [123] and miR-1, targeting BDNF [124].

A study by Viader [125] analysed miRNA expression in the distal stump of injured nerves in mice, largely constituted by SCs, and identified 48 dysregulated miRNAs. Bioinformatic analysis showed that 31 of the dysregulated miRNAs' predicted targets are involved in SC de-differentiation and proliferation. Additionally, deletion of Dicer resulted in a delay in the proliferation and remyelination cycle. A closer look at the identified miRNAs revealed that miR-34 is downregulated sharply following nerve injury and targets Notch1 and Ccnd1, positive regulators of SC proliferation. Interestingly, miR-140, which is downregulated until day 7 post-injury, was shown to target Egr2, a transcription factor directing myelination, in in silico and cell culture systems; however, their expression in vivo is positively correlated. This could point to miR-140's role in fine-tuning Erb2 expression, or it could indicate that in vivo interaction does not actually occur to a significant extent.

Several studies have investigated the role of miRNA expressed in SCs in nerve regeneration following injury; however, studies focused on miRNA in SCs that contribute to the establishment or persistence of neuropathic pain are lacking. Given the role that SCs play in nerve regeneration, it is difficult to distinguish between adaptive changes that promote regeneration and maladaptive ones that lead to chronic pain. The comparison between neuropathic models characterised by different pain intensities, such as the one presented by Norcini, et al. [126], or the comparison between genetic lines with different susceptibilities to pain, as shown in Bali, et al. [127], could be used to overcome this hurdle.

3.4.3. Lymphocyte Differentiation Is Altered by miRNA Expression

Lymphocytes, in particular, T cells, are recruited to the injury site following nerve damage where they secrete pro-inflammatory cytokines. They also infiltrate the spinal cord and promote astrocytic activation [118].

A study using blood samples collected from patients suffering from a variety of neuropathic pain conditions (polyneuropathy, postherpetic neuralgia and trigeminal neuralgia) identified two differentially expressed miRNAs compared to healthy individuals: miR-124a and -155. They are both involved in the differentiation of regulatory T cells (Tregs). miR-124a and -155 directly repress histone deacetylase sirtuin1 (SIRT1), which is a negative regulator of Foxp3, a master regulator of the development of Tregs. Increased levels of miR-124a and miR-155 in neuropathic pain promote Tregs differentiation, which have an anti-inflammatory role [90].

In a mouse model for type II diabetes-induced peripheral neuropathy, miR-590-3p was found to be downregulated in the dorsal root ganglia, alongside an increase in CD4 immunolabelling compared to non-diabetic mice, indicating increased T cell infiltration. Overexpression of miR-590 attenuated the behavioural responses indicative of pain. The validated target RAP1A was shown to promote T cell viability and migration in isolated T cells, indicating that neuropathic pain in diabetic mice might be exacerbated by RAP1A-induced T cell infiltration, enabled by the downregulation of miR-590-3p [51].

3.4.4. Microglial Activation Is Regulated by miRNA

Microglia are essentially CNS-specific macrophages and play an important role in inflammation and nociception in the spinal cord. Following nerve injury, they show increased activation in the spinal cord, characterised by increased phosphorylation of p38 and ERK1/2, increased expression of M1 markers (MHC Class II, CD45, integrins) and a morphological change [118].

MicroRNA-124 has been identified as an important regulator of the transition to the activated pro-inflammatory phenotype of microglia. Its expression is highest in non-activated microglia and its knockdown results in in vivo microglial activation [123]. This plays a role in the transition from acute to persistent hyperalgesia: downregulation of miR-124 in isolated spinal cord microglia following plantar IL-1β injection is observed concomitantly with an increase in M1 markers. Additionally, the injection of miR-124 reverses mechanical allodynia in mice following spared nerve injury [103]. Similarly, miR-451, which is downregulated during inflammatory pain, prevents microglial activation by targeting TLR4, a receptor on microglial surface responsible for cytokine release [72].

Regulation of microglial activity by miRNA in neuropathic pain has been also shown to occur through autophagy impairment. Increased miR-195 in spinal microglia is correlated with a decrease in autophagy activation following peripheral nerve injury. In particular, miR-195 targets ATG14, involved in the autophagy pathway. Impairment of autophagy leads to further accumulation of pro-inflammatory cytokines and exacerbation of hyperalgesia [12].

3.4.5. Astrocytic Activation and Cytokine Production Is Influenced by miRNA

Astrocyte activation in the spinal cord is observed with some delay compared to the microglial response, but its increase is sustained for up to 5 months following nerve injury. A role for miRNA-mediated communication between glia and neurons has been reported [18], in which miR-186, CXCL13 and its receptor CXCR5 trigger astrocytic activation. Following spinal nerve ligation (SNL), CXCL13 expression is increased in neurites, whilst miR-186 is downregulated. miR-186 inhibition in naïve mice elicits behavioural responses to a lower threshold of mechanical stimulation, which is reversed by CXCL13 neutralising antibody injection. Additionally, CXCR5, a known CXCL13 receptor expressed in astrocytes, is upregulated following SNL and its inhibition leads to reduced SNL-induced pain hypersensitivity for up to 91 days. In CXCR5 KO mice, decreased glial activation is observed. This indicates that CXCL13 expression in neurons is controlled by miR-186 and leads to CXCR5 activation in astrocytes, which triggers glial activation through the ERK signalling pathway.

Once astrocytes are activated, miR-146 plays a role in establishing the balance in pro-inflammatory molecule production. Inflammatory mediators such as TNFα and IL-1β, which stimulate astrocytic activation, lead to a sharp increase in TRAF6 followed by a delayed miR-146 increase. miR-146 targets TRAF6 mRNA, inhibiting its downstream targets JNK and CCL2. Simultaneously, LPS treatment enhances AP-1 (downstream of JNK) binding site for miR-146, promoting its transcription. It emerges that miR-146 is at the centre of a negative feedback loop in astrocytes to fine-tune the production of pro-inflammatory signalling molecules such as JNK and CCL2 [129].

4. A Closer Look at miRNA Regulation and Function

In this review, several examples of how miRNA dysregulation contributes to the development of neuropathic pain are summarised. Typically, this involves the downregulation of miRNAs that target molecules which promote excitability and inflammation. But how is miRNA expression altered following nerve damage?

A study by Leung [130] found that in conditions of cellular stress, which lead to the formation of stress granules, miRNA-induced repression of translation is decreased five-fold. Additionally, Ago2, part of the RISC complex, is co-immunoprecipitated with PARP-13, a component of stress granules. This indicates that following stress, Ago2 bound to miRNA might be sequestered to stress granules and prevented from repressing its mRNA targets. Similar evidence was found in the context of neuropathic pain. Aldrich, et al. [131] identified a miRNA cluster–miR-96/182/183–which is downregulated following nerve injury and localised at the periphery of cell bodies. In contrast, miR-96/182/183 displayed an even localisation throughout the cell bodies of uninjured animals. In injured neurons, the miRNA cluster was also co-localised with a stress granule protein (TIA1), which is commonly found in apoptotic neurons. Co-immunoprecipitation and reporter assays are necessary to establish if direct interaction between the miRNA cluster or RISC complexes and TIA1 occurs. However, this provides a potential mechanism through which miRNA regulation takes place during the development of chronic pain, whereby miRNAs are sequestered by stress granules at the periphery of the cell. The author suggests two possible strategies on how this occurs: miRNAs bound to stress granules might become translational activators, or their compartmentalisation at the periphery might result in increased cytoplasmic volume free of translational repressors.

Another way through which miRNAs are sequestered in neuropathic pain is through "sponging" by long non-coding RNA (lncRNA). This process has also been observed in cancer, as several lncRNAs have been shown to bind to miRNAs in order to derepress their mRNA targets [132]. This is also relevant in the development of neuropathic pain, as reviewed in Song, et al. [133]: examples include miR-381, negatively regulated by lncRNA NEAT1 [31], miR-150 and miR-154 by XIST [73], miR-206 and miR-129 by MALAT1 [27,81], and miR-124 and miR-141 by SNHG16 [36]. A study by Wang, et al. [134] investigated the network of interactions between lncRNAs, miRNAs and mRNAs in Schwann cells cultured from rats affected by diabetic peripheral neuropathy. The expression of thousands of transcripts was analysed with RNA sequencing. The resulting competing endogenous RNA (ceRNA) network was calculated using co-expression similarity and target prediction algorithms and included 38 lncRNAs, 10 miRNAs and 702 mRNAs. This complex network of interaction should be validated experimentally; however, the interaction between one of the miRNAs involved (miR-212-5p) and its predicted target Gucy1a3 was verified in a cell-line. ceRNA networks were also investigated in trigeminal neuropathic pain in mice by Fang, et al. [135]. Total RNA sequencing identified 67 miRNAs, 216 lncRNAs, 14 circRNA and 595 mRNA that were dysregulated following infraorbital CCI compared to sham-operated mice. Computational analysis identified a complex network of interactions, involving several previously identified pain-related transcripts. It is perhaps unlikely that the network of interactions will be exactly replicated in humans; however, studies of this kind are invaluable to identify master regulators that dictate molecular changes leading to neuronal hyperexcitability in chronic neuropathic pain, helping to identify a set of targets that can then be investigated in humans.

The complexity surrounding miRNA regulation does not end here. The conventional modality of action of miRNA consists in translational repression of mRNA targets. However, an alternative mechanism of action has emerged, which involves the direct interaction between miRNA and a protein, resulting in its activation. Lehmann, et al. [105] found that let-7b can be secreted extracellularly by dying neurons and induce further neuronal cell death through TLR7 activation. In the context of pain, let-7b induces nociception through direct interaction with TLR7, which elicits TRPA1-mediated currents. Let-7b has been observed to be co-localised on the cell membrane with TRPA1 and TLR7, but not in TLR7 deficient cells, indicating that let-7b directly binds to TLR7 and promotes TRPA1 activation [136]. In other words, let-7b has a positive effect on TRPA1 through direct interaction with TLR7's amino acid sequence. Mir-21 and miR-29a also bind to human TLR8 and murine TLR7 in non-small cell lung cancer, increasing the secretion of pro-inflammatory cytokines [137]. Indeed, miR-21 is upregulated in mouse following SNL and targets TLR8, causing ERK activation [74].

Another miRNA acting in a similar way is miR-711, which directly interacts with the extracellular loop of TRPA1 to elicit pruritus. miR-711 cheek injection is sufficient to cause pruritus in mice, and this requires the presence of TRPA1 and the core miR-711 sequence (GGGACCC). Calcium imaging of cultured DRG neurons show that extracellular miR-711 administration is sufficient to elicit currents in a subset of neurons, whilst the presence of a TRPA1 inhibitor prevents this. Again, this indicates that miR-711 directly interacts with TRPA1 peptide sequence causing its activation [138].

This mode of miRNA interaction presents an additional opportunity to harness with pathways involved in chronic pain and inflammation that could be exploited in drug discovery. It also provides a fascinating insight on the regulatory capabilities of noncoding RNA molecules. Further research is needed to identify which other miRNAs (or other noncoding RNA), if any, act in a similar way and how the interaction causes receptor activation.

5. Potential Clinical Application of miRNA Studies

MicroRNA expression appears to be dynamic, changing extensively according to the pain model, time frame and animal studied. In a systematic study by Guo, et al. [139], data from 37 different papers on miRNA expression in rat neuropathic pain models (SCI, CCI and SNL) were compared. Despite the use of similar pain models, few studies showed overlapping expression patterns. Only five dysregulated miRNAs (rno-miR-183/96, rno-miR-30b, rno-miR-150 and rno-miR-206) were observed in two or more studies, suggesting that various factors including variations in the animal weight, age, time after injury, injury model and handling could influence significantly miRNA expression. This entails a significant obstacle in the application of miRNA research to the clinic. However, it could contribute to the development of strategies to stratify patients, as particular miRNA signatures could be associated with a better response to particular drugs and treatments or with chronic pain of different origins.

An example of this is presented by Dayer, et al. [89], who performed a study on circulating miRNAs in plasma of patients affected by chronic pain following orthopaedic trauma. The pain symptoms were classified into neuropathic, nociceptive, mixed and CPRS through a DN4 questionnaire, clinical history investigation and assessment by physiotherapists and physicians. Two circulating plasma miRNAs (miR-320 and miR-98) were found to successfully classify patients suffering from neuropathic or nociceptive pain in 70% of the cases.

If more miRNAs are identified, possibly through wider RNA-sequencing screening, the accuracy might increase, leading to faster diagnosis, earlier start of appropriate treatment and a more robust and efficient cohort selection in clinical trials.

The role of circulating miR-320 in chronic post-traumatic pain in humans has also been elucidated by Linnstaedt, et al. [140], pointing to an alternative approach to stratify patients based on genetic variants. A riboSNitch (i.e., a regulatory element in an RNA transcript with a function that is disrupted by a specific SNP) in the 3'UTR of the FKBP5 gene was linked to increased vulnerability to chronic post-traumatic pain by decreasing the affinity of miR-320 to its binding region. Individuals with the minor allele were more likely to report symptoms of musculoskeletal pain 6 weeks post-trauma if they experienced high levels of peritraumatic distress, while the level of distress in individuals with the major allele had little impact on the development of chronic pain. This riboSNitch was found to affect the secondary structure of FKBP5 3'UTR, causing the miR-320 binding site to become inaccessible, leading to increased FKBP5 translation, glucocorticoid resistance and susceptibility to chronic pain. This evidence shows how a deeper understanding of the regulatory networks involving miRNA–mRNA interactions could lead to new strategies to identify patients who are at higher risk of developing chronic pain.

Another fundamental question when translating animal studies to humans is whether miRNA function is conserved across different organisms. Studies on human DRG and spinal cord are lacking due to the inaccessibility of the tissues, which makes it challenging to translate the role of miRNAs characterised in animal studies to human disease. Some studies have been performed on blood samples in CRPS patients [83,84] and a variety of neuropathic pain conditions [90], which have been discussed in previous paragraphs.

Interesting translational insights on miRNAs and neuropathic pain come from Leinders, et al. [91]. MicroRNA expression was analysed in WBCs and sural nerve biopsies of patients affected by a variety of peripheral neuropathies. It was found that miR-132-3p was significantly increased in WBCs of neuropathic pain patients compared to healthy controls, and that miR-132-3p expression in the sural nerve was correlated with pain intensity in patients with peripheral neuropathies. Experiments on animal models identified the same miRNA to be altered in the spinal cord of rats 10 days following SNI. Additionally, daily injections of miR-132-3p antagonist caused an increase in mechanical withdrawal thresholds following SNI, indicative of reduced allodynia, compared to rats treated with scrambled control injections. This work highlighted the importance of this particular miRNA, which is altered in both nerve and WBCs of human patients and was shown to affect the behavioural responses to pain in a pre-clinical animal model. Interestingly, miR-132 was also found to be upregulated in plasma of patients affected by peripheral neuropathies in a different study [92]. This type of study is invaluable to understand the local and systemic impact of the development of peripheral neuropathies on gene expression, while the comparison with pre-clinical models allows a more in-depth analysis of the molecular mechanisms that drive the transition to chronic pain.

Similarly, a study by Tavares-Ferreira, et al. [88] used lingual neuroma tissues from patients with lingual nerve injury and pre-clinical models to identify changes in miRNA expression following nerve injury. Lingual nerve injury can occur during routine dental practices such as anaesthetic injections and third molar removal. Following nerve damage, the injured axon undergoes extensive sprouting in the attempt to regenerate, supported by proliferating Schwann cells. However, this process may lead to the formation of a swollen mass—classified as a neuroma—constituted by the accumulation of fibroblasts, immune cells, Schwann cells and collagen fibres. The patient is often left with altered sensation and hyperalgesia, with symptoms including anaesthesia, discomfort, tingling, burning or sharp shooting pain. Repairing the nerve, which involves dissecting the neuroma out and micro-surgically re-joining the two nerve ends, promotes functional recovery in most patients [141]. Investigation of these neuromas revealed two miRNAs (hsa-miR-29a and hsa-miR-500a) that were differentially expressed in painful and non-painful human lingual nerve neuromas, and significant correlations between miRNA expression and the pain VAS score for both miR-29 and miR-500. This comparison allows the identification of factors which are associated with pain intensity, rather than positive adaptive changes, such as factors promoting nerve regeneration.

The study also investigated miRNA expression when a similar type of injury was replicated in rat, which will enable further investigation of the molecular basis of miRNA function. Chronic constriction injury was performed on the rat lingual nerve: two miRNAs were identified (rno-miR-667 and rno-miR-138) that were correlated with altered behaviour indicative of allodynia. Bioinformatics analysis showed several common potential targets, involved in inflammation, chemotaxis and ion channel activity. Despite the difference in the miRNAs identified, the shared potential targets hint that miRNA investigation is useful to identify important pathways involved in the establishment of chronic neuropathic pain.

6. Conclusions

Neuropathic pain results from various pathophysiological processes following nerve injury, including inflammation, neuronal death, altered excitability and long-term synaptic alterations, which take place from the periphery of nociceptors to central circuits involved in pain processing. Being such a complex and subjective phenomenon, the mechanisms underlying its development are not fully understood.

The study of microRNAs provides new insights into pathways involved in the development and persistence of neuropathic pain. Several miRNAs have been shown to induce analgesia or hypersensitivity in animal models, through targeting various pathways linked with neuronal excitability, intracellular signalling and communication with glial and immune cells. These molecules can exert their effect in various ways, with the most conventional being through mRNA repression, whilst direct protein activation has also been observed. The study of mechanisms that cause miRNA depletion during neuropathic pain, such as long non-coding RNA sponging and stress granule sequestration, has provided valuable insights on how translational homeostasis is achieved in health and disrupted in disease.

As the current treatments available are not satisfactory for long-term management of neuropathic pain, new targets are needed in order to develop better therapeutics. MicroRNAs could potentially be targeted to achieve analgesia, being theoretically capable of influencing several molecules involved in various pathways. While several miRNA-based therapeutics are in phase I/II clinical trials, none have reached phase III clinical trials yet. Challenges include RNA degradation, low tissue permeability and low specificity [142]. Chemical modifications can increase RNA stability, while issues concerning tissue permeability and specificity can be addressed by designing drug delivery systems that target specific cell types [143].

MicroRNAs also offer the opportunity to investigate phenotypic subtyping, in order to stratify patients into groups that are more or less likely to respond to a certain treatment by their miRNA signature. Finally, the study of miRNAs is critical to develop further understanding of the pathophysiology of neuropathic pain and may benefit several other conditions that share common pathways such as inflammation, neuronal cell death and alterations in intracellular signalling.

Overall, a stronger focus on the use of human tissue in the field of miRNAs and neuropathic pain is needed in order to identify clinically relevant biomarkers and drug targets. With the advent of new technologies and the reduction in sequencing costs, investigation of patients' samples is increasingly more accessible and represents the most promising route to advance the field and benefit patients, while animal models remain a great tool to discover the mechanisms underlying miRNAs' action in the context of pain.

Author Contributions: Conceptualization, F.M.B., D.W.L. and M.M.; writing—original draft preparation, M.M.; writing—review and editing, M.M., F.M.B., E.S. and D.W.L.; supervision, F.M.B., D.W.L., D.A.C. and E.S.; funding acquisition, F.M.B., D.W.L., D.A.C. and E.S. All authors have read and agreed to the published version of the manuscript.

Funding: This research was funded by BBSRC, grant number BB/T508159/1 and Eli Lilly.

Institutional Review Board Statement: Not applicable.

Data Availability Statement: Not applicable.

Conflicts of Interest: The authors declare no conflict of interest.

References

1. Finnerup, N.B.; Attal, N.; Haroutounian, S.; McNicol, E.; Baron, R.; Dworkin, R.H.; Gilron, I.; Haanpää, M.; Hansson, P.; Jensen, T.S.; et al. Pharmacotherapy for neuropathic pain in adults: A systematic review and meta-analysis. *Lancet Neurol.* **2015**, *14*, 162–173. [CrossRef] [PubMed]
2. Giovannini, S.; Coraci, D.; Brau, F.; Galluzzo, V.; Loreti, C.; Caliandro, P.; Padua, L.; Maccauro, G.; Biscotti, L.; Bernabei, R. Neuropathic Pain in the Elderly. *Diagnostics* **2021**, *11*, 613. [CrossRef] [PubMed]
3. Rupaimoole, R.; Slack, F.J. MicroRNA therapeutics: Towards a new era for the management of cancer and other diseases. *Nat. Rev. Drug Discov.* **2017**, *16*, 203–222. [CrossRef] [PubMed]
4. Kristen, A.V.; Ajroud-Driss, S.; Conceição, I.; Gorevic, P.; Kyriakides, T.; Obici, L. Patisiran, an RNAi therapeutic for the treatment of hereditary transthyretin-mediated amyloidosis. *Neurodegener. Dis. Manag.* **2019**, *9*, 5–23. [CrossRef] [PubMed]
5. Andersen, H.H.; Duroux, M.; Gazerani, P. MicroRNAs as modulators and biomarkers of inflammatory and neuropathic pain conditions. *Neurobiol. Dis.* **2014**, *71*, 159–168. [CrossRef]
6. López-González, M.J.; Landry, M.; Favereaux, A. MicroRNA and chronic pain: From mechanisms to therapeutic potential. *Pharmacol. Ther.* **2017**, *180*, 1–15. [CrossRef]
7. Bai, G.; Ambalavanar, R.; Wei, D.; Dessem, D. Downregulation of Selective microRNAs in Trigeminal Ganglion Neurons Following Inflammatory Muscle Pain. *Mol. Pain* **2007**, *3*, 15. [CrossRef]
8. Zhao, J.; Lee, M.-C.; Momin, A.; Cendan, C.-M.; Shepherd, S.T.; Baker, M.D.; Asante, C.; Bee, L.; Bethry, A.; Perkins, J.R.; et al. Small RNAs Control Sodium Channel Expression, Nociceptor Excitability, and Pain Thresholds. *J. Neurosci.* **2010**, *30*, 10860–10871. [CrossRef]
9. Kuhn, D.E.; Martin, M.M.; Feldman, D.S.; Terry, A.V.; Nuovo, G.J.; Elton, T.S. Experimental validation of miRNA targets. *Methods* **2008**, *44*, 47–54. [CrossRef]
10. Cai, W.; Zhang, Y.; Liu, Y.; Liu, H.; Zhang, Z.; Su, Z. Effects of miR-150 on neuropathic pain process via targeting AKT3. *Biochem. Biophys. Res. Commun.* **2019**, *517*, 532–537. [CrossRef]
11. You, H.; Zhang, L.; Chen, Z.; Liu, W.; Wang, H.; He, H. MiR-20b-5p relieves neuropathic pain by targeting Akt3 in a chronic constriction injury rat model. *Synapse* **2019**, *73*, e22125. [CrossRef]
12. Shi, G.; Shi, J.; Liu, K.; Liu, N.; Wang, Y.; Fu, Z.; Ding, J.; Jia, L.; Yuan, W. Increased miR-195 aggravates neuropathic pain by inhibiting autophagy following peripheral nerve injury. *Glia* **2013**, *61*, 504–512. [CrossRef]
13. Zhang, Y.; Liu, J.; Wang, X.; Zhang, J.; Xie, C. Extracellular vesicle-encapsulated microRNA-23a from dorsal root ganglia neurons binds to A20 and promotes inflammatory macrophage polarization following peripheral nerve injury. *Aging* **2021**, *13*, 6752–6764. [CrossRef]
14. Li, X.; Wang, S.; Yang, X.; Chu, H. miR-142-3p targets AC9 to regulate sciatic nerve injury-induced neuropathic pain by regulating the cAMP/AMPK signalling pathway. *Int. J. Mol. Med.* **2021**, *47*, 561–572. [CrossRef]
15. Gandla, J.; Lomada, S.K.; Lu, J.; Kuner, R.; Bali, K.K. miR-34c-5p functions as pronociceptive microRNA in cancer pain by targeting Cav2.3 containing calcium channels. *Pain* **2017**, *158*, 1765–1779. [CrossRef]
16. Pan, Z.; Zhu, L.-J.; Li, Y.-Q.; Hao, L.-Y.; Yin, C.; Yang, J.-X.; Guo, Y.; Zhang, S.; Hua, L.; Xue, Z.-Y.; et al. Epigenetic Modification of Spinal miR-219 Expression Regulates Chronic Inflammation Pain by Targeting CaMKII gamma. *J. Neurosci.* **2014**, *34*, 9476–9483. [CrossRef]
17. Favereaux, A.; Thoumine, O.; Bouali-Benazzouz, R.; Roques, V.; Papon, M.-A.; Salam, S.A.; Drutel, G.; Léger, C.; Calas, A.; Nagy, F.; et al. Bidirectional integrative regulation of Cav1.2 calcium channel by microRNA miR-103: Role in pain. *EMBO J.* **2011**, *30*, 3830–3841. [CrossRef]
18. Jiang, B.-C.; Cao, D.-L.; Zhang, X.; Zhang, Z.-J.; He, L.-N.; Li, C.-H.; Zhang, W.-W.; Wu, X.-B.; Berta, T.; Ji, R.-R.; et al. CXCL13 drives spinal astrocyte activation and neuropathic pain via CXCR5. *J. Clin. Investig.* **2016**, *126*, 745–761. [CrossRef]
19. Pan, Z.; Shan, Q.; Gu, P.; Wang, X.M.; Tai, L.W.; Sun, M.; Luo, X.; Sun, L.; Cheung, C.W. miRNA-23a/CXCR4 regulates neuropathic pain via directly targeting TXNIP/NLRP3 inflammasome axis. *J. Neuroinflamm.* **2018**, *15*, 29. [CrossRef]
20. Jiang, M.; Zhang, X.; Wang, X.; Xu, F.; Zhang, J.; Li, L.; Xie, X.; Wang, L.; Yang, Y.; Xu, J. MicroRNA-124-3p attenuates the development of nerve injury–induced neuropathic pain by targeting early growth response 1 in the dorsal root ganglia and spinal dorsal horn. *J. Neurochem.* **2021**, *158*, 928–942. [CrossRef]
21. Tan, M.; Shen, L.; Hou, Y. Epigenetic modification of BDNF mediates neuropathic pain via miR-30a-3p/EP300 axis in CCI rats. *Biosci. Rep.* **2020**, *40*. [CrossRef] [PubMed]
22. Sun, L.; Zhou, J.; Sun, C. MicroRNA-211-5p Enhances Analgesic Effect of Dexmedetomidine on Inflammatory Visceral Pain in Rats by Suppressing ERK Signaling. *J. Mol. Neurosci.* **2019**, *68*, 19–28. [CrossRef] [PubMed]

23. Zhang, Y.; Liu, H.; An, L.; Li, L.; Wei, M.; Ge, D.; Su, Z. miR-124-3p attenuates neuropathic pain induced by chronic sciatic nerve injury in rats via targeting EZH2. *J. Cell. Biochem.* **2018**, *120*, 5747–5755. [CrossRef] [PubMed]
24. Zhang, X.; Chen, Q.; Shen, J.; Wang, L.; Cai, Y.; Zhu, K. miR-194 relieve neuropathic pain and prevent neuroinflammation via targeting FOXA1. *J. Cell. Biochem.* **2020**, *121*, 3278–3285. [CrossRef]
25. Huang, Z.-Z.; Wei, J.-Y.; Ou-Yang, H.-D.; Li, D.; Xu, T.; Wu, S.-L.; Zhang, X.-L.; Liu, C.-C.; Ma, C.; Xin, W.-J. mir-500-Mediated GAD67 Downregulation Contributes to Neuropathic Pain. *J. Neurosci.* **2016**, *36*, 6321–6331. [CrossRef]
26. Li, T.; Wan, Y.; Sun, L.; Tao, S.; Chen, P.; Liu, C.; Wang, K.; Zhou, C.; Zhao, G. Inhibition of MicroRNA-15a/16 Expression Alleviates Neuropathic Pain Development through Upregulation of G Protein-Coupled Receptor Kinase 2. *Biomol. Ther.* **2019**, *27*, 414–422. [CrossRef]
27. Ma, X.; Wang, H.; Song, T.; Wang, W.; Zhang, Z. lncRNA MALAT1 contributes to neuropathic pain development through regulating miR-129-5p/HMGB1 axis in a rat model of chronic constriction injury. *Int. J. Neurosci.* **2020**, *130*, 1215–1224. [CrossRef]
28. Zhang, J.; Zhang, H.; Zi, T. Overexpression of microRNA-141 relieves chronic constriction injury-induced neuropathic pain via targeting high-mobility group box 1. *Int. J. Mol. Med.* **2015**, *36*, 1433–1439. [CrossRef]
29. Zhang, Y.; Mou, J.; Cao, L.; Zhen, S.; Huang, H.; Bao, H. MicroRNA-142-3p relieves neuropathic pain by targeting high mobility group box 1. *Int. J. Mol. Med.* **2017**, *41*, 501–510. [CrossRef]
30. Wu, B.; Guo, Y.; Chen, Q.; Xiong, Q.; Min, S. MicroRNA-193a Downregulates HMGB1 to Alleviate Diabetic Neuropathic Pain in a Mouse Model. *Neuroimmunomodulation* **2019**, *26*, 250–257. [CrossRef]
31. Xia, L.-X.; Ke, C.; Lu, J.-M. NEAT1 contributes to neuropathic pain development through targeting miR-381/HMGB1 axis in CCI rat models. *J. Cell. Physiol.* **2018**, *233*, 7103–7111. [CrossRef]
32. Zhan, L.-Y.; Lei, S.-Q.; Zhang, B.-H.; Li, W.-L.; Wang, H.-X.; Zhao, B.; Cui, S.-S.; Ding, H.; Huang, Q.-M. Overexpression of miR-381 relieves neuropathic pain development via targeting HMGB1 and CXCR4. *Biomed. Pharmacother.* **2018**, *107*, 818–823. [CrossRef]
33. Liu, C.C.; Cheng, J.T.; Li, T.Y.; Tan, P.H. Integrated analysis of microRNA and mRNA expression profiles in the rat spinal cord under inflammatory pain conditions. *Eur. J. Neurosci.* **2017**, *46*, 2713–2728. [CrossRef]
34. Wang, Z.; Liu, F.; Wei, M.; Qiu, Y.; Ma, C.; Shen, L.; Huang, Y. Chronic constriction injury-induced microRNA-146a-5p alleviates neuropathic pain through suppression of IRAK1/TRAF6 signaling pathway. *J. Neuroinflamm.* **2018**, *15*, 179. [CrossRef]
35. Sun, Q.; Zeng, J.; Liu, Y.; Chen, J.; Zeng, Q.-C.; Tu, L.-L.; Chen, P.; Yang, F.; Zhang, M. microRNA-9 and -29a regulate the progression of diabetic peripheral neuropathy via ISL1-mediated sonic hedgehog signaling pathway. *Aging* **2020**, *12*, 11446–11465. [CrossRef]
36. Li, H.; Fan, L.; Zhang, Y.; Cao, Y.; Liu, X. SNHG16 aggravates chronic constriction injury-induced neuropathic pain in rats via binding with miR-124-3p and miR-141-3p to upregulate JAG1. *Brain Res. Bull.* **2020**, *165*, 228–237. [CrossRef]
37. Sakai, A.; Saitow, F.; Maruyama, M.; Miyake, N.; Miyake, K.; Shimada, T.; Okada, T.; Suzuki, H. MicroRNA cluster miR-17-92 regulates multiple functionally related voltage-gated potassium channels in chronic neuropathic pain. *Nat. Commun.* **2017**, *8*, 16079. [CrossRef]
38. Zhang, J.; Rong, L.; Shao, J.; Zhang, Y.; Liu, Y.; Zhao, S.; Li, L.; Yu, W.; Zhang, M.; Ren, X.; et al. Epigenetic restoration of voltage-gated potassium channel Kv1.2 alleviates nerve injury-induced neuropathic pain. *J. Neurochem.* **2021**, *156*, 367–378. [CrossRef]
39. Wang, W.; Li, R. MiR-216a-5p alleviates chronic constriction injury-induced neuropathic pain in rats by targeting KDM3A and inactivating Wnt/β-catenin signaling pathway. *Neurosci. Res.* **2020**, *170*, 255–264. [CrossRef]
40. Tozaki-Saitoh, H.; Masuda, J.; Kawada, R.; Kojima, C.; Yoneda, S.; Masuda, T.; Inoue, K.; Tsuda, M. Transcription factor MafB contributes to the activation of spinal microglia underlying neuropathic pain development. *Glia* **2018**, *67*, 729–740. [CrossRef]
41. Zhang, Y.; Su, Z.; Liu, H.-L.; Li, L.; Wei, M.; Ge, D.-J.; Zhang, Z.-J. Effects of miR-26a-5p on neuropathic pain development by targeting MAPK6 in in CCI rat models. *Biomed. Pharmacother.* **2018**, *107*, 644–649. [CrossRef] [PubMed]
42. Huang, B.; Guo, S.; Zhang, Y.; Lin, P.; Lin, C.; Chen, M.; Zhu, S.; Huang, L.; He, J.; Zhang, L.; et al. MiR-223-3p alleviates trigeminal neuropathic pain in the male mouse by targeting MKNK2 and MAPK/ERK signaling. *Brain Behav.* **2022**, *12*, e2634. [CrossRef] [PubMed]
43. Qiu, S.; Liu, B.; Mo, Y.; Wang, X.; Zhong, L.; Han, X.; Mi, F. MiR-101 promotes pain hypersensitivity in rats with chronic constriction injury via the MKP-1 mediated MAPK pathway. *J. Cell. Mol. Med.* **2020**, *24*, 8986–8997. [CrossRef] [PubMed]
44. Xie, X.; Ma, L.; Xi, K.; Zhang, W.; Fan, D. MicroRNA-183 Suppresses Neuropathic Pain and Expression of AMPA Receptors by Targeting mTOR/VEGF Signaling Pathway. *Cell. Physiol. Biochem.* **2017**, *41*, 181–192. [CrossRef] [PubMed]
45. Dong, Y.; Li, P.; Ni, Y.; Zhao, J.; Liu, Z. Decreased MicroRNA-125a-3p Contributes to Upregulation of p38 MAPK in Rat Trigeminal Ganglions with Orofacial Inflammatory Pain. *PLoS ONE* **2014**, *9*, e111594. [CrossRef]
46. Wang, X.; Wang, H.; Zhang, T.; He, M.; Liang, H.; Wang, H.; Xu, L.; Chen, S.; Xu, M. Inhibition of MicroRNA-195 Alleviates Neuropathic Pain by Targeting Patched1 and Inhibiting SHH Signaling Pathway Activation. *Neurochem. Res.* **2019**, *44*, 1690–1702. [CrossRef]
47. Wan, Y.; Su, Z.; Li, F.; Gao, P.; Zhang, X. MiR-122-5p suppresses neuropathic pain development by targeting PDK4. *Neurochem. Res.* **2021**, *46*, 957–963. [CrossRef]
48. Pan, Z.; Li, G.-F.; Sun, M.-L.; Xie, L.; Liu, D.; Zhang, Q.; Yang, X.-X.; Xia, S.; Liu, X.; Zhou, H.; et al. MicroRNA-1224 Splicing CircularRNA-Filip1l in an Ago2-Dependent Manner Regulates Chronic Inflammatory Pain via Targeting Ubr5. *J. Neurosci.* **2019**, *39*, 2125–2143. [CrossRef]

49. Chen, W.; Guo, S.; Wang, S. MicroRNA-16 Alleviates Inflammatory Pain by Targeting Ras-Related Protein 23 (RAB23) and Inhibiting p38 MAPK Activation. *Experiment* **2016**, *22*, 3894–3901. [CrossRef]
50. Fang, B.; Wei, L.; Dong, K.; Niu, X.; Sui, X.; Zhang, H. miR-202 modulates the progression of neuropathic pain through targeting RAP1A. *J. Cell. Biochem.* **2018**, *120*, 2973–2982. [CrossRef]
51. Wu, Y.; Gu, Y.; Shi, B. miR-590-3p Alleviates diabetic peripheral neuropathic pain by targeting RAP1A and suppressing infiltration by the T cells. *Acta Biochim. Pol.* **2020**, *67*, 587–593. [CrossRef] [PubMed]
52. Zhang, X.; Guo, H.; Xie, A.; Liao, O.; Ju, F.; Zhou, Y. MicroRNA-144 relieves chronic constriction injury-induced neuropathic pain via targeting RASA. *Biotechnol. Appl. Biochem.* **2019**, *67*, 294–302. [CrossRef] [PubMed]
53. Li, J.; Zhu, Y.; Ma, Z.; Liu, Y.; Sun, Z.; Wu, Y. miR-140 ameliorates neuropathic pain in CCI rats by targeting S1PR1. *J. Recept. Signal Transduct. Res.* **2020**, *41*, 401–407. [CrossRef] [PubMed]
54. Chen, H.-P.; Zhou, W.; Kang, L.-M.; Yan, H.; Zhang, L.; Xu, B.-H.; Cai, W.-H. Intrathecal miR-96 Inhibits Nav1.3 Expression and Alleviates Neuropathic Pain in Rat Following Chronic Construction Injury. *Neurochem. Res.* **2013**, *39*, 76–83. [CrossRef] [PubMed]
55. Ye, G.; Zhang, Y.; Zhao, J.; Chen, Y.; Kong, L.; Sheng, C.; Yuan, L. miR-384-5p ameliorates neuropathic pain by targeting SCN3A in a rat model of chronic constriction injury. *Neurol. Res.* **2020**, *42*, 299–307. [CrossRef]
56. Jia, Q.; Dong, W.; Zhang, L.; Yang, X. Activating Sirt1 by resveratrol suppresses Nav1.7 expression in DRG through miR-182 and alleviates neuropathic pain in rats. *Channels* **2020**, *14*, 69–78. [CrossRef]
57. Cai, W.; Zhao, Q.; Shao, J.; Zhang, J.; Li, L.; Ren, X.; Su, S.; Bai, Q.; Li, M.; Chen, X.; et al. MicroRNA-182 Alleviates Neuropathic Pain by Regulating Nav1.7 Following Spared Nerve Injury in Rats. *Sci. Rep.* **2018**, *8*, 16750. [CrossRef]
58. Shao, J.; Cao, J.; Wang, J.; Ren, X.; Su, S.; Li, M.; Li, Z.; Zhao, Q.; Zang, W. MicroRNA-30b regulates expression of the sodium channel Nav1.7 in nerve injury-induced neuropathic pain in the rat. *Mol. Pain* **2016**, *12*, 671523. [CrossRef]
59. Chen, S.; Gu, Y.; Dai, Q.; He, Y.; Wang, J. Spinal miR-34a regulates inflammatory pain by targeting SIRT1 in complete Freund's adjuvant mice. *Biochem. Biophys. Res. Commun.* **2019**, *516*, 1196–1203. [CrossRef]
60. Chu, Y.; Ge, W.; Wang, X. MicroRNA-448 modulates the progression of neuropathic pain by targeting sirtuin 1. *Exp. Ther. Med.* **2019**, *18*, 4665–4672. [CrossRef]
61. Yang, D.; Yang, Q.; Wei, X.; Liu, Y.; Ma, D.; Li, J.; Wan, Y.; Luo, Y. The role of miR-190a-5p contributes to diabetic neuropathic pain via targeting SLC17A6. *J. Pain Res.* **2017**, *10*, 2395–2403. [CrossRef]
62. Zhou, X.G.; He, H.; Wang, P. A critical role for miR-135a-5p-mediated regulation of SLC24A2 in neuropathic pain. *Mol. Med. Rep.* **2020**, *22*, 2115–2122. [CrossRef]
63. Tan, Y.; Yang, J.; Xiang, K.; Tan, Q.; Guo, Q. Suppression of MicroRNA-155 Attenuates Neuropathic Pain by Regulating SOCS1 Signalling Pathway. *Neurochem. Res.* **2014**, *40*, 550–560. [CrossRef]
64. Xia, L.; Zhang, Y.; Dong, T. Inhibition of MicroRNA-221 Alleviates Neuropathic Pain Through Targeting Suppressor of Cytokine Signaling 1. *J. Mol. Neurosci.* **2016**, *59*, 411–420. [CrossRef]
65. Li, L.; Zhao, G. Downregulation of microRNA-218 relieves neuropathic pain by regulating suppressor of cytokine signaling International 3. *J. Mol. Med.* **2016**, *37*, 851–858. [CrossRef]
66. Yan, X.-T.; Ji, L.-J.; Wang, Z.; Wu, X.; Wang, Q.; Sun, S.; Lu, J.-M.; Zhang, Y. MicroRNA-93 alleviates neuropathic pain through targeting signal transducer and activator of transcription 3. *Int. Immunopharmacol.* **2017**, *46*, 156–162. [CrossRef]
67. Zhong, L.; Fu, K.; Xiao, W.; Wang, F.; Shen, L. Overexpression of miR-98 attenuates neuropathic pain development via targeting STAT3 in CCI rat models. *J. Cell. Biochem.* **2018**, *120*, 7989–7997. [CrossRef]
68. Jin, H.; Du, X.; Zhao, Y.; Xia, D. XIST/miR-544 axis induces neuropathic pain by activating STAT3 in a rat model. *J. Cell. Physiol.* **2018**, *233*, 5847–5855. [CrossRef]
69. Elramah, S.; López-González, M.J.; Bastide, M.; Dixmérias, F.; Roca-Lapirot, O.; Wielanek-Bachelet, A.C.; Vital, A.; Leste-Lasserre, T.; Brochard, A.; Landry, M.; et al. Spinal miRNA-124 regulates synaptopodin and nociception in an animal model of bone cancer pain. *Sci. Rep.* **2017**, *7*, 10949. [CrossRef]
70. Bao, Y.; Wang, S.; Xie, Y.; Jin, K.; Bai, Y.; Shan, S. MiR-28-5p relieves neuropathic pain by targeting Zeb1 in CCI rat models. *J. Cell. Biochem.* **2018**, *119*, 8555–8563. [CrossRef]
71. Tramullas, M.; Francés, R.; de la Fuente, R.; Velategui, S.; Carcelén, M.; García, R.; Llorca, J.; Hurlé, M.A. MicroRNA-30c-5p modulates neuropathic pain in rodents. *Sci. Transl. Med.* **2018**, *10*, eaao6299. [CrossRef] [PubMed]
72. Sun, X.; Zhang, H. miR-451 elevation relieves inflammatory pain by suppressing microglial activation-evoked inflammatory response via targeting TLR4. *Cell Tissue Res.* **2018**, *374*, 487–495. [CrossRef] [PubMed]
73. Wei, M.; Li, L.; Zhang, Y.; Zhang, Z.; Liu, H.; Bao, H. LncRNA X inactive specific transcript contributes to neuropathic pain development by sponging miR-154-5p via inducing toll-like receptor 5 in CCI rat models. *J. Cell. Biochem.* **2018**, *120*, 1271–1281. [CrossRef] [PubMed]
74. Zhang, Z.-J.; Guo, J.-S.; Li, S.-S.; Wu, X.-B.; Cao, D.-L.; Jiang, B.-C.; Jing, P.-B.; Bai, X.-Q.; Li, C.-H.; Wu, Z.-H.; et al. TLR8 and its endogenous ligand miR-21 contribute to neuropathic pain in murine DRG. *J. Exp. Med.* **2018**, *215*, 3019–3037. [CrossRef]
75. Shi, D.-N.; Yuan, Y.-T.; Ye, D.; Kang, L.-M.; Wen, J.; Chen, H.-P. MiR-183-5p Alleviates Chronic Constriction Injury-Induced Neuropathic Pain Through Inhibition of TREK-1. *Neurochem. Res.* **2018**, *43*, 1143–1149. [CrossRef]
76. Miao, J.; Zhou, X.; Ji, T.; Chen, G. NF-κB p65-dependent transcriptional regulation of histone deacetylase 2 contributes to the chronic constriction injury-induced neuropathic pain via the microRNA-183/TXNIP/NLRP3 axis. *J Neuroinflamm.* **2020**, *17*, 225. [CrossRef]

77. Ji, L.-J.; Su, J.; Xu, A.-L.; Pang, B.; Huang, Q.-M. MiR-134-5p attenuates neuropathic pain progression through targeting Twist1. *J. Cell. Biochem.* **2019**, *120*, 1694–1701. [CrossRef]
78. Brandenburger, T.; Johannsen, L.; Prassek, V.; Kuebart, A.; Raile, J.; Wohlfromm, S.; Köhrer, K.; Huhn, R.; Hollmann, M.W.; Hermanns, H. MiR-34a is differentially expressed in dorsal root ganglia in a rat model of chronic neuropathic pain. *Neurosci. Lett.* **2019**, *708*, 134365. [CrossRef]
79. Zhang, X.; Zhang, Y.; Cai, W.; Liu, Y.; Liu, H.; Zhang, Z.; Su, Z. MicroRNA-128-3p Alleviates Neuropathic Pain Through Targeting ZEB1. *Neurosci. Lett.* **2020**, *729*, 134946. [CrossRef]
80. Yan, X.; Lu, J.; Wang, Y.; Cheng, X.; He, X.; Zheng, W.; Chen, H.; Wang, Y. XIST accelerates neuropathic pain progression through regulation of miR-150 and ZEB1 in CCI rat models. *J. Cell. Physiol.* **2018**, *233*, 6098–6106. [CrossRef]
81. Chen, Z.-L.; Liu, J.-Y.; Wang, F.; Jing, X. Suppression of MALAT1 ameliorates chronic constriction injury-induced neuropathic pain in rats via modulating miR-206 and ZEB2. *J. Cell. Physiol.* **2019**, *234*, 15647–15653. [CrossRef]
82. Łuczkowska, K.; Rogińska, D.; Ulańczyk, Z.; Safranow, K.; Paczkowska, E.; Baumert, B.; Milczarek, S.; Osękowska, B.; Górska, M.; Borowiecka, E.; et al. microRNAs as the biomarkers of chemotherapy-induced peripheral neuropathy in patients with multiple myeloma. *Leuk Lymphoma* **2021**, *62*, 2768–2776. [CrossRef]
83. McDonald, M.K.; Tian, Y.; Qureshi, R.A.; Gormley, M.; Ertel, A.; Gao, R.; Lopez, E.A.; Alexander, G.M.; Sacan, A.; Fortina, P.; et al. Functional significance of macrophage-derived exosomes in inflammation and pain. *Pain* **2014**, *155*, 1527–1539. [CrossRef]
84. Orlova, I.A.; Alexander, G.M.; Qureshi, R.A.; Sacan, A.; Graziano, A.; Barrett, J.E.; Schwartzman, R.J.; Ajit, S.K. MicroRNA modulation in complex regional pain syndrome. *J. Transl. Med.* **2011**, *9*, 195. [CrossRef]
85. Ciccacci, C.; Latini, A.; Colantuono, A.; Politi, C.; D'Amato, C.; Greco, C.; Rinaldi, M.E.; Lauro, D.; Novelli, G.; Spallone, V.; et al. Expression study of candidate miRNAs and evaluation of their potential use as biomarkers of diabetic neuropathy. *Epigenomics* **2020**, *12*, 575–585. [CrossRef]
86. Li, Y.B.; Wu, Q.; Liu, J.; Fan, Y.Z.; Yu, K.F.; Cai, Y. miR-199a-3p is involved in the pathogenesis and progression of diabetic neuropathy through downregulation of SerpinE2. *Mol. Med. Rep.* **2017**, *16*, 2417–2424. [CrossRef]
87. Asahchop, E.L.; Branton, W.G.; Krishnan, A.; Chen, P.A.; Yang, D.; Kong, L.L.; Zochodne, D.W.; Brew, B.; John, G.M.; Power, D.C. HIV-associated sensory polyneuropathy and neuronal injury are associated with miRNA–455-3p induction. *J. Clin. Investig.* **2018**, *3*. [CrossRef]
88. Tavares-Ferreira, D.; Lawless, N.; Bird, E.V.; Atkins, S.; Collier, D.; Sher, E.; Malki, K.; Lambert, D.W.; Boissonade, F.M. Correlation of miRNA expression with intensity of neuropathic pain in man. *Mol. Pain* **2019**, *15*. [CrossRef]
89. Dayer, C.F.; Luthi, F.; Le Carré, J.; Vuistiner, P.; Terrier, P.; Benaim, C.; Giacobino, J.-P.; Léger, B. Differences in the miRNA signatures of chronic musculoskeletal pain patients from neuropathic or nociceptive origins. *PLoS ONE* **2019**, *14*, e0219311. [CrossRef]
90. Heyn, J.; Luchting, B.; Hinske, L.C.; Hübner, M.; Azad, S.C.; Kreth, S. miR-124a and miR-155 enhance differentiation of regulatory T cells in patients with neuropathic pain. *J. Neuroinflamm.* **2016**, *13*, 248. [CrossRef]
91. Leinders, M.; Üçeyler, N.; Pritchard, R.; Sommer, C.; Sorkin, L. Increased miR-132-3p expression is associated with chronic neuropathic pain. *Exp. Neurol.* **2016**, *283*, 276–286. [CrossRef] [PubMed]
92. Liu, J.C.; Xue, D.F.; Wang, X.Q.; Ai, D.B.; Qin, P.J. MiR-101 relates to chronic peripheral neuropathic pain through targeting KPNB1 and regulating NF-κB signaling. *Kaohsiung J. Med. Sci.* **2019**, *35*, 139–145. [CrossRef] [PubMed]
93. Leinders, M.; Üçeyler, N.; Thomann, A.; Sommer, C. Aberrant microRNA expression in patients with painful peripheral neuropathies. *J. Neurol. Sci.* **2017**, *380*, 242–249. [CrossRef] [PubMed]
94. Li, X.; Wang, D.; Zhou, J.; Yan, Y.; Chen, L. Evaluation of circulating microRNA expression in patients with trigeminal neuralgia: An observational study. *Medicine* **2020**, *99*, e22972. [CrossRef]
95. Li, Z.; Zhou, Y.; Li, Z. NFKB1 Signalling Activation Contributes to TRPV1 Over-expression via Repressing MiR-375 and MiR-455: A Study on Neuropathic Low Back Pain. *Folia Biol. (Praha)* **2022**, *68*, 105–111.
96. Ha, M.; Kim, V.N. Regulation of microRNA biogenesis. *Nat. Rev. Mol. Cell Biol.* **2014**, *15*, 509–524. [CrossRef]
97. Kosik, K.S. The neuronal microRNA system. *Nat. Rev. Neurosci.* **2006**, *7*, 911–920. [CrossRef]
98. Stavast, C.; Erkeland, S. The Non-Canonical Aspects of MicroRNAs: Many Roads to Gene Regulation. *Cells* **2019**, *8*, 1465. [CrossRef]
99. Sakai, A.; Saitow, F.; Miyake, N.; Miyake, K.; Shimada, T.; Suzuki, H. miR-7a alleviates the maintenance of neuropathic pain through regulation of neuronal excitability. *Brain* **2013**, *136*, 2738–2750. [CrossRef]
100. Wang, J.-J.; Li, Y. KCNQ potassium channels in sensory system and neural circuits. *Acta Pharmacol. Sin.* **2015**, *37*, 25–33. [CrossRef]
101. Alloui, A.; Zimmermann, K.; Mamet, J.; Duprat, F.; Noël, J.; Chemin, J.; Guy, N.; Blondeau, N.; Voilley, N.; Rubat-Coudert, C.; et al. TREK-1, a K$^+$ channel involved in polymodal pain perception. *EMBO J.* **2006**, *25*, 2368–2376. [CrossRef]
102. Perret, D.; Luo, Z.D. Targeting voltage-gated calcium channels for neuropathic pain management. *Neurotherapeutics* **2009**, *6*, 679–692. [CrossRef]
103. Willemen, H.L.D.M.; Huo, X.-J.; Mao-Ying, Q.-L.; Zijlstra, J.; Heijnen, C.J.; Kavelaars, A. MicroRNA-124 as a novel treatment for persistent hyperalgesia. *J. Neuroinflamm.* **2012**, *9*, 143. [CrossRef]
104. Scholz, J.; Broom, D.C.; Youn, D.-H.; Mills, C.D.; Kohno, T.; Suter, M.R.; Moore, K.A.; Decosterd, I.; Coggeshall, R.E.; Woolf, C.J. Blocking Caspase Activity Prevents Transsynaptic Neuronal Apoptosis and the Loss of Inhibition in Lamina II of the Dorsal Horn after Peripheral Nerve Injury. *J. Neurosci.* **2005**, *25*, 7317–7323. [CrossRef]

105. Lehmann, S.M.; Krüger, C.; Park, B.; Derkow, K.; Rosenberger, K.; Baumgart, J.; Trimbuch, T.; Eom, G.; Hinz, M.; Kaul, D.; et al. An unconventional role for miRNA: Let-7 activates Toll-like receptor 7 and causes neurodegeneration. *Nat. Neurosci.* **2012**, *15*, 827–835. [CrossRef]
106. Chen, Y.; Stallings, R.L. Differential Patterns of MicroRNA Expression in Neuroblastoma Are Correlated with Prognosis, Differentiation, and Apoptosis. *Cancer Res.* **2007**, *67*, 976–983. [CrossRef]
107. Yin, K.-J.; Deng, Z.; Huang, H.; Hamblin, M.; Xie, C.; Zhang, J.; Chen, Y.E. miR-497 regulates neuronal death in mouse brain after transient focal cerebral ischemia. *Neurobiol. Dis.* **2010**, *38*, 17–26. [CrossRef]
108. Cheng, J.-K.; Ji, R.-R. Intracellular Signaling in Primary Sensory Neurons and Persistent Pain. *Neurochem. Res.* **2008**, *33*, 1970–1978. [CrossRef]
109. Ji, R.-R.; Gereau, R.W.; Malcangio, M.; Strichartz, G.R. MAP kinase and pain. *Brain Res. Rev.* **2009**, *60*, 135–148. [CrossRef]
110. Yang, Q.; Liu, Z.; Chang, Y. Downregulation of miR-206 contributes to neuropathic pain in rats by enhancing RASA1 expression. *Int. J. Clin. Exp. Med.* **2016**, *9*, 3146–3152.
111. Sun, W.; Zhang, L.; Li, R. Overexpression of miR-206 ameliorates chronic constriction injury-induced neuropathic pain in rats via the MEK/ERK pathway by targeting brain-derived neurotrophic factor. *Neurosci. Lett.* **2017**, *646*, 68–74. [CrossRef] [PubMed]
112. Ji, R.-R.; Suter, M. p38 MAPK, microglial signaling, and neuropathic pain. *Mol. Pain* **2007**, *3*, 33. [CrossRef] [PubMed]
113. Duan, Z.; Zhang, J.; Li, J.; Pang, X.; Wang, H. Inhibition of microRNA-155 Reduces Neuropathic Pain During Chemotherapeutic Bortezomib via Engagement of Neuroinflammation. *Front. Oncol.* **2020**, *10*, 416. [CrossRef]
114. Gao, Y.-J.; Ji, R.-R. Activation of JNK pathway in persistent pain. *Neurosci. Lett.* **2008**, *437*, 180–183. [CrossRef] [PubMed]
115. Yang, F.-R.; Chen, J.; Yi, H.; Peng, L.-Y.; Hu, X.-L.; Guo, Q.-L. MicroRNA-7a ameliorates neuropathic pain in a rat model of spinal nerve ligation via the neurofilament light polypeptide-dependent signal transducer and activator of transcription signaling pathway. *Mol. Pain* **2019**, *15*, 842464. [CrossRef]
116. Zhou, S.; Yu, B.; Qian, T.; Yao, D.; Wang, Y.; Ding, F.; Gu, X. Early changes of microRNAs expression in the dorsal root ganglia following rat sciatic nerve transection. *Neurosci. Lett.* **2011**, *494*, 89–93. [CrossRef]
117. Ji, R.-R.; Chamessian, A.; Zhang, Y.-Q. Pain regulation by non-neuronal cells and inflammation. *Science* **2016**, *354*, 572–577. [CrossRef]
118. Calvo, M.; Dawes, J.M.; Bennett, D.L. The role of the immune system in the generation of neuropathic pain. *Lancet Neurol.* **2012**, *11*, 629–642. [CrossRef]
119. Simeoli, R.; Montague, K.; Jones, H.R.; Castaldi, L.; Chambers, D.; Kelleher, J.H.; Vacca, V.; Pitcher, T.; Grist, J.; Al-Ahdal, H.; et al. Exosomal cargo including microRNA regulates sensory neuron to macrophage communication after nerve trauma. *Nat. Commun.* **2017**, *8*, 1778. [CrossRef]
120. Bhatheja, K.; Field, J. Schwann cells: Origins and role in axonal maintenance and regeneration. *Int. J. Biochem. Cell Biol.* **2006**, *38*, 1995–1999. [CrossRef]
121. Scholz, J.; Woolf, C.J. The neuropathic pain triad: Neurons, immune cells and glia. *Nat. Neurosci.* **2007**, *10*, 1361–1368. [CrossRef]
122. Sohn, E.J.; Park, H.T. MicroRNA Mediated Regulation of Schwann Cell Migration and Proliferation in Peripheral Nerve Injury. *BioMed Res. Int.* **2018**, *2018*, 8198365. [CrossRef]
123. Li, S.; Wang, X.; Gu, Y.; Chen, C.; Wang, Y.; Liu, J.; Hu, W.; Yu, B.; Wang, Y.; Ding, F.; et al. Let-7 microRNAs Regenerate Peripheral Nerve Regeneration by Targeting Nerve Growth Factor. *Mol. Ther.* **2015**, *23*, 423–433. [CrossRef]
124. Yi, S.; Yuan, Y.; Chen, Q.; Wang, X.; Gong, L.; Liu, J.; Gu, X.; Li, S. Regulation of Schwann cell proliferation and migration by miR-1 targeting brain-derived neurotrophic factor after peripheral nerve injury. *Sci. Rep.* **2016**, *6*, 29121. [CrossRef]
125. Viader, A.; Chang, L.-W.; Fahrner, T.; Nagarajan, R.; Milbrandt, J. MicroRNAs Modulate Schwann Cell Response to Nerve Injury by Reinforcing Transcriptional Silencing of Dedifferentiation-Related Genes. *J. Neurosci.* **2011**, *31*, 17358–17369. [CrossRef]
126. Norcini, M.; Sideris, A.; Hernandez, L.A.M.; Zhang, J.; Blanck, T.J.J.; Recio-Pinto, E. An approach to identify microRNAs involved in neuropathic pain following a peripheral nerve injury. *Front. Neurosci.* **2014**, *8*, 266. [CrossRef]
127. Bali, K.K.; Hackenberg, M.; Lubin, A.; Kuner, R.; Devor, M. Sources of Individual Variability: Mirnas That Predispose to Neuropathic Pain Identified Using Genome-Wide Sequencing. *Mol. Pain* **2014**, *10*, 22. [CrossRef]
128. Ponomarev, E.D.; Veremeyko, T.; Barteneva, N.; Krichevsky, A.M.; Weiner, H.L. MicroRNA-124 promotes microglia quiescence and suppresses EAE by deactivating macrophages via the C/EBP-α–PU.1 pathway. *Nat. Med.* **2011**, *17*, 64–70. [CrossRef]
129. Lu, Y.; Cao, D.-L.; Jiang, B.-C.; Yang, T.; Gao, Y.-J. MicroRNA-146a-5p attenuates neuropathic pain via suppressing TRAF6 signaling in the spinal cord. *Brain Behav. Immun.* **2015**, *49*, 119–129. [CrossRef]
130. Leung, A.K.; Vyas, S.; Rood, J.E.; Bhutkar, A.; Sharp, P.A.; Chang, P. Poly(ADP-Ribose) Regulates Stress Responses and MicroRNA Activity in the Cytoplasm. *Mol. Cell* **2011**, *42*, 489–499. [CrossRef]
131. Aldrich, B.; Frakes, E.; Kasuya, J.; Hammond, D.; Kitamoto, T. Changes in expression of sensory organ-specific microRNAs in rat dorsal root ganglia in association with mechanical hypersensitivity induced by spinal nerve ligation. *Neuroscience* **2009**, *164*, 711–723. [CrossRef] [PubMed]
132. Ergun, S.; Oztuzcu, S. Oncocers: ceRNA-mediated cross-talk by sponging miRNAs in oncogenic pathways. *Tumour Biol.* **2015**, *36*, 3129–3136. [CrossRef] [PubMed]
133. Song, G.; Yang, Z.; Guo, J.; Zheng, Y.; Su, X.; Wang, X. Interactions Among lncRNAs/circRNAs, miRNAs, and mRNAs in Neuropathic Pain. *Neurotherapeutics* **2020**, *17*, 917–931. [CrossRef] [PubMed]

134. Wang, C.; Xu, X.; Chen, J.; Kang, Y.; Guo, J.; Duscher, D.; Yang, X.; Guo, G.; Ren, S.; Xiong, H.; et al. The Construction and Analysis of lncRNA-miRNA-mRNA Competing Endogenous RNA Network of Schwann Cells in Diabetic Peripheral Neuropathy. *Front. Bioeng. Biotechnol.* **2020**, *8*, 490. [CrossRef] [PubMed]
135. Fang, Z.H.; Liao, H.L.; Tang, Q.F.; Liu, Y.J.; Zhang, Y.Y.; Lin, J.; Yu, H.P.; Zhou, C.; Li, C.J.; Liu, F.; et al. Interactions among Non-Coding RNAs and mRNAs in the Trigeminal Ganglion Associated with Neuropathic Pain. *J. Pain Res.* **2022**, *15*, 2967–2988. [CrossRef]
136. Park, C.-K.; Xu, Z.-Z.; Berta, T.; Han, Q.; Chen, G.; Liu, X.-J.; Ji, R.-R. Extracellular microRNAs activate nociceptor neurons to elicit pain via TLR7 and TRPA1. *Neuron* **2014**, *82*, 47–54. [CrossRef]
137. Fabbri, M. TLRs as miRNA Receptors. *Cancer Res.* **2012**, *72*, 6333–6337. [CrossRef]
138. Han, Q.; Liu, D.; Convertino, M.; Wang, Z.; Jiang, C.; Kim, Y.H.; Luo, X.; Zhang, X.; Nackley, A.; Dokholyan, N.V.; et al. miRNA-711 Binds and Activates TRPA1 Extracellularly to Evoke Acute and Chronic Pruritus. *Neuron* **2018**, *99*, 449–463. [CrossRef]
139. Guo, J.-B.; Zhu, Y.; Chen, B.-L.; Song, G.; Peng, M.-S.; Hu, H.-Y.; Zheng, Y.-L.; Chen, C.-C.; Yang, J.-Z.; Chen, P.-J.; et al. Network and pathway-based analysis of microRNA role in neuropathic pain in rat models. *J. Cell. Mol. Med.* **2019**, *23*, 4534–4544. [CrossRef]
140. Linnstaedt, S.D.; Riker, K.D.; Rueckeis, C.A.; Kutchko, K.M.; Lackey, L.; McCarthy, K.R.; Tsai, Y.-H.; Parker, J.S.; Kurz, M.C.; Hendry, P.L.; et al. A Functional riboSNitch in the 3′ Untranslated Region of *FKBP5* Alters MicroRNA-320a Binding Efficiency and Mediates Vulnerability to Chronic Post-Traumatic Pain. *J. Neurosci.* **2018**, *38*, 8407–8420. [CrossRef]
141. Atkins, S.; Kyriakidou, E. Clinical outcomes of lingual nerve repair. *Br. J. Oral Maxillofac. Surg.* **2021**, *59*, 39–45. [CrossRef]
142. Dasgupta, I.; Chatterjee, A. Recent Advances in miRNA Delivery Systems. *Methods Protoc.* **2021**, *4*, 10. [CrossRef]
143. Paunovska, K.; Loughrey, D.; Dahlman, J.E. Drug delivery systems for RNA therapeutics. *Nat. Rev. Genet.* **2022**, *23*, 265–280. [CrossRef]

Disclaimer/Publisher's Note: The statements, opinions and data contained in all publications are solely those of the individual author(s) and contributor(s) and not of MDPI and/or the editor(s). MDPI and/or the editor(s) disclaim responsibility for any injury to people or property resulting from any ideas, methods, instructions or products referred to in the content.

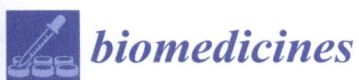

Systematic Review

The Effects of Non-Pharmacological Interventions in Fibromyalgia: A Systematic Review and Metanalysis of Predominants Outcomes

Isabel Hong-Baik [1], Edurne Úbeda-D'Ocasar [1], Eduardo Cimadevilla-Fernández-Pola [1], Victor Jiménez-Díaz-Benito [2] and Juan Pablo Hervás-Pérez [1,*]

[1] Department of Physiotherapy, Faculty of Health, Camilo José Cela University, 28692 Villanueva de la Cañada, Madrid, Spain; isabel.hong@alumno.ucjc.edu (I.H.-B.); eubeda@ucjc.edu (E.Ú.-D.); ecimadevilla@ucjc.edu (E.C.-F.-P.)

[2] Department of Sport Sciences, Faculty of Physical Activity and Sport Sciences, Universidad Europea de Madrid, 28670 Villaviciosa de Odón, Madrid, Spain; victorjimenezdb@gmail.com

* Correspondence: jphervas@ucjc.edu; Tel.: +34-91-815-31-31

Abstract: (1) Fibromyalgia (FM) is a chronic musculoskeletal condition with multiple symptoms primarily affecting women. An imbalance in cytokine levels has been observed, suggesting a chronic low-grade inflammation. The main aim of the meta-analysis was to examine the effect of multimodal rehabilitation on cytokine levels and other predominant variables in patients with FM. Furthermore, to examine which non-pharmacological tools have been used to investigate the effects that these can have on cytokines in FM patients. (2) Methods: Searches were conducted in PubMed, Scopus, Web of Science, Cochrane, and ScienceDirect databases. This systematic review and metanalysis followed the PRISMA statement protocol. The methodological quality of the studies was assessed using the PEDro scale, the risk of bias followed the Cochrane Manual 5.0.1, and the GRADE system was used for rating the certainty of evidence. (3) Results: Of 318 studies found, eight were finally selected, with a sample size of 320 women with a mean age of 57 ± 20. The proinflammatory cytokines IL-1β, IL-6, IL-8 and TNF-α were the most studied. Resistance exercise, aquatic exercise, dynamic contractions, cycling, treadmill, and infrared therapy were the main non-pharmacological tools used. (4) Conclusions: The systematic review with meta-analysis found evidence of elevated cytokine levels in patients with FM, suggesting low chronic inflammation and a possible contribution to central sensitization and chronic pain. However, the effects of physiotherapeutic interventions on cytokine levels are variable, highlighting the importance of considering different factors and the need for further research.

Keywords: cytokines; fibromyalgia; physiotherapy; metanalysis

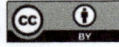

1. Introduction

Fibromyalgia (FM) is characterized by chronic, widespread musculoskeletal pain with multiple tender points and generalized tenderness with muscle stiffness, joint stiffness, sleep disturbances, fatigue, mood, cognitive dysfunction, anxiety, depression, general tenderness, and inability to perform daily life activities. Regarding prevalence, it is estimated that 4% of the world's population is affected by FM, mainly in women aged 20–55 years [1].

The diagnosis is only clinical and consists of a complete assessment based on the 1990 American College of Rheumatology (ACR) criteria of three consecutive months of widespread pain and "tender points" of pain on palpation. In 2010, the ACR updated the criteria with two new parameters, and in 2016, the criteria were further revised to decrease the likelihood of misdiagnosis [2].

FM is a syndrome with a multifactorial etiology that develops depending on genetic predisposition, personal experiences, emotional and cognitive factors, and the individual's ability to cope with stress [3].

Although FM is traditionally a non-inflammatory condition, current evidence suggests that other factors contribute to its pathogenesis, such as inflammatory, immunological, and endocrine factors [4]. In FM, there is increasing evidence of inflammatory mechanisms of neurogenic origin in peripheral tissues, the spinal cord, and the brain. Cytokines/chemokines, lipid mediators, oxidative stress and various plasma-derived factors underlie the inflammatory state in fibromyalgia [1].

This inflammation is closely related to the activation of both the innate and adaptive immune systems that produce an inflammatory cascade of neuropeptides, cytokines, and chemokines, which may play an essential role in the pathophysiology of FM [5]. Cytokines function as messengers of the immune system and have a regulatory role in inflammation and are essential in a brief form; the problem comes when there is prolonged exposure to them, leading to chronic low-grade inflammation. Cytokines are classified into proinflammatory and anti-inflammatory cytokines. The central proinflammatory cytokines are IL-1, IL-2, IL-6, IL-8, IL-12, TNF-α, and IFN, while the central anti-inflammatory cytokines are IL-4, IL-10, IL-13, and TGF. The proinflammatory to anti-inflammatory cytokines ratio is vital in determining disease outcomes [4]. Current research has shown that cytokine levels are imbalanced in the human body and that the proinflammatory to anti-inflammatory cytokines ratio is critical in determining disease outcomes [4].

Current research has shown that cytokine levels are imbalanced in FM patients. There is an imbalance between proinflammatory and anti-inflammatory cytokines, with more proinflammatory cytokines such as TNF-α, IL-1RA, IL-6, and IL-8 [6].

Various non-pharmacology tools and their efficacy in treating patients with FM have been examined in the scientific literature, including strength exercise, aerobic exercise, aquatic exercise, and flexibility exercise. However, the latter is used as part of the warm-up. Therapeutic massage has also been studied, and techniques such as myofascial release, connective tissue massage, lymphatic drainage, and Shiatsu have been explored. In addition, electrotherapy has been incorporated into treatment protocols due to its efficacy and safety profile, including techniques such as Transcutaneous electrical nerve stimulation, transcranial magnetic stimulation, transcranial direct current, and laser [7]. Other tools that have been evaluated include balneotherapy, dry needling, acupuncture, and patient education. Current recommendations for the treatment of FM stress the importance of including patient education and the use of physiotherapy tools as part of the primary treatment [8]. Research on physiotherapy tools is aimed at analyzing whether they can generate effects on proinflammatory and anti-inflammatory cytokine levels in patients with FM [9,10].

This set of specific inflammatory and biochemical markers could help diagnose FM, so research is directed toward studying inflammatory markers to achieve a more objective diagnosis of FM [2]. Recent reviews with metanalysis [11] revealed that individual biomarkers may play a relevant role in identifying pathologies coexisting with FM. However, new research could make it possible to offer the predominant instruments and parameters depending on the type of intervention carried out. Once these parameters were classified, a grouping of predominant outcomes was carried out from the original data of the articles whenever these data were offered. The main aim of the meta-analysis was to examine the effect of multimodal rehabilitation on cytokine levels and other predominant variables in patients with FM. Additionally, the principal purpose of the present study was to analyze women with FM since, at present, the rate of diagnosis is still higher in women than in men, which undoubtedly represents a limitation to being able to draw conclusions about this disease in the male gender.

2. Materials and Methods

2.1. Acquisition of Evidence

For this systematic review, we followed the protocol according to the standards and guidelines of the PRISMA statement [12] for systematic reviews and meta-analyses, which aims to improve the reporting of future systematic reviews. The methodological protocol was registered after the present work (protocol number: INPLASY202370033).

2.2. Eligibility Criteria

The components described in the PICO framework were applied to achieve appropriate results (P—patients with FM according to ACR 1990; I—physiotherapy intervention tool; C—comparison of healthy group vs. FM group (same intervention). FM group vs. FM group (physiotherapy and relaxation intervention); O—results ... levels of proinflammatory and anti-inflammatory cytokines. In the control group and experimental group.

Articles that met the following inclusion criteria were included: (a) publications in the last ten years (from 2013 to 2023); (b) written in English or Spanish; (c) clinical trials and randomized controlled clinical trials using a placebo or control group; (d) subjects with a diagnosis of FM according to the ACR 1990; (e) women of working age (an intervention group performing a physiotherapeutic intervention; (f) cytokine analysis. Exclusion criteria were: (i) subjects with pathologies other than FM; (ii) clinical trials with no results or not completed.

2.3. Sources of Information

The databases Pubmed, Scopus, Web of Science, Cochrane Register, and ScienceDirect were searched. A search was also made in second-line sources, doctoral theses, journal articles, etc., in Dialnet; and Teseo, but there were no results.

These searches were carried out from December 2022 to March 2023.

2.4. Search Strategies

Before starting the present systematic review, a search of different databases was carried out to verify the existence of recent reviews on the topic in question. Subsequently, several searches were performed using different combinations of the key terms, including "cytokines AND fibromyalgia" and "cytokines AND fibromyalgia AND physiotherapy". It used the search equation ("cytokines and Fibromyalgia and Physiotherapy") to focus the search on studies that used physiotherapy tools as an intervention and analyzed their possible effects on cytokines in FM patients. The same Medical Subject Headings (MeSH) terms were used to improve the specificity of the search.

A series of filters were established and included in each database to perform the current searches, which are detailed in Section 2.2 eligibility criteria.

The flow diagram below graphically shows the selection of the articles included in this systematic review and metanalysis.

2.5. Study Selection Process

In the present systematic review and metanalysis, the assessment of potentially relevant studies was performed based on their title and abstracts. The independent variables included in each of the selected studies were the number of patients, the number of withdrawals in each group, the clinical variables of the participants, the measurement tools evaluated, and the characteristics of the intervention applied. The primary dependent variable analyzed was the presence of proinflammatory and anti-inflammatory cytokines in plasma and muscle, regardless of the tool used to measure them. The secondary variables analyzed were the non-pharmacological techniques used. In total, eight studies were included in the systematic review and metanalysis.

2.6. Data Extraction Process

An exhaustive reading and evaluation of the eight studies finally selected were carried out, to which the PEDro scale was applied to assess their methodological quality, evaluating the design of the study, the source of obtaining the subjects, whether the study was randomized, whether there was concealment, whether there was blinding and what the outcome of the study was like. The PEDro scale of the synthesis results can be found in more detail in (Figure 1).

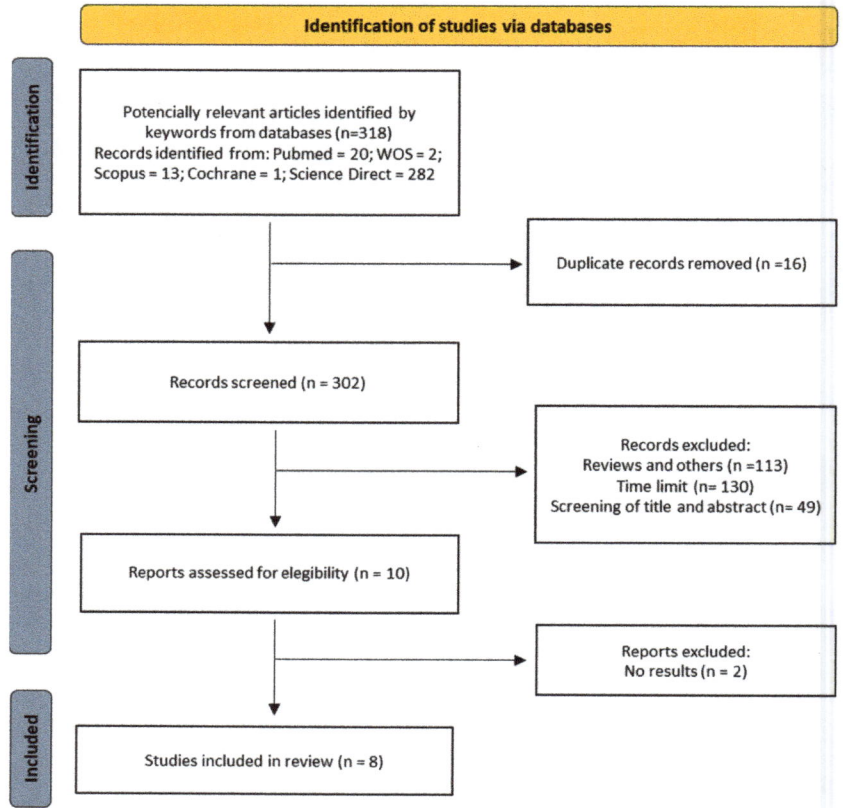

Figure 1. Flow diagram according to the PRISMA declaration.

Also, the PRISMA 2020 checklist [12] was used to collect the most relevant data from each of the studies, author and year, type of study, sample characteristics, objectives, type of intervention, intervention time, number of sessions, frequency of sessions, session time, measures assessing the impact of FM, pain, fatigue, quality of life, depression, anxiety, physical capacity, blood tests to measure the different cytokines, results, conclusions, limitations of the study and the follow-up. The results of the data extraction will be presented in (Supplementary Materials Table S1).

A reviewer working independently carried out both the study selection process and the data extraction process for each of the final articles. Subsequently, the results obtained were analyzed by two independent reviewers (IHB and EUD). In case of doubt or disagreement between the reviewers, they were jointly assessed until a consensus was reached.

2.7. List of Data

The (Supplementary Materials Table S2) presents the table of the most studied cytokines, clearly identifying the most investigated and analyzed cytokines in the studies included in this review. On the other hand, (Supplementary Materials Table S3) contains a comparative table of cytokine levels between the control group of healthy subjects and the experimental group of subjects with FM, which will provide a more accurate and understandable picture of the differences between the two groups.

2.8. Risk of Bias Assessment of Individual Studies

Risk of bias is a tool developed by the Cochrane Collaboration to assess the methodology of scientific evidence. It is useful in systematic reviews for the individual analysis of included CTs and RCTs. In this sense, the present systematic review has followed the Cochrane Handbook 5.1.0 [13] to assess the risk of bias.

The Cochrane Handbook 5.1.0 presents six levels of bias: selection bias, conduct bias, detection bias, attrition bias, reporting bias, and other bias. Each level has one or more specific items in a Risk of Bias table, and each item includes a description of what happened in the study and an assessment where the assignment of "low risk", "high risk", or "unclear risk" of bias is included [13]. The risk of bias assessment for each included study can be found in (Supplementary Materials Table S4) of this systematic review.

2.9. Synthesis Methods

The synthesis methods used in the present review are the eligibility criteria that were determined in Section 2.2 of material and methods and the analysis of methodological quality using the PEDro scale, which is based on the Delphi checklist developed by Verhagen [14]. The checklist has a total of 11 items. The first item refers to external validity and is not considered for the final score; items 2–9 refer to internal validity, and items 10 and 11 indicate whether the statistical information provided by the authors allows for an adequate interpretation of the results.

Therefore, the maximum score is 10 points, and the minimum is 0. Only items that are answered affirmatively are scored. Studies with a score of 9–10 were of excellent methodological quality, 6–8 were of good quality, and 5 were of fair or acceptable quality. The PEDro scale can be found in more detail in Section 3.5 Results of the Synthesis.

Further to the synthesis measures, we assessed whether the studies included in the analysis met their objectives set at the start of the study. Of the eight studies included in this review, all of them met the objectives proposed at the outset. Regarding the homogeneity of the experimental and control groups of the studies, it was observed that in six of the eight articles [15–20], the groups were homogeneous, and the subjects were matched. However, in one of the studies [21], participants were not matched according to BMI, and the experimental group had higher BMI and blood pressure than the control group, and some participants had concomitant metabolic syndrome. In another study [22], the plasma analysis performed on the participants was not homogeneous, as the experimental group consisted of 75 subjects, while the control group had only 25 subjects. This information can be found in the descriptive tables in (Supplementary Materials Table S1).

2.10. Assessment of the Certainty of the Evidence

The GRADE system [23] was followed to measure the assessment of the certainty of the evidence, which defines the quality of evidence as the degree of confidence we have that the estimate of an effect is adequate to make a recommendation. In classifying the quality of evidence, the GRADE system establishes four categories: high, moderate, low, and very low. From the present systematic review, five of the eight studies have a high quality of evidence [17–19,21,22], and three studies have a moderate quality [15,16,20]. These results can be seen in more detail in Section 3.6 Certainty of evidence.

2.11. Data Synthesis and Statistical Analysis

Statistical analysis of the meta-analysis was performed using the Review Manager software (RevMan 5.4; Cochrane Collaboration, Oxford, UK). A meta-analysis of the predominant variables using the same parameter and measurement scale was carried out using the random effects model, in which it was assumed that the effect of the treatments was not the same in all the studies included in the model. For this, the original values of each study (Mean and Standard Deviation or Median and interquartile range) were taken as reference. The effects of the experimental interventions against the comparison groups (controls, placebo, relaxation therapy, and healthy women without fibromyalgia) were presented as mean differences and their confidence intervals, taking a 95% CI as reference. The heterogeneity of the studies was evaluated using the I^2 statistic, where values greater than 35% were heterogeneous. The variance between studies was calculated using Tau-square (Tau2) [24]. The significance level was set at 0.05 for statistically significant effects.

For the calculation of the effect size in cytokines, the predominant cytokine parameters at plasma levels (pg/mL) were selected and pooled from the original data of the different trials when a minimum N was obtained in two studies. Several trials reported median and interquartile ranges in their study. To combine the results of these studies, the mean and standard deviation of the sample were estimated using the method of Wan et al. [25]. This method, less effective than the method proposed by Hozo et al. [26], was more suitable for such an estimate. In cases where studies reported only p value greater than 0.05 or mean difference (Δ) in inter- and intragroup pre- and post-test value change, estimated values were taken from the original study data. Once all the necessary scores were obtained, the effect size of each parameter was calculated according to the method proposed by Lipsey and Wilson [27]. When the hypothesis testing of the original trial employed nonparametric techniques or more than two means were compared, Eta squared, or Eta squared partial (η^2) was calculated directly or from Cohen's d using the method of Lenhard et al. [28]. In some cases, the z-contrast statistic was calculated from the p-value offered in the trial. The cytokine meta-analysis model was random-effects based on the standardized mean difference and standard error of each study, also previously calculated [27]. The size of the effect on cytokines was considered small around 0.01, about 0.06 was considered a medium effect, and greater than 0.14 a large effect, this being negligible when 0 was found in the CI [29].

3. Results

3.1. Selection of Studies

During the initial stage of the search, 318 studies were identified from different databases. After removing duplicates, 302 studies remained.

To refine the selection, we applied date filters (2013–2023) and chose to select only clinical trials and randomized clinical trials, which were available in English or Spanish. After reviewing the titles and abstracts, 49 studies that did not fit the study topic were discarded, leaving ten studies for analysis. Of these, after a detailed reading, two studies were eliminated for inconclusive results, leaving a total of eight studies that met the inclusion criteria and were subjected to a qualitative analysis.

To carry out date and study type filters, we used database filters. To search for duplicates and perform the inclusion or exclusion of studies, we used an intelligent research collaboration platform called Rayyan, which optimizes efficiency in elaborating systematic reviews by facilitating the organization and classification of relevant studies to be considered.

3.2. Characteristics of the Studies

Of the total articles included in this review, 12.5% were published in 2013 [16], 25% in 2014 [15,20], 12.5% in 2015 [17], 12.5% in 2016 [18], 12.5% in 2018 [21] and 25% in 2019 [19,22]. A total of 575 individuals participated, all of whom were women with age ranges between 35 and 66 years; the median age was around 50. All FM patients were diagnosed by ACR 1990 criteria.

All articles were clinical trials or randomized clinical trials, presenting baseline measures, and comparing them with post-intervention. Of the eight studies included in this systematic review, seven present an experimental group including subjects diagnosed with FM and a control group composed of healthy subjects [15–18,20–22]; within these seven studies, there are two that also compare two types of interventions [exercise and relaxation] in subjects with FM [21,22]. A single study focuses on comparing the experimental group and a placebo group, while two studies compare two types of interventions (exercise and relaxation) in subjects with FM [19]. More detailed information can be found in the descriptive table for each of the studies in (Supplementary Materials Table S1).

3.3. Risk of Bias in Individual Studies

A risk of bias assessment of the individual studies was performed, allowing a more accurate picture of the quality of the available evidence and the reliability of the results obtained. More detailed information on the risk of bias assessment of each of the studies included in this systematic review can be found in the tables in (Supplementary Materials Table S4).

The risk of bias assessment figures for each study included in this systematic review are shown below. Each figure will show the result of the risk of bias assessment for each domain assessed, allowing us to identify the strengths and weaknesses of each study. In this way, we will gain a more detailed understanding of the quality of the included studies and their impact on the overall results of the systematic review.

In the risk of bias graph (Figure 2), it can be seen that in the blinding of participants and staff, blinding of assessors, incomplete short- and long-term outcome data, and selective reporting is 100% low risk whereas, in the generation of the randomized sequence, the risk of bias is 100% low, while randomized sequence generation, allocation concealment and other sources of bias are 70% low risk, 62.5% low risk and 37.5% high risk.

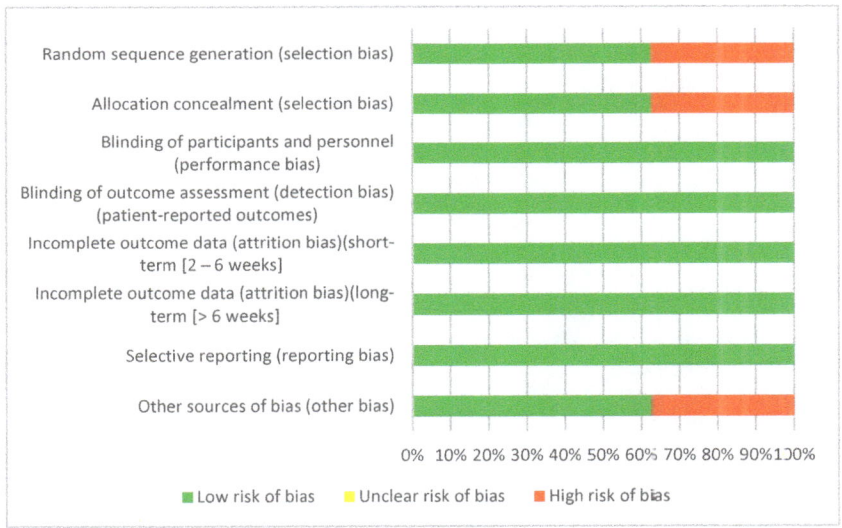

Figure 2. Risk of bias.

Furthermore, in the risk of bias summary (Figure 3), it can be seen which author and item has a low risk, unclear risk, and high risk. In the present review, clearly, those with the highest risk of bias are the non-randomized clinical trial studies [15,16,20], for the items of random sequence generation and allocation concealment, compared to the randomized clinical trial studies [17–19,21,22], which have in this case a low risk. Another item where a high risk of bias was found in three of the articles was in other sources of bias. In two of the studies [18,20], it was by allowing participants to continue taking the medication they were taking and controls to take medication during the intervention which could condition the results; in another study [21] it was by not matching subjects in the experimental group with subjects in the control group.

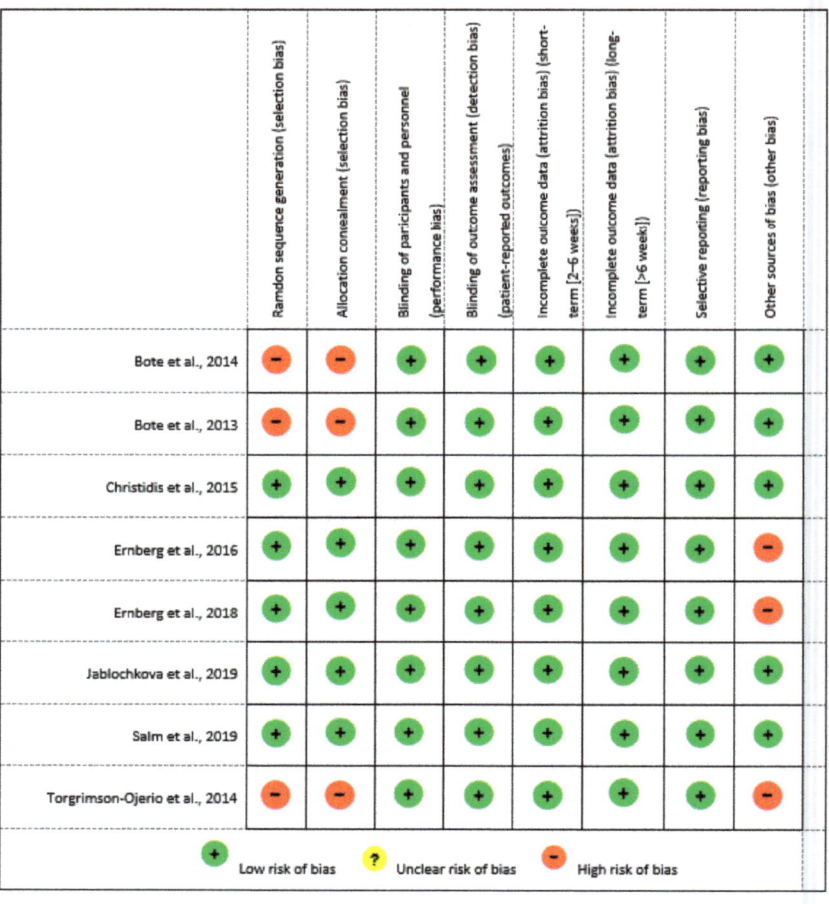

Figure 3. Risk of bias summary [15–22].

3.4. Results of Individual Studies

The results were obtained from the types of intervention; it was observed that different physiotherapy tools were used. Cycling was used in 12.5% [16]; aquatic exercise in 25% [15,19]; dynamic contractions in 25% [17,18,21]; strength exercise in 37.5% [18,21,22], a treadmill in 12.5% [20] and infrared in 12.5% [19].

In addition, each of the interventions used different durations and frequencies. They ranged from one-time sessions lasting 45 min, 20 min, or until exhaustion [16,17,20] to 6-week interventions, with three sessions per week, lasting 18–50 min per session [19], 15 weeks, with two sessions per week of 60 min [18,21,22] or eight months, with two sessions per week of 60 min per session [15]. Next, the most assessed variables were cytokine analysis, which was performed in all included studies [100%], followed by pain in 87.5% of the studies, fatigue, depression, physical capacity, and quality of life studied in 62.5% of the studies and anxiety and other variables in 50%. The tools used to measure variables such as FM were: FIQ [15,16,19–22] in 62.5%, FIQR [20] in 12.5%, SIQR [20] in 12.5%; the algometer (PPT) [18,20–22] was used to measure pain in 50% of the studies, VAS [17–19,22] in 50%, VAS [17,19,21] in 37.5%, PCS [21,22] in 25%, while SF-MPQ [19], MTPS [20], FTPS [20] and PDI in 12.5% of the studies; for fatigue, the Borg Scale [17,18] was used in 37.5% and the MFI [21,22] in 25%, for measuring the quality of life the SF-36 [16–18,21,22] in 62.5%

and the SF-36-PSC [17,18,21,22], SF-36-MSC [17,18,21,22] in 50% of the studies. The HADS test [17,18,21,22] was used in 50% and the BDI-R [20] in 12.5% to measure anxiety and depression; for the measurement of physical capacity, the dynamometer [18,21] was used in 37.5%, the Rpar-Q [15,16] in 25%, the manual pressure force [21], the VO2 test [20], pulse rate [20] and blood pressure [20] in 12.5%; and the 6MWT [15,18,21] in 37.5% of the studies; for blood analysis muscle micro-dialysis [17,18] was used in 25% of the studies and venipuncture blood analysis in 100% [15–22]; other variables such as lifestyle, medication, and other diseases [15,16,20] were studied in 37.5% and finally, infrared thermography [19] in 12.5% of the studies.

Notably, the most studied variable was the blood test and cytokine expression before and after the intervention (in 100% of the studies). For this reason, a table was made to analyze the most studied cytokines in the studies we are concerned with here. In the evaluation of cytokines in blood obtained by venous puncture, it was observed that, of the 10 cytokines studied, seven were proinflammatory cytokines: IL-1β, IL-2, IL-6, IL-8, IL-17A, IL-18, and TNF-α, among these, IL-6 [16–22], IL-8 [15–18,20–22] and TNF-α [16–22] were studied in 87.5% of the studies, while IL-1β [16–18,20–22] was examined in 75% of them (Supplementary Materials Table S2). IL-2 and IL-17A in 25% [21,22], and the least studied proinflammatory cytokine was IL-18 in 12.5% [16] of the studies. In contrast, only three anti-inflammatory cytokines were studied: IL-1ra, IL-4, and IL-10, with IL-10 being the most studied in 62.5% of studies [16,19–22], followed by IL-1ra in 37.5% [20–22] and IL-4 in only 25% of trials [21,22]. For muscle micro-dialysis, only the proinflammatory cytokine responses of IL-1β, IL-6, IL-8, and TNF-α were examined, and this measurement was performed in only 25% of studies [17,18] Supplementary Materials Table S2. An additional table has been developed to compare cytokine levels between the control group of healthy subjects and the experimental group of subjects with fibromyalgia. In two studies [15,19], no data were obtained because the intervention was between groups of subjects with fibromyalgia. In two other studies [21,22], only a comparison of circulating cytokine levels between the control group and experimental groups was performed without applying any intervention, so we only have the baseline data. The most relevant finding in this table is that the cytokine levels in the control group of healthy subjects are lower than in the experimental group of fibromyalgia patients.

3.5. Results of the Synthesis

The articles included in the review were assessed using the PEDro methodological quality scale, shown below in Table 1. The final score obtained ranged from 5 to 10. Two studies were classified as being of excellent quality, three of good quality, and three of fair or fair quality. The studies achieved a mean value of 7.12 ± 2.88.

Table 1. Methodological assessment PEDro scale.

Reference	Type of Study	PEDro											TOTAL	Conflict of Interests
		1	2	3	4	5	6	7	8	9	10	11		
Bote et al., 2014 [15]	Clinical trial	+	−	−	+	−	−	−	+	+	+	+	5/10	N/A
Bote et al., 2013 [16]	Clinical trial	+	−	−	+	−	−	−	+	+	+	+	5/10	N/A
Christidis et al., 2015 [19]	Ramdomized clinical trial multicenter	+	+	+	+	+	+	+	+	+	+	+	10/10	N/A
Ernberg et al., 2016 [17]	Ramdomized clinical trial multicenter	+	+	+	+	+	+	−	−	+	+	+	8/10	NO
Ernberg et al., 2018 [20]	Ramdomized clinical trial multicenter	+	+	+	+	+	−	+	−	−	+	+	7/10	NO
Jablochkova et al., 2019 [21]	Ramdomized clinical trial	+	+	+	−	+	+	+	−	+	+	+	8/10	NO
Salm et al., 2019 [18]	Double-blind, ramdomized, placebo-controlled study	+	+	+	+	+	−	+	+	+	+	+	9/10	NO
Torgrimson-Ojerio et al., 2014 [22]	Clinical trial	−	−	−	+	−	−	+	+	+	+	−	5/10	N/A

1: elegibility criteria were specified; 2: subjects were ramdomly allocated to groups; 3: allocation was concealed; 4: the groups were similar at baseline regarding the most important prognostic indicators; 5: blinding of all subjects; 6: blinding of all therapist who administered the therapy; 7: blinding of all assessors who measured at least one key outcome; 8: >85% outcomes of the subjets initially allocated to groups; 9: data for at least one key outcome by "intention to treat"; 10: between-group statistical comparisons; 11: point measures and measures of variability; N/A: not available.

3.6. Certainty of Evidence

The GRADE system [23] has been used to classify the studies included in this review to determine the certainty of the evidence, five of the eight studies have a high quality of evidence [17–19,21,22], and three studies a moderate quality [15,16,20], and can be visualized more clearly in the following Table 2.

Table 2. GRADE system.

Author, Year and Reference	Type of Study	Evidence Quality
Bote et al., 2014 [15]	Clinical trial	Moderate
Bote et al., 2013 [16]	Clinical trial	Moderate
Christidis et al., 2015 [19]	Ramdomized clinical trial	High
Ernberg et al., 2016 [17]	Ramdomized clinical trial	High
Ernberg et al., 2018 [20]	Ramdomized clinical trial	High
Jablochkova et al., 2019 [21]	Ramdomized clinical trial	High
Salm et al., 2019 [18]	Ramdomized clinical trial	High
Torgrimson-Ojerio et al., 2014 [22]	Clinical trial	Moderate

3.7. Metanalysis Results

Figure 4 shows the effects of the treatments versus the comparison group on the outcome measures. Ernberg et al. [20] showed a reduction of 7.1 points in the FIQ instrument. The treatments were effective in combination with the study by Slam et al. 19] [IV = -7.84 (-13.09 to -2.60); z = 2.93; p = 0.003]. Figure 5 shows the effects of the treatment compared to the comparison group on the algometry (PPT) in the left and right limbs. The study by Jablochkova et al. [21] found no statistically significant differences in the Algometer measurement in favor of the resistance program versus relaxation therapy (z = 0.19; p = 0.85), not observing intragroup effects on this variable in the original study. No heterogeneity was observed in either of the two analyses ($\chi^2(1)$ = 0.89; I^2 = 0% and ($\chi^2(1)$ = 0.86; I^2 = 0% respectively).

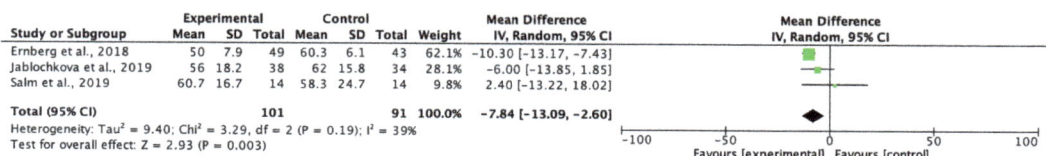

Figure 4. Effects of treatment versus the comparison group on the "Fibromyalgia Impact Questionnaire" (FIQ) [18,20,21].

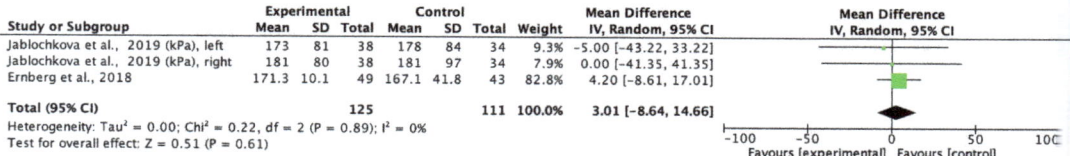

Figure 5. Effects of the treatment compared to the comparison group on the Algometry (PPT) in the left and right limb [20,21].

Likewise, a change of 2.5 points was found in the mental component of the SF-36 scale in favor of the group that underwent 15 weeks of progressive resistance exercise and in the overall combination in favor of treatment in the SF-36, the pain, and the variable Static strength knee extension force (Figure 6). No heterogeneity was observed in either of the FIQ, PPT, SF-36, and HADS analyses ($I^2 = 0\%$), however, heterogeneity was observed from $\chi^2(2) = 196.33$; $p < 0.01$; $I^2 = 99\%$ for the pain variable; $\chi^2(2) = 196.33$; $p < 0.01$; $I^2 = 99\%$; for elbow flexion force and $\chi^2(2) = 4.88$; $p = 0.09$; $I^2 = 59\%$ for the outcome knee extension force. Figure 6 shows the effects of treatment versus comparison group on the QoL (SF-36-PSC, SF-36-MSC and combined effects). Ernberg et al. [20] found a significant increase in the mental component of the quality of life of these patients after treatment (IV = −6.90 (−11.52 to −2.28)). The treatments were effective in combination with the study by Jablochkova et al. [21] (IV = −6.67 (−10.65 to −2.68); z = 3.23; $p = 0.001$). No statistically significant changes were found in the combination of values from the pre to post-test in quality of life in its physical dimension in any of the studies examined ($p > 0.05$) (Figure 7).

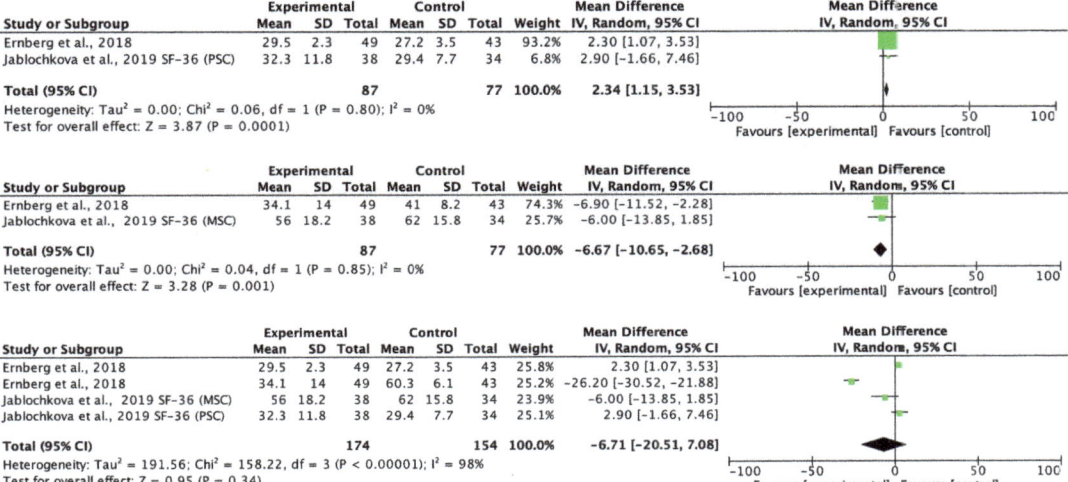

Figure 6. Effects of treatment versus comparison group on the QoL (SF-36-PSC, SF-36-MSC and combined effects) [20,21].

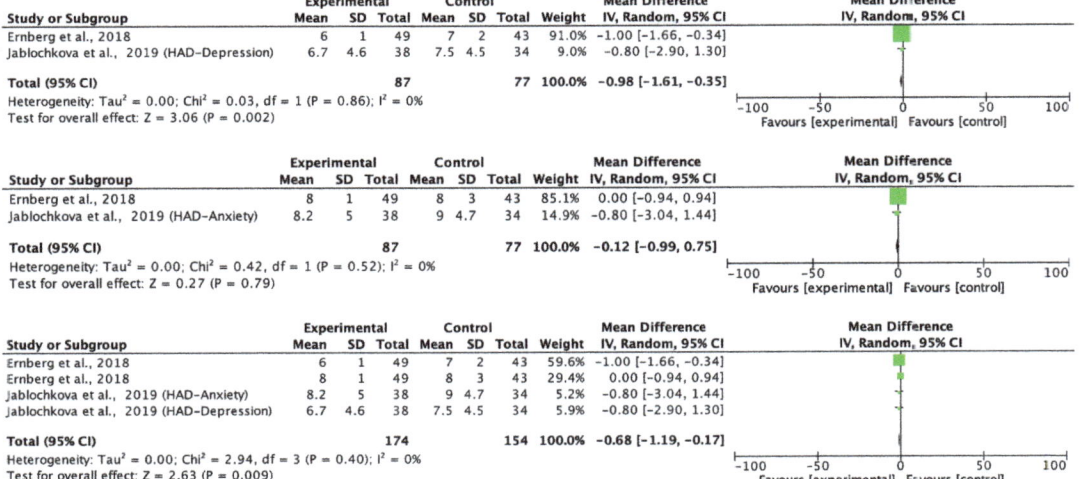

Figure 7. Effects of treatment versus comparison group on the "Anxiety and Depression Scale" Depression (HADS)-Depression, Anxiety, and combined effects [20,21].

The studies by Ernberg et al. [17] and Jablochkova et al. [21] found a significant reduction in pain in favor of the experimental group IV = −20.00 (−22.64 to −17.36) and IV = 16.80 (−26.88 to −6.72); $p < 0.05$, respectively. However, no statistically significant differences were found in the overall analysis of both studies (Figure 8).

Study or Subgroup	Experimental Mean	SD	Total	Control Mean	SD	Total	Weight	Mean Difference IV, Random, 95% CI
Enberg et al., 2016	50	23.5	24	0	2	27	33.2%	50.00 [40.57, 59.43]
Ernberg et al., 2018	34	4	49	54	8	43	33.7%	-20.00 [-22.64, -17.36]
Jablochkova et al., 2019	37.2	23.7	38	54	19.9	34	33.1%	-16.80 [-26.88, -6.72]
Total (95% CI)			**111**			**104**	**100.0%**	**4.29 [-37.20, 45.77]**

Heterogeneity: Tau² = 1327.10; Chi² = 196.33, df = 2 (P < 0.00001); I² = 99%
Test for overall effect: Z = 0.20 (P = 0.84)

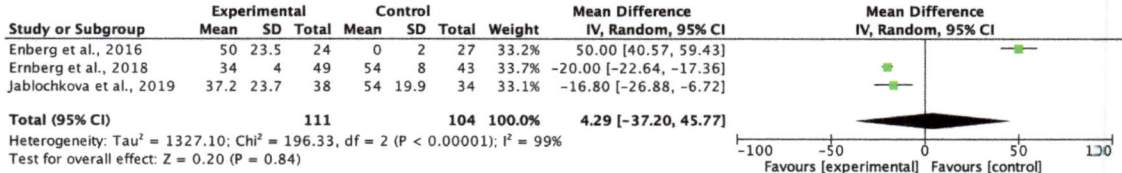

Figure 8. Effects of treatment versus comparison group on Pain (0–100) [20,21].

Regarding the effects of treatment versus comparison group on Static strength elbow flexion force, no statistically significant changes were found in the combination of values from pre to post-test in the results presented by right and left in any of the studies examined ($p > 0.05$) (Figures 9 and 10).

Study or Subgroup	Experimental Mean	SD	Total	Control Mean	SD	Total	Weight	Mean Difference IV, Random, 95% CI
Enberg et al., 2016	14.3	6.7	24	16.9	6.3	27	26.0%	-2.60 [-6.18, 0.98]
Enberg et al., 2016	14.2	7.4	24	17.3	4.3	27	27.4%	-3.10 [-6.48, 0.28]
Ernberg et al., 2018	10.3	1.8	49	9.8	1.7	43	46.6%	0.50 [-0.22, 1.22]
Total (95% CI)			**97**			**97**	**100.0%**	**-1.29 [-3.98, 1.40]**

Heterogeneity: Tau² = 3.91; Chi² = 6.68, df = 2 (P = 0.04); I² = 70%
Test for overall effect: Z = 0.94 (P = 0.35)

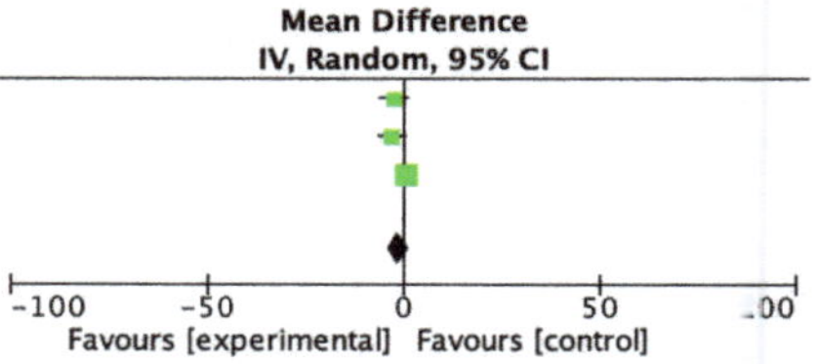

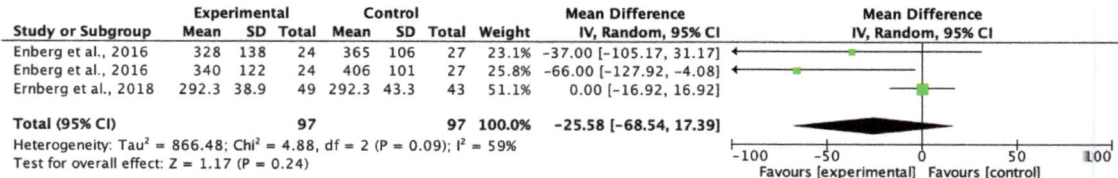

Figure 9. Effects of treatment versus comparison group on Static strength elbow flexion force (Kg)—Presented by right and left [17,20].

Study or Subgroup	Experimental Mean	SD	Total	Control Mean	SD	Total	Weight	Mean Difference IV, Random, 95% CI
Enberg et al., 2016	328	138	24	365	106	27	23.1%	-37.00 [-105.17, 31.17]
Enberg et al., 2016	340	122	24	406	101	27	25.8%	-66.00 [-127.92, -4.08]
Ernberg et al., 2018	292.3	38.9	49	292.3	43.3	43	51.1%	0.00 [-16.92, 16.92]
Total (95% CI)			**97**			**97**	**100.0%**	**-25.58 [-68.54, 17.39]**

Heterogeneity: Tau² = 866.48; Chi² = 4.88, df = 2 (P = 0.09); I² = 59%
Test for overall effect: Z = 1.17 (P = 0.24)

Figure 10. Effects of treatment versus comparison group on Static strength knee extension force (N)—Presented by right and left [17,20].

Analysis of treatment effects was not significant in our IL-8 analyses. In the second study by Ernberg et al. [20], no intergroup effects were observed (Exercise treatment vs. Relaxaxion group) because 0 was found in IQ ($p > 0.05$), although there was a trend in favor of treatment in the original study (Figure 11).

No statistically significant differences were observed in the analysis of the effect of the studies on cortisol. Bote's trial [16] found a difference of 0.38, but it was not significant ($p > 0.05$), as was the TNF variable (Figures 12 and 13). The studies that examined the IL-1β variable found negligible effects in the trials included in the overall analysis conducted ($p > 0.05$) (Figure 14).

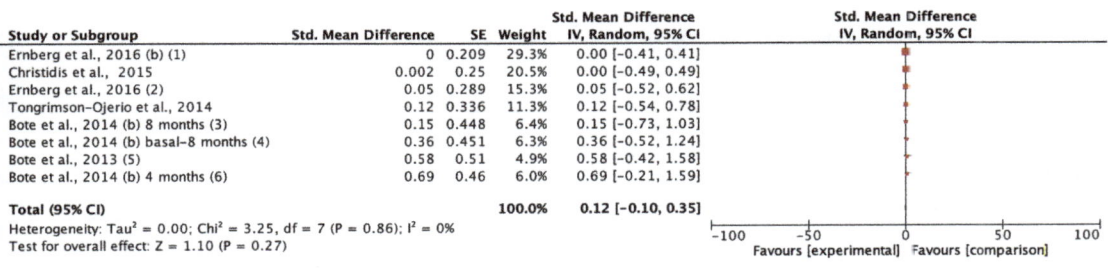

Figure 11. Effects of treatment versus comparison on IL-8 (pg/mL). b: second measurement of this outcome in the original study [15–17,19,22].

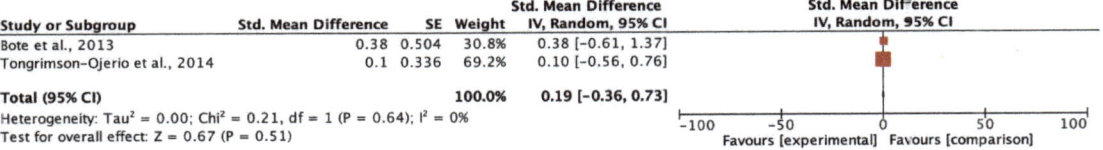

Figure 12. Effects of treatment versus comparison on Cortisol (pg/mL) [16,22].

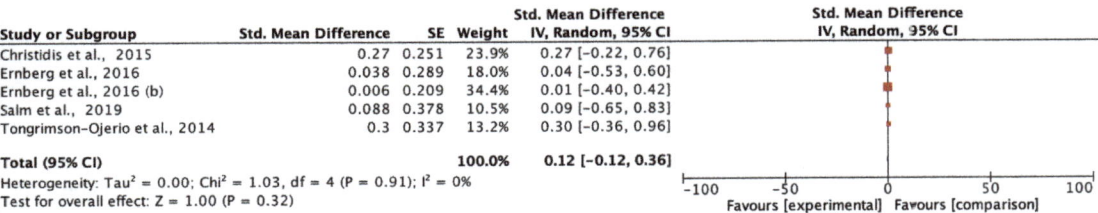

Figure 13. Effects of treatment versus comparison on TFN (pg/mL). b: second measurement of this outcome in the original study [17–19,21,22].

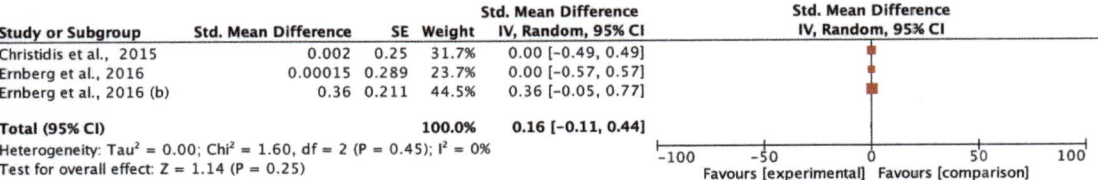

Figure 14. Effects of treatment versus comparison on IL-1β (pg/mL). b: second measurement of this outcome in the original study [17,19].

However, a statistically significant effect size was found in the study by Ernberg et al. [20] in favor of relaxation treatment on IL-6 (SMD = 0.50 (0.08 to 0.92; $p < 0.05$) (Figure 15).

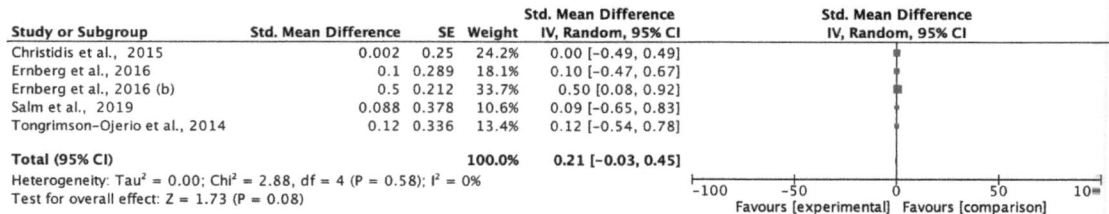

Figure 15. Effects of treatment versus comparison on IL-6 (pg/mL). b: second measurement of this outcome in the original study. b: second measurement of this outcome in the original study [17–19,22].

4. Discussion

The main aim of the meta-analysis was to examine the effect of multimodal rehabilitation on cytokine levels and other predominant variables in patients with FM. The intervention by Ernberg et al. [20] significantly decreased the scores of the FIQ in favor of the relaxation group, but the two fibromyalgia groups examined did not find functional and clinical differences in the change in values from pre to post-test. Other studies showed differences in variables in favor of the control group in pain ratios applying programs of 15 weeks of strength exercise 2 sessions/week 1 session/60 min 10 min warm-up 50 min and lower limb strength, however, this intervention did not normalize a chronic inflammation profile nor did it have any effect on the anti-inflammatory effect in patients with FM symptoms on the clinical and functional variables examined [17,20,21].

Furthermore, the response of cytokine levels to intervention was found to differ between the groups. While in the healthy group, cytokine levels are low and increase during the intervention, in the experimental group, cytokine levels are elevated and decrease during the intervention. This observation suggests the presence of chronic inflammation in FM patients, which supports the hypothesis that inflammation and altered immune response may play a role in the development and maintenance of FM symptoms [4]. In addition, it also provides a possible explanation for many of the symptoms experienced by FM patients. For example, elevated concentrations of IL-6 and IL-8 have been shown to have additive or synergistic effects on the perpetuation of chronic pain in these patients [30]. IL-6 induces pain, fatigue, and psychiatric disorders such as depression and stress [4], while IL-8 is associated with pain and sleep disorders [16]. Consequently, an imbalance between proinflammatory and anti-inflammatory cytokines contributes to chronic peripheral sensitization of the nervous system and pain processing [2,4]. Another study also points to an imbalance between proinflammatory and anti-inflammatory cytokines, with higher levels of proinflammatory cytokines such as TNF-α, IL-1ra, IL-6, and IL-8 [6]. These results support the hypothesis that inflammation and immune responses are altered in the FM group.

Although the heterogeneity associated with the processes, techniques, and instruments for the detection of cytokines in different body fluids represents an underlying factor in the literature, we highlight the importance of using the mean difference technique. standardized in the meta-analysis. The study had difficulties in making Forrest plots regarding cytokines and the correlation with exercise in the study, as the authors did not show sufficient data to calculate the effect size from the original individual trial data. Our work showed a high methodological and statistical heterogeneity of the studies. The lack of data made it impossible to analyze all the variables, which is a limitation when it comes to quantifying the effects. This could affect the results of the meta-analysis, as some effects found were negligible in the meta-analytic model. However, a qualitative description of the effects of these variables has been made.

Proinflammatory cytokines are products of lymphocytes that are activated not only by injury but also by glial and neuronal cells. The main proinflammatory cytokines include IL-1, IL-2, IL-6, IL-8, IL-12, TNF-α, INF-α and IFN-α, while the main anti-inflammatory cytokines are IL-4, IL-10, IL-13, and TGF-α [4]. In the studies reviewed, mainly 1) cytokines were analyzed, with IL-1β, IL-6, IL-8, and TNF-α standing out as proinflammatory cytokines. However, there was a lack of investigation and analysis of anti-inflammatory cytokines, both at the muscle level [17,18], which only investigated the levels of proinflammatory cytokines, and at the plasma level where, for example, IL-13 was not analyzed in any of the studies.

According to investigate the cytokines present in the muscle tissue and plasma of patients with FM. In the present systematic review, only 25% of the studies [17,18] employed the micro-dialysis technique in muscle tissue and revealed no significant difference in the release of inflammatory cytokines between the groups in terms of IL-1β, IL-6, IL-8. However, an increase in the cytokine TNF-α was observed only in the control group. These findings align with the conclusions of other studies suggesting that physical exercise affects the metabolic profile of muscle but does not impact the plasma immune profile of FM patients [17,22].

The final specific objective was to examine the physical therapy tools used to investigate the effects of such interventions on cytokine levels in FM patients. In the studies that evaluated the effects of exercise on cytokines, variable results were found. Regarding the study of anti-inflammatory cytokines, we identified that in three studies, no analysis of these cytokines was performed [15,17,18]. In the other trials where they were analyzed, three found no evidence of an anti-inflammatory effect after the intervention, with no significant changes observed [20–22]. However, in three other studies, there was an anti-inflammatory effect [15,16,19]. Significantly, this effect was not directly attributed to the action of anti-inflammatory cytokines but to the reduction of pro-inflammatory cytokines, suggesting a possible inhibition of some anti-inflammatory cytokines, such as IL-10 [20]. For example, in one of the studies, after a moderate cycling session, an anti-inflammatory effect was found due to a slight decrease in IL-10 in the experimental group, but what made the difference was a significant reduction in IL-8 levels, attributed to a lower release of pro-inflammatory cytokines by monocytes and lower activation of neutrophils [16]. In another study, a combination of exercise and infrared therapy was used, and a reduction in IL-6 levels was observed, exerting an anti-inflammatory effect, and improving pain and quality of life in FM subjects [19]. However, after a 15-week strength exercise intervention, no anti-inflammatory effect was found on any FM symptoms [21]. From the methodological point of view of the meta-analysis, only a few studies could be analyzed. When the data distribution is symmetrical, the median can be used in meta-analyses. This criterion was adopted methodologically with the studies by Enberg et al. [17,20], so it would have been indicated to meta-analyze these studies using the probability of superiority (PS) as an index of effect size given the non-parametric analysis used (Mann-Whitney U test) [31,32]. Future lines of research could aim to carry out an analysis of the real impact of the size of the effect that is unknown by calculating the non-overlapping percentage of the population in order not to adopt risks. Likewise, in future research, it would be interesting to carry out a meta-regression that considered cytokines and the MFI (0–20) fatigue scale [33].

An important point of discussion that could be taken up in the future would be the probable association of virus infection with cytokines levels or immune responses in patients with FM. However, among the interests of the present study was to analyze the presence of anti-inflammatory and proinflammatory cytokines, but not to relate it to the probable viral association, since this hypothesis has been dismissed on some occasions. For example, what could be analyzed in the future is the possible relationship of FM symptoms with COVID-19 symptoms opening new etiopathogenetic horizons, but this objective will be pursued later.

The type of exercise, its duration, and intensity are also essential factors in the results obtained. For example, in a study of warm water aquatic exercise performed for eight months, two sessions per week, and 60 min per session, it was observed that after four months no anti-inflammatory effects were obtained. However, after eight months they were [15]. Although we know that all patients with chronic pain and FM have low-grade systemic inflammation, our meta-analysis was unable to demonstrate that blood biomarkers are specific or diagnostic for FM. The fact of having few studies and being very heterogeneous among themselves, does not provide sufficient scientific evidence to establish the cause-effect relationship of the treatments on the levels of cytokines and FM, for all this new research that analyzes the heterogeneity and seeks to carry out synthesis of results in a homogeneous way will be able to demonstrate the effect of the type of intervention carried out. In this case, it would be convenient to explore the moderate effect related to the participants and the characteristics of the intervention using regression techniques with confounding outcomes [11].

In another study of aquatic exercise in a heated pool, which lasted six weeks, three times per week and 50 min per session, together with thermotherapy, a decrease in IL-6 levels and improvements in pain and quality of life were observed in the FM group [19]. According to future research lines, we recommended examining continuous covariates that could be subjected to individual and pooled meta-regression in a random-effects meta-regression model taking into account the mean age of the women with FM, weight, height, study durations (weeks or months), sessions, days a week, number of exercises or treatment content, and even the method of blood extraction or cytokine measurement as predictor variables. Subgroups could also be used and analyzed for effects for categorical variables (women with fibromyalgia and healthy controls).

Therefore, although it was the same type of exercise, differences were observed in the duration of the intervention, the number of sessions per week, the duration of each session, and the addition of another physiotherapy tool.

5. Conclusions

In this systematic review, we found evidence to support elevated levels of proinflammatory and anti-inflammatory cytokines in patients with fibromyalgia compared to healthy subjects. These findings suggest the existence of chronic inflammation that may be responsible for an altered immune response and play a role in fibromyalgia symptoms, as well as developmental and nervous system sensitization to chronic pain. The most studied and analyzed cytokines were IL-1β, IL-6, IL-8, and TNF-α, while there was a lack of investigation of anti-inflammatory cytokines such as IL-4, IL-10, and IL-13. It was found through microanalyses that exercise affects the metabolic profile of muscle tissue but has no significant effect on the immune profile in the plasma of FM patients. Furthermore, results on the impact of exercise on cytokine levels have been variable, so it is essential to consider factors such as type of exercise, duration, intensity, and combination with other physiotherapeutic tools. These aspects are fundamental to formulating recommendations and intervention strategies for managing FM. However, our meta-analysis has reported a state-of-the-art, but the reported evidence is very low due to problems with the study design, the small number of participants, and the low certainty of the results after the effects of physiotherapy on cytokine levels.

Supplementary Materials: The following supporting information can be downloaded at: https://www.mdpi.com/article/10.3390/biomedicines11092367/s1, Table S1: Descriptive table; Table S2: Studied cytokines; Table S3: Analysis of the studied cytokines in groups of healthy subjects and subjects with FM; Table S4: Rick of bias assessment.

Author Contributions: Conceptualization, I.H.-B. and E.Ú.-D.; methodology, V.J.-D.-B., J.P.H.-P. and E.C.-F.-P.; software, V.J.-D.-B. and I.H.-B.; validation, E.Ú.-D., E.C.-F.-P. and J.P.H.-P.; formal analysis, V.J.-D.-B. and J.P.H.-P.; investigation, I.H.-B., V.J.-D.-B., E.Ú.-D., E.C.-F.-P. and J.P.H.-P.; resources, I.H.-B., E.Ú.-D., E.C.-F.-P. and J.P.H.-P.; data curation, E.Ú.-D., E.C.-F.-P. and J.P.H.-P.; writing—original draft preparation, I.H.-B. and E.Ú.-D.; writing—review and editing, V.J.-D.-B., I.H.-B. and E.Ú.-D.; visualization, I.H.-B., J.P.H.-P. and E.Ú.-D.; supervision, V.J.-D.-B., E.Ú.-D. and J.P.H.-P. All authors have read and agreed to the published version of the manuscript.

Funding: This research received no external funding.

Institutional Review Board Statement: Not applicable.

Informed Consent Statement: Not applicable.

Data Availability Statement: Data used for this manuscript are available on request.

Conflicts of Interest: The authors declare no conflict of interest.

References

1. Sánchez, A.I.; Goya Nakakaneku, M.; Miró, E.; Pilar Martínez, M.; de Personalidad, D.; Psicológico, T. Tratamiento multidisciplinar para la fibromialgia y el síndrome de fatiga crónica: Una revisión sistemática 1. *Behav. Psychol. Psicol. Conduct.* **2021**, *29*, 455–488. [CrossRef]
2. Siracusa, R.; Paola, R.D.; Cuzzocrea, S.; Impellizzeri, D. Fibromyalgia: Pathogenesis, mechanisms, diagnosis and treatment options update. *Int. J. Mol. Sci.* **2021**, *22*, 3891. [CrossRef]
3. Sarzi-Puttini, P.; Giorgi, V.; Marotto, D.; Atzeni, F. Fibromyalgia: An update on clinical characteristics, aetiopathogenesis and treatment. *Nat. Rev. Rheumatol.* **2020**, *16*, 645–660. [CrossRef] [PubMed]
4. Rodríguez-Pintó, I.; Agmon-Levin, N.; Howard, A.; Shoenfeld, Y. Fibromyalgia and cytokines. *Immunol. Lett.* **2014**, *161*, 200–203. [CrossRef] [PubMed]
5. Littlejohn, G.; Guymer, E. Neurogenic inflammation in fibromyalgia. *Semin. Immunopathol.* **2018**, *40*, 291–300. [CrossRef]
6. Surendran, S.; Mithun, C.; Chandran, V.; Balan, S.; Tiwari, A. Serum interleukin-6, interleukin-8, and interleukin-1 receptor antagonist levels in South Indian fibromyalgia patients and its correlation with disease severity. *Indian J. Rheumatol.* **2021**, *16*, 381–387. [CrossRef]
7. Antunes, M.D.; Marques, A.P. The role of physiotherapy in fibromyalgia: Current and future perspectives. *Front. Physiol.* **2022**, *13*, 968292. [CrossRef]
8. Hernando-Garijo, I.; Jiménez-Del-Barrio, S.; Mingo-Gómez, T.; Medrano-De-La-Fuente, R.; Ceballos-Laita, L. Effectiveness of non-pharmacological conservative therapies in adults with fibromyalgia: A systematic review of high-quality clinical trials. *J. Back Musculoskelet. Rehabil.* **2022**, *35*, 3–20. [CrossRef]
9. Kundakci, B.; Kaur, J.; Goh, S.L.; Hall, M.; Doherty, M.; Zhang, W.; Abhishek, A. Efficacy of nonpharmacological interventions for individual features of fibromyalgia: A systematic review and meta-analysis of randomised controlled trials. *Pain* **2022**, *163*, 1432–1445. [CrossRef]
10. Sanada, K.; Díez, M.A.; Valero, M.S.; Pérez-Yus, M.C.; Demarzo, M.M.P.; García-Toro, M.; García-Campayo, J. Effects of non-pharmacological interventions on inflammatory biomarker expression in patients with fibromyalgia: A systematic review. *Arthritis Res. Ther.* **2015**, *17*, 272. [CrossRef] [PubMed]
11. Kumbhare, D.; Hassan, S.; Diep, D.; Duarte, F.C.K.; Hung, J.; Damodara, S.; West, D.W.D.; Selvaganapathy, P.R. Potential role of blood biomarkers in patients with fibromyalgia: A systematic review with meta-analysis. *Pain* **2022**, *163*, 1232–1253. [CrossRef] [PubMed]
12. Yepes-Nuñez, J.J.; Urrútia, G.; Romero-García, M.; Alonso-Fernández, S. Declaración PRISMA 2020: Una guía actualizada para la publicación de revisiones sistemáticas. *Rev. Esp. Cardiol.* **2021**, *74*, 790–799. [CrossRef]
13. Centro Cochrane Iberoamericano. *(Translators) Manual Cochrane de Revisiones Sistemáticas de Intervenciones, Versión 5.1.0* Centro Cochrane Iberoamericano: Barcelona, Spain, 2011; Volume 8, pp. 207–218. Available online: https://es.cochrane.org/sites/es.cochrane.org/files/uploads/Manual_Cochrane_510_reduit.pdf (accessed on 12 February 2023).
14. Verhagen, A.P.; De Vet, H.C.W.; De Bie, R.A.; Kessels, A.G.H.; Boers, M.; Bouter, L.M.; Knipschild, P.G. The Delphi list: A criteria list for quality assessment of randomized clinical trials for conducting systematic reviews developed by Delphi consensus. *J. Clin. Epidemiol.* **1998**, *51*, 1235–1241. [CrossRef]
15. Bote, M.E.; García, J.J.; Hinchado, M.D.; Ortega, E. An exploratory study of the effect of regular aquatic exercise on the function of neutrophils from women with fibromyalgia: Role of IL-8 and noradrenaline. *Brain Behav. Immun.* **2014**, *39*, 107–112. [CrossRef] [PubMed]
16. Bote, M.E.; Garcia, J.J.; Hinchado, M.D.; Ortega, E. Fibromyalgia: Anti-inflammatory and stress responses after acute moderate exercise. *PLoS ONE* **2013**, *8*, e74524. [CrossRef]
17. Ernberg, M.; Christidis, N.; Ghafouri, B.; Bileviciute-Ljungar, I.; Löfgren, M.; Larsson, A.; Palstam, A.; Bjersing, J.; Mannerkorpi, K.; Kosek, E.; et al. Effects of 15 weeks of resistance exercise on pro-inflammatory cytokine levels in the vastus lateralis muscle of patients with fibromyalgia. *Arthritis Res. Ther.* **2016**, *18*, 137. [CrossRef] [PubMed]
18. Salm, D.C.; Belmonte, L.A.O.; Emer, A.A.; Leonel, L.D.S.; de Brito, R.N.; da Rocha, C.C.; Martins, T.C.; dos Reis, D.C; Moro, A.R.P.; Mazzardo-Martins, L.; et al. Aquatic exercise and Far Infrared (FIR) modulates pain and blood cytokines in fibromyalgia patients: A double-blind, randomized, placebo-controlled pilot study. *J. Neuroimmunol.* **2019**, *337*, 577077. [CrossRef]
19. Christidis, N.; Ghafouri, B.; Larsson, A.; Palstam, A.; Mannerkorpi, K.; Bileviciute-Ljungar, I.; Löfgren, M.; Bjersing, J.; Kosek, E.; Gerdle, B.; et al. Comparison of the levels of pro-inflammatory cytokines released in the Vastus lateralis muscle of patients with fibromyalgia and healthy controls during contractions of the quadriceps muscle—A microdialysis study. *PLoS ONE* **2015**, *10*, e0143856. [CrossRef] [PubMed]
20. Ernberg, M.; Christidis, N.; Ghafouri, B.; Bileviciute-Ljungar, I.; Löfgren, M.; Bjersing, J.; Palstam, A.; Larsson, A.; Mannerkorpi, K.; Gerdle, B.; et al. Plasma cytokine levels in fibromyalgia and their response to 15 weeks of progressive resistance exercise or relaxation therapy. *Mediat. Inflamm.* **2018**, *2018*, 3985154. [CrossRef]

21. Jablochkova, A.; Bäckryd, E.; Kosek, E.; Mannerkorpi, K.; Ernberg, M.; Gerdle, B.; Ghafouri, B. Unaltered low nerve growth factor and high brain-derived neurotrophic factor levels in plasma from patients with fibromyalgia after a 15-week progressive resistance exercise. *J. Rehabil. Med.* **2019**, *51*, 779–787. [CrossRef]
22. Torgrimson-Ojerio, B.; Ross, R.L.; Dieckmann, N.F.; Avery, S.; Bennett, R.M.; Jones, K.D.; Guarino, A.J.; Wood, L.J. Preliminary evidence of a blunted anti-inflammatory response to exhaustive exercise in fibromyalgia. *J. Neuroimmunol.* **2014**, *277*, 160–167. [CrossRef]
23. Aguayo-Albasini, J.L.; Flores-Pastor, B.; Soria-Aledo, V. Sistema GRADE: Clasificación de la calidad de la evidencia y graduación de la fuerza de la recomendación. *Cir. Esp.* **2014**, *92*, 82–88. [CrossRef]
24. Higgins, J.P.; Thompson, S.G.; Deeks, J.J.; Altman, D.G. Measuring inconsistency in meta-analyses. *BMJ* **2003**, *327*, 557–560. [CrossRef] [PubMed]
25. Wan, X.; Wang, W.; Liu, J.; Tong, T. Estimating the sample mean and standard deviation from the sample size, median, range and/or interquartile range. *BMC Med. Res. Methodol.* **2014**, *14*, 135. [CrossRef] [PubMed]
26. Hozo, S.P.; Djulbegovic, B.; Hozo, I. Estimating the mean and variance from the median, range, and the size of a sample. *BMC Med. Res. Methodol.* **2005**, *5*, 13. [CrossRef]
27. Lipsey, M.W.; Wilson, D.B. *Practical Meta-Analysis*; Applied Social Research Methods Series; Sage Publications: Thousand Oaks, CA, USA, 2001; ISBN 978-0-7619-2167-7.
28. Lenhard, W.; Lenhard, A. Computation of Effect Sizes. Psychometrica. 2016. Available online: https://www.psychometrica.de/effect_size.html (accessed on 30 July 2023).
29. Cohen, J. *Statistical Power Analysis for the Behavioral Sciences*, 2nd ed.; Lawrence Erlbaum Associates: Hillsdale, NJ, USA, 1988.
30. Mendieta, D.; De la Cruz-Aguilera, D.L.; Barrera-Villalpando, M.I.; Becerril-Villanueva, E.; Arreola, R.; Hernández-Ferreira, E.; Pérez-Tapia, S.M.; Pérez-Sánchez, G.; Garcés-Alvarez, M.E.; Aguirre-Cruz, L.; et al. IL-8 and IL-6 primarily mediate the inflammatory response in fibromyalgia patients. *J. Neuroimmunol.* **2016**, *290*, 22–25. [CrossRef] [PubMed]
31. Grissom, R.; Kim, J. *Effect Sizes for Research*; Lawrence Erlbaum Associates: Mahwah, NJ, USA, 2005.
32. Ruscio, J.; Mullen, T. Confidence intervals for the probability of superiority effect size measure and the area under a receiver operating characteristic curve. *Multivar. Behav. Res* **2012**, *47*, 201–223. [CrossRef] [PubMed]
33. Casado, A.; Prieto, L.; Alonso, J. The effect size of the difference between two means: Statistically significant or clinically relevant? *Med. Clin.* **1999**, *15*, 584–588.

Disclaimer/Publisher's Note: The statements, opinions and data contained in all publications are solely those of the individual author(s) and contributor(s) and not of MDPI and/or the editor(s). MDPI and/or the editor(s) disclaim responsibility for any injury to people or property resulting from any ideas, methods, instructions or products referred to in the content.

MDPI
St. Alban-Anlage 66
4052 Basel
Switzerland
www.mdpi.com

Biomedicines Editorial Office
E-mail: biomedicines@mdpi.com
www.mdpi.com/journal/biomedicines

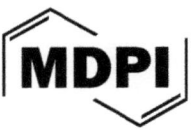

Disclaimer/Publisher's Note: The statements, opinions and data contained in all publications are solely those of the individual author(s) and contributor(s) and not of MDPI and/or the editor(s). MDPI and/or the editor(s) disclaim responsibility for any injury to people or property resulting from any ideas, methods, instructions or products referred to in the content.

www.ingramcontent.com/pod-product-compliance
Lightning Source LLC
LaVergne TN
LVHW070621100526
838202LV00012B/696